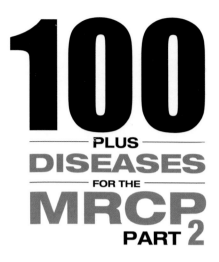

100
PLUS
DISEASES
FOR THE
MRCP
PART 2

Commissioning Editor: *Pauline Graham*
Project Development Manager: *Lulu Stader*
Project Manager: *Morven Dean*
Design: *Charles Gray*

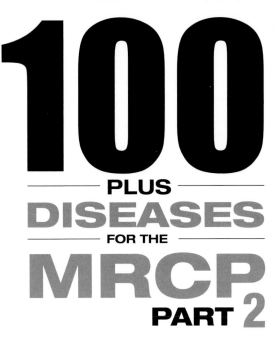

100 PLUS DISEASES FOR THE MRCP PART 2

SECOND EDITION

Miles Witham BM BCh PhD MRCP

Clinical Lecturer
Section of Ageing and Health
University of Dundee
Ninewells Hospital
Dundee, UK

Mudher Al-Khairalla MBChB MRCP(UK)

Chest Unit
Ninewells Hospital
Dundee, UK

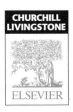

EDINBURGH LONDON NEW YORK OXFORD PHILADELPHIA ST LOUIS SYDNEY TORONTO 2008

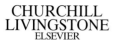

CHURCHILL
LIVINGSTONE
ELSEVIER

An Imprint of Elsevier Limited

First edition 2002
Reprinted 2003, 2004, 2006
Second edition 2008
Reprinted 2009

ISBN 9780443103759

British Library Cataloguing in Publication Data
A catalogue record for this book is available from the British Library

Library of Congress Cataloging in Publication Data
A catalog record for this book is available from the Library of Congress

---

Notice

Knowledge and best practice in this field are constantly changing. As new research and experience broaden our knowledge, changes in practice, treatment and drug therapy may become necessary or appropriate. Readers are advised to check the most current information provided (i) on procedures featured or (ii) by the manufacturer of each product to be administered, to verify the recommended dose or formula, the method and duration of administration, and contraindications. It is the responsibility of the practitioner, relying on their own experience and knowledge of the patient, to make diagnoses, to determine dosages and the best treatment for each individual patient, and to take all appropriate safety precautions. To the fullest extent of the law, neither the Publisher nor the Authors assume any liability for any injury and/or damage to persons or property arising out or related to any use of the material contained in this book.

The Publisher

Printed in China

 your source for books,
journals and multimedia
in the health sciences
www.elsevierhealth.com

Working together to grow
libraries in developing countries

www.elsevier.com | www.bookaid.org | www.sabre.org

ELSEVIER   BOOK AID International   Sabre Foundation

The publisher's policy is to use **paper manufactured from sustainable forests**

PREFACE

There are many MRCP books on the market. Most still use the question-based classical format, but the success of the first edition of this book confirms our belief that basing an MRCP book around diseases offers a complementary approach to revising for the exam.

In response to feedback we received from the first edition and taking into account some of the changes in structure of the MRCP exam that have occurred recently, we have extensively revised the text to include more diseases – hence the name '100 Plus Diseases'! We have also included more pictures and more questions reformatted in the contemporary best-of-five format, with answers and concise explanations.

We hope that these changes will maintain the book as a relevant and valuable resource for all of you attempting the MRCP – not only for part 2 but for the other components of the exam as well.

We would like to thank Justine Davies and Zayneb Al-Khairalla for their long-standing and continued patience, support and encouragement. Thanks are also due to Tim Gray for coauthoring the first edition, to Sanjay, Emer, Richard and Rebecca for their help with radiographic images, and to Lulu Stader for managing her unenviable task of being our editor with patience and persistence.

Miles Witham
Mudher Al-Khairalla

CONTENTS

CARDIOLOGY

1

AORTIC VALVE DISEASE

Aortic valve disease encompasses aortic stenosis, aortic regurgitation and mixed aortic valve disease. Aortic stenosis occurs as a result of calcific or degenerative processes, presence of a bicuspid valve, rheumatic fever or congenital stenosis. Aortic regurgitation can occur because of aortic root dilatation (e.g. hypertension, dissection, syphilis, seronegative spondyloarthropathy), trauma, endocarditis or rheumatic fever. Degeneration of the valve also occurs in collagen vascular disease and mucopolysaccharidoses.

SYMPTOMS
Aortic stenosis
Tiredness
Breathlessness
Exertional syncope
Chest pain

Aortic regurgitation
Tiredness
Breathlessness
Often asymptomatic until disease is advanced

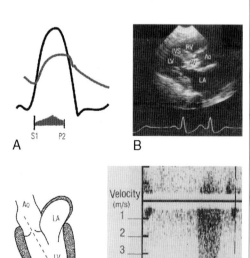

Figure 1.1 Doppler echo showing high-velocity flow across a stenosed aortic valve. (Reproduced with permission from Souhami, Moxham (2002) *Textbook of Medicine*, 4th edn. Churchill Livingstone.)

SIGNS
Aortic stenosis
Slow rising pulse
Narrow pulse pressure
Soft second heart sound
Ejection click
Ejection systolic murmur
Bibasal crackles, raised JVP, ankle oedema if heart failure has been precipitated

Aortic regurgitation
Collapsing pulse
Eponymous peripheral signs (Durozier's, Quincke's, pistol-shot femorals)
Wide pulse pressure
Both heart sounds may be soft or inaudible
Early diastolic murmur
Ejection systolic flow murmur
Mid-diastolic murmur may be present (Austin–Flint murmur)
Bibasal crackles, raised JVP, ankle oedema if heart failure has been precipitated
Mixed valve disease may produce a bisferiens (double) pulse

INVESTIGATIONS
FBC
Normal

U + Es
Urea and creatinine ↑ if congestive cardiac failure

LFTs
Abnormal if congestive cardiac failure

Clotting
Normal

ECG
Aortic stenosis
Typically shows high voltage complexes (LVH), often with lateral T-wave inversion (strain)

Aortic regurgitation
May also show LVH; poor R-wave progression as ventricle dilates

CXR
May show pulmonary oedema if decompensated cardiac failure

2

Cardiac enlargement in advanced disease
May also show aortic root dilatation as a cause of aortic regurgitation

DIAGNOSIS
Echocardiography
Allows quantification of valve gradient, and semiquantitative estimation of the degree of regurgitation. Also gives information on valve morphology, aortic root diameter, ventricular function and left ventricular end-diastolic volume

Angiography
Allows accurate estimation of the valve gradient by comparing pressure in the LV with pressure in the aorta ('pull-back' gradient). Also allows estimation of LV function, may delineate paravalvular leaks and delineates coronary anatomy if surgery is considered.

DIFFERENTIAL DIAGNOSIS
Aortic stenosis
Consider other causes of systolic murmurs:
Hypertrophic cardiomyopathy
Aortic flow murmur
Calcified aortic valve
VSD
Mitral regurgitation

Aortic regurgitation
Occasionally confused with mitral stenosis, but the murmur is quite different. Differential usually focuses on the underlying cause for the aortic regurgitation

Mixed valve disease
Patent ductus arteriosus (continuous murmur)

COMPLICATIONS
Endocarditis – prophylaxis required
Declining LV function with cardiac failure
For aortic stenosis: sudden death

TREATMENT
Is with valve replacement. Vasodilators (including ACE inhibitors) may retard ventricular dilatation in aortic regurgitation

Indications in aortic stenosis
Onset of symptoms necessitates consideration of surgery
Asymptomatic patients with severe stenosis and a positive exercise test may also benefit from surgery

Indications in aortic regurgitation
Acute severe aortic regurgitation (e.g. endocarditis)
Symptomatic severe regurgitation
Asymptomatic, but ejection fraction < 55%, LV end-systolic diameter > 55 mm or LV end-diastolic diameter > 75 mm

PROGNOSIS
Untreated symptomatic aortic stenosis median survival: 2 years
Untreated aortic regurgitation may remain asymptomatic for years, before a more rapid decline once the left ventricle fails and chronic heart failure develops

QUESTION SPOTTING
The presence of aortic valve disease will usually be clear from the history. You are more likely to be asked about the underlying cause (especially for aortic regurgitation) or about investigation and management.

MITRAL VALVE DISEASE

Mitral valve disease encompasses mitral stenosis and mitral regurgitation, including mitral valve prolapse. Mitral stenosis usually occurs almost exclusively as a result of rheumatic fever, although congenital stenosis does occur. Mitral regurgitation can occur because of left ventricular dilatation seen in heart failure. Disease can affect the valve leaflets themselves, e.g. trauma, endocarditis, rheumatic fever, myxomatous degeneration. Alteration of the subvalvar apparatus (chordal rupture, papillary muscle dysfunction due to ischaemia) also causes mitral regurgitation.

SYMPTOMS
Mitral stenosis
Tiredness
Breathlessness – on exertion, orthopnoea, paroxysmal nocturnal dysnoea
Chest pain
Haemoptysis
Cough
Dysphagia⎫
Dysphonia⎭ from enlarged left atrium

Mitral regurgitation
Tiredness
Breathlessness – on exertion, orthopnoea,
Cough

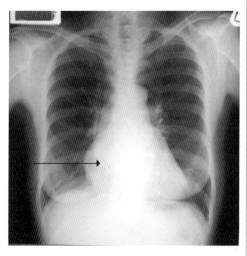

Figure 1.2 Chest X-ray from a patient with mitral valve disease. Note the double shadow on the right side of the heart, caused by left atrial enlargement (arrow).

Dysphagia⎫
Dysphonia⎭ from enlarged left atrium
Often asymptomatic until disease is advanced

SIGNS
Mitral stenosis
Low-volume pulse (usually AF)
Undisplaced apex; tapping if valve leaflets mobile
Loud first heart sound (if valve leaflets mobile)
Opening snap in diastole
Mid-diastolic murmur – presystolic accentuation if in sinus rhythm
Parasternal heave; loud P2
Bibasal crackles, raised JVP, ankle oedema if heart failure has been precipitated
Mitral facies
May develop giant V-waves (tricuspid regurgitation) due to pulmonary hypertension

Mitral regurgitation
Pulse and BP usually normal. May be in AF
Displaced, volume-overloaded apex
Second heart sound may be inaudible
Third heart sound
Pansystolic murmur at apex – may radiate to axilla or to left sternal edge
Parasternal heave and loud P2 (if pulmonary hypertension)
May develop giant V-waves (tricuspid regurgitation) due to pulmonary hypertension

Mitral valve prolapse
Mid-systolic click
Late systolic murmur. Loudest in apical area

INVESTIGATIONS
FBC
Hb – may be ↑ if pulmonary hypertension and cyanosis

U + Es
Urea and creatinine ↑ if congestive cardiac failure

LFTs
Abnormal if congestive cardiac failure

Clotting

Normal

ECG
Mitral stenosis
P mitrale (if in sinus rhythm); otherwise AF
RVH and right axis deviation

Mitral regurgitation
P mitrale (if in sinus rhythm); otherwise AF
RVH and right axis deviation (pulmonary
  hypertension)
Poor R-wave progression as ventricle dilates

CXR
Large left atrial bulge; pulmonary oedema may
be seen. Heart size often normal in mitral
stenosis, but large in mitral regurgitation

DIAGNOSIS
Echocardiography
Allows quantification of valve gradient via
pressure half-time; the valve orifice area may be
measured directly. Mitral regurgitation can be
estimated semiquantitatively with colour flow
Doppler. Also gives information on valve
calcification, whether the leaflets move,
pulmonary artery pressure, ventricular function
and left ventricular end-diastolic volume.

Angiography
Not necessary for diagnosis, but allows
estimation of LV function; may delineate
paravalvular leaks and delineates coronary
anatomy if surgery is considered. RV pressures
are often measured at the same time; severe
pulmonary hypertension or poor LV function
makes valve replacement riskier.

DIFFERENTIAL DIAGNOSIS
Mitral stenosis
Aortic regurgitation with Austin–Flint murmur
Atrial myxoma
Acute rheumatic fever

Mitral regurgitation
Aortic stenosis/sclerosis
VSD
HCM
Tricuspid regurgitation

COMPLICATIONS
Endocarditis – prophylaxis required
Declining LV function with cardiac failure
Pulmonary hypertension and right ventricular
  failure
Stroke and other arterial emboli
Dysphonia and dysphagia from left atrial
  dilatation

TREATMENT
Mitral stenosis
Anticoagulation – even in sinus rhythm if severe
  stenosis, spontaneous contrast or large LA
Beta-blockers (to prolong diastole and give time
  for LV to fill); diuretics
If symptomatic and mitral valve area < 1.5 cm:
Balloon valvotomy – if valve is not heavily
  calcified and no significant mitral regorgitation
Mitral valve replacement

Mitral regurgitation
Anticoagulation if in AF
ACE inhibitors; diuretics

Consider surgery if severe MR with symptoms,
or asymptomatic patients with progressive LV
dysfunction; choice is between mitral valve
repair and replacement

QUESTION SPOTTING
The presence of mitral valve disease will usually
be clear from the history, although the presence
of an atrial myxoma may cause confusion. You
are more likely to be asked about the underlying
cause (especially for mitral regurgitation) or
about investigation and management.

HYPERTROPHIC CARDIOMYOPATHY

HCM is an umbrella term for a group of inherited diseases affecting myocardial development. The disorders are usually inherited in an autosomal-dominant manner with incomplete penetrance. Several of the genes involved in HCM code for myocardial proteins, e.g. titin, myosin heavy chain and tropomyosin. The key pathological lesion is asymmetic hypertrophy, usually of the septum. This causes narrowing of the LV outflow tract, setting up a pressure gradient. Derangements of myocardial structure also provide a substrate for ventricular arrhythmias.

SYMPTOMS
HCM is often asymptomatic
Chest pain
Breathlessness
Palpitations
Dizziness on exertion
Loss of consciousness
Sudden death

SIGNS
Jerky pulse
Double impulse at apex
Third and fourth heart sounds
Ejection systolic murmur, louder when standing, quieter when squatting
Pansystolic murmur

INVESTIGATIONS
FBC
Normal

U + Es
Normal

LFTs
Normal

Clotting
Normal

ECG
Usually shows high-voltage complexes (LVH) and T-wave inversion
May also show atrial fibrillation
Wolff–Parkinson–White syndrome (short PR interval, delta wave) may be associated

CXR
Usually normal unless cardiac failure present

DIAGNOSIS
Is via transthoracic echocardiography. Asymmetric septal hypertrophy is present, with a gradient detectable between the left ventricular cavity and the aorta. The mitral valve apparatus is often seen to move anteriorly during systole. Doppler studies may demonstrate mitral regurgitation.

DIFFERENTIAL DIAGNOSIS
Aortic stenosis. There is no change in murmur with posture in AS, and HCM does not exhibit an ejection click
Subvalvular or supravalvular stenosis
Left ventricular hypertrophy (e.g. due to hypertension)

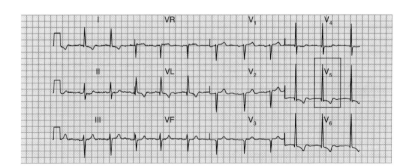

Figure 1.3 ECG showing typical high-voltage QRS and deep inverted T-waves of HCM. (Reproduced with permission from Hampton (2003) *The ECG in Practice*, 4th edn. Churchill Livingstone.)

VSD
Mitral regurgitation

COMPLICATIONS

Angina: this may occur even with normal
  coronary arteries and reflects poor endocardial
  blood supply to the grossly thickened ventricle
Sudden death, either from ventricular
  arrhythmias or from pump failure
Atrial fibrillation: the stiff LV does not tolerate
  AF well, and the onset of AF may lead to
  striking breathlessness and signs of heart
  failure
Ventricular tachycardia
Ventricular fibrillation – may occur due to rapid
  conduction of AF down an accessory pathway
Bradycardia – sick-sinus syndrome may occur

TREATMENT

Drugs. Beta-blockers can treat associated angina,
and can reduce the outflow tract gradient.
Nitrates and other vasodilators increase the
gradient and should be avoided. Atrial
fibrillation should be cardioverted electrically or
with amiodarone. Digoxin should be used with
caution – especially in those with WPW.

Septal ablation – either surgical or more
commonly via catheter ablation to infarct the
hypertrophied segment. Useful for reducing
the outflow gradient, and may help reduce the
incidence of heart failure.

Dual-chamber pacing. This can be used to
reduce the outflow gradient by altering septal
motion relative to the LV free wall.

Implantable cardioverter-defibrillator. May
be useful in patients with documented VT,
or with a strong family history of sudden death
from HCM.

PROGNOSIS

Is highly variable. Overall death rate is
approximately 4% per year, but some mutations
are associated with near-normal life
expectancy, whereas others carry a much
higher rate of sudden death. Not all
genotypes produce obstructive and arrhythmic
sequelae.

QUESTION SPOTTING

Look out for young people with ejection systolic
murmurs, especially if there is a family history of
sudden death or a history of syncope. A change
in the murmur with a change in afterload or
preload may help to differentiate HCM from
aortic stenosis. Also consider the condition if
Wolff–Parkinson–White syndrome is present.

VENTRICULAR SEPTAL DEFECT

A VSD is a defect in the interventricular septum, allowing communication between the left and right ventricles. Such a defect can be congenital, or can be acquired, usually as the result of myocardial infarction or trauma. VSDs account for 30–40% of congenital heart defects. Flow initially proceeds from left to right and, if significant, leads to RV hypertrophy, increased pulmonary pressures and pulmonary hypertension. Eventually, if RV pressure matches or exceeds LV pressure, the Eisenmenger syndrome may occur.

SYMPTOMS
Tiredness
Breathlessness
Failure to thrive (infants and children)

SIGNS
Apex beat may be forceful (pressure overload)
Parasternal heave with large VSDs
Second heart sound often obscured; P2 may be
 loud however
Pansystolic murmur loudest at left sternal edge.
 May have an associated thrill
Early diastolic murmur in pulmonary area or left
 sternal edge (pulmonary regurgitation if pulmonary hypertension; aortic regurgitation if
 lesion is close to the aortic valve)
Mid-diastolic flow murmur in mitral area
Note that the murmur becomes softer as RV
 pressure approaches LV pressure

INVESTIGATIONS
Biochemistry
Normal

Haematology
Normal unless Eisenmenger's syndrome develops

CXR
Pulmonary congestion with enlarged pulmonary arteries. Heart may appear large with large VSDs

ECG
May show LVH, and, with large VSDs, RVH as well.

DIAGNOSIS
Is by echocardiography. The defect may be
 visible, and colour Doppler will show blood
 flow across the defect, together with the way
 the shunt is flowing.
Cardiac catheterization will also allow
 delineation of the site of the shunt, both with
 dye and via saturations.

DIFFERENTIAL DIAGNOSIS
Atrial septal defect (in cases of Eisenmenger's
 syndrome)
Mitral regurgitation
Pulmonary stenosis
HCM
Complex congenital defects (e.g. Fallot's
 tetralogy)

COMPLICATIONS
Acute
Pulmonary oedema
Cardiogenic shock
Ventricular arrhythmias

Chronic
Pulmonary hypertension, leading to Eisenmenger
 syndrome

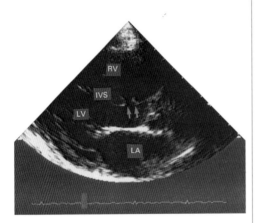

Figure 1.4 Transoesophageal echo showing ventricular septal defect after inferior myocardial infarction. (Reproduced with permission from Kumar, Clarke (2001) *Clinical Medicine*, 5th edn. Saunders.)

TREATMENT

In acute cases, the treatment is emergency surgery if the patient's comorbid state allows it; the defect is repaired with a woven patch.

In chronic cases, small defects usually close spontaneously. Moderate or larger defects (especially if causing pulmonary hypertension or if pulmonary flow is twice systemic flow) require surgery to close them, using an artificial patch. For some VSDs in the apical (muscular) septum, percutaneous closure devices can be used.

If surgery cannot be attempted, medical management of heart failure (e.g. with diuretics) is necessary.

PROGNOSIS

30–50% of congenital VSDs close spontaneously. The larger the VSD, the less likely closure is.

VSDs due to myocardial infarction carry a poor prognosis – emergency cardiac surgery can be life-saving, however, if the patient is otherwise fit. A few patients survive the acute period and can undergo later surgery to patch the defect.

QUESTION SPOTTING

Congenital VSDs usually present in childhood; a question involving an adult will either have had a diagnosis made years ago, or will present as Eisenmenger syndrome. Consider especially in patients with Down's syndrome.

Consider VSD in patients who suddenly become unwell a few days after myocardial infarction – they often present with pulmonary oedema or cardiogenic shock.

Also consider as an uncommon substrate for endocarditis.

FALLOT'S TETRALOGY

Fallot's tetralogy is one of the commoner causes of cyanotic congenital heart disease. It accounts for approximately 5–10% of all congenital heart defects. The tetralogy is:

Pulmonary stenosis (or subpulmonary stenosis)
Right ventricular hypertrophy
Ventricular septal defect
Overriding aorta (aortic outflow tract receives blood from left and right ventricles)

Other cardiac malformations may be associated, e.g. ASD, anomalous pulmonary venous drainage, bicuspid pulmonary valve, coronary artery abnormalities. RV hypertrophy leads to increased left-to-right shunting and consequent biventricular failure. Cyanosis occurs because of the VSD shunt and the overriding aorta draining RV and LV.

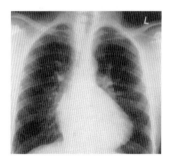

Figure 1.5 CXR of a patient with Fallot's tetralogy. (Reproduced with permission from Souhami, Moxham (2002) *Textbook of Medicine*, 4th edn. Churchill Livingstone.)

SYMPTOMS

Poor appetite and feeding
Breathlessness, especially on exertion
Cyanotic attacks, ending in syncope if severe. Precipitated by exertion or stress
Squatting (to relieve breathlessness or cyanotic attacks)
Note that symptoms may take several weeks to develop after birth

SIGNS

Small for age
Cyanosis – may only occur during acute attacks
Plethora
Clubbing
Parasternal heave
Loud second heart sound
Ejection systolic murmur to pulmonary area (may have accompanying thrill). May become quieter during acute attacks
Continuous murmur in back (due to collaterals)

INVESTIGATIONS
FBC

Hb ↑
Hct ↑
WCC normal
Platelets normal or ↑

U + Es

Urea and creatinine raised if congestive cardiac failure

LFTs

Abnormal if congestive cardiac failure
Clotting usually normal

ECG

RBBB

RV hypertrophy

CXR

Boot-shaped heart

Small pulmonary arteries; oligaemic lung fields

Right-sided aortic knuckle in 25%

DIAGNOSIS

Is by echocardiography and, more definitively, by right and left cardiac catheterization. This shows the VSD, aortic position and pulmonary stenosis and demonstrates the pulmonary vessels, allowing detailed planning for surgery.

DIFFERENTIAL DIAGNOSIS

Other causes of cyanotic congenital heart disease:

Transposition of the great arteries

Total anomalous pulmonary venous drainage

Also consider Eisenmenger's syndrome (especially due to VSD)

TREATMENT

Definitive treatment is by surgical repair – closure of VSD and correction of pulmonary stenosis. 2–5% perioperative mortality. Usually carried out in first 2–3 years of life.

Shunting (e.g. Blalock–Taussig shunt) may be performed in severe disease in the first year of life, pending definitive surgical correction at a later date.

Morphine, beta-blockers or phenylephrine can be used to reduce the severity of cyanotic attacks.

COMPLICATIONS

Ventricular arrhythmias

Syncopal/cyanotic attacks; may lead to cerebral damage if very severe

Uncorrected, Fallot's leads to RV and LV failure

Even after total surgical correction, late-onset heart failure, pulmonary regurgitation, AV block and ventricular arrhythmias may occur

Endocarditis

Cerebral abscess

Paradoxical embolism

Arterial and venous thrombosis

Gout

PROGNOSIS

Excellent after surgery. Survival into adulthood is very rare (and only in mild cases) without intervention

QUESTION SPOTTING

Fallot's will usually be a consideration in children only. However, incompletely corrected Fallot's may present in adulthood; look for a history of cardiac surgery as a child, the presence of cyanosis, and prominent RV features on CXR and ECG.

EISENMENGER'S SYNDROME

Eisenmenger's syndrome occurs when there is significant communication between pulmonary and systemic circulation. The syndrome occurs when the blood flow reverses direction (flow from right to left) due to increased right-sided pressures. The site of the defect is usually divided into pre- and posttricuspid, and this determines the presentation.

Pretricuspid defects (e.g. ASD, single atrium and sinus venosum defects)
The left and right ventricles at birth are the same size and the right ventricle usually regresses with the reduction of right-sided pressures at birth. In pretricuspid defect cases, although there is increased flow (often 3:1+), the right ventricle regresses normally and dilates to accommodate the increased flow and protect the pulmonary vasculature. The shunt by definition bypasses the left ventricle, which is usually normal. Eisenmenger's in this situation is unusual, is often atypical, occurs late (90% present in adulthood) and heart failure is rare.

Posttricuspid defects (e.g. VSD, single ventricle and patent ductus arteriosus)
High flow rates (3:1–5:1) and high pressure from birth in the right ventricle stop the normal right ventricular regression. Pulmonary artery smooth-muscular hypertrophy occurs with reduced lung compliance, and increased work of breathing. This causes right ventricular failure and obliterative pulmonary changes. 80% present in infancy.

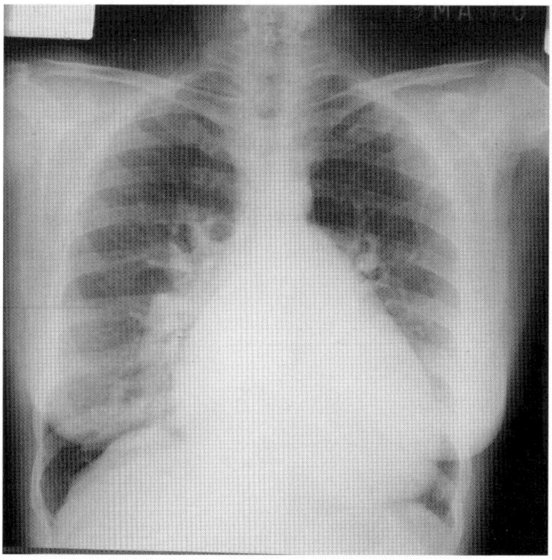

SYMPTOMS
Dyspnoea, fatigue, syncope from low-output state
Headache, dizziness, visual disturbance from hyperviscosity
Palpitations
Haemoptysis and excessive bleeding
Stroke from hyperviscosity, paradoxical embolus and cerebral abscess

SIGNS
Cyanosis and clubbing (feet only if PDA)
Parasternal heave
Lungs are typically clear
Ankle swelling

Heart sounds
Loud pulmonary component of second heart sound (sometimes palpable)
Right-sided S4
Single S2 in VSD or wide and fixed in ASD
Pulmonary regurgitation murmur (Graham Steell)
Pulmonary ejection click and murmur
Peripheral oedema if RV failure
No murmur of VSD or PDA

INVESTIGATIONS
FBC
Hb ↑
Hct ↑
WCC normal
Platelets normal or ↓

U + Es
Urea and creatinine ↑ if congestive cardiac failure

LFTs
Abnormal if congestive cardiac failure

ESR ↓
Clotting normal or prolonged
Urate ↑

Figure 1.6 Chest X-ray showing cardiomegaly, large pulmonary arteries and peripheral pruning in Eisenmenger's syndrome.

ECG

P pulmonale
↑ RV ± LV hypertrophy
Atrial arrhythmias

CXR

↑ PA with oligaemic lung fields – 'pruning'
May see calcification of the PA
Cardiomegaly in ASD but normal heart size
typical of VSD/PDA

DIAGNOSIS
Echocardiography

Identifies defects and valve abnormalities
Colour mapping may show flow across the shunt
TOE better for visualization of ASD or PDA.
Cardiac MRI can also be used to delineate the
anatomy.

Cardiac catheter

Shows high RV pressure, and can locate site of
defect using angiography and saturation
measurements. Degree of shunt can also be
estimated.

DIFFERENTIAL DIAGNOSIS

Primary pulmonary hypertension
Pulmonary vascular obstruction
Pulmonary vascular disease
Lung disease, e.g. restrictive interstitial lung
disease
Left atrial hypertension
Left ventricular diastolic dysfunction

COMPLICATIONS

Endocarditis
Hyperviscosity and CVAs
Haemostatic abnormalities with reduced clotting
factors and platelets
Cholelithiasis
Hypertrophic osteoarthropathy
Hyperuricaemia and gout
Renal dysfunction
Haemoptysis

TREATMENT

Avoidance of calcium-channel blockers (reduce
systemic blood pressure and so increase shunt),
antiplatelet and anticoagulant drugs due to
increased risk of bleeding
Antibiotic prophylaxis against endocarditis
Isovolaemic phlebotomy (only if symptomatic or
if Hct > 0.65 with a bleeding diathesis). If
symptoms persist despite phlebotomy, then
consider iron-deficiency state
Transplant – heart/lung or lung with repair of
defect if normal LV function and no coronary
disease

PROGNOSIS

80% 10-year, 77% 15-year and 42% 25-year
survival
Death mostly due to arrhythmia; also heart
failure, haemoptysis, brain abscess, embolism
Transplant survival: 70% 1-year, 50% 5-year,
30% 10-year survival
Pregnancy mortality 45%, with 50% being
premature and 40% spontaneous abortion rate
Up to 19% mortality rate with non-cardiac
surgery so best avoided if possible

QUESTION SPOTTING

A new presentation of Eisenmenger's in an adult
is almost always due to an ASD and is less likely
to present with heart failure, and more likely with
arrhythmia or hyperviscosity syndrome. Being
asked about pregnancy in a woman with
Eisenmenger's is a possibility.
Also consider Eisenmenger's in young to
middle-aged patients with any of:

Cyanosis
Clubbing
Stroke/cerebral abscess
Polycythaemia

INFECTIVE ENDOCARDITIS

Microbial infection of the endothelial surface of the heart. This is usually bacterial, but may be fungal or an atypical organism. The disease usually occurs on the heart valves (in order of mitral, aortic, tricuspid and pulmonary) but may also affect septal defects, cardiac tendinae and shunts, including patent ductus arteriosus and coarctation. The vegetations consist of fibrin, collagen, platelets, red and white blood cells and bacteria. These cause destruction of cardiac tissue, leading to valvular incompetence, chordae rupture and abscess formation; embolization of vegetation leads to septic foci in distal organs such as CNS, lungs, kidneys and spleen, and immune-complex vasculitis, especially affecting the kidneys. Most common organisms can be seen in Table 1.1.

Risk factors

No known predisposing factors in 20–40%. Predisposing factors include rheumatic heart disease, congenital heart disease, mitral valve prolapse with mitral regurgitation, degenerative heart disease, intravenous drug abuse, hypertrophic cardiomyopathy, prosthetic valves and previous endocarditis.

SYMPTOMS

Fever
Sweats
Weight loss
Fatigue
Anorexia
Dyspnoea
Cough
Stroke
Headache

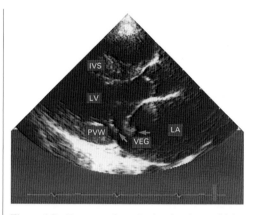

Figure 1.7 Transoesophageal echo showing multiple small vegetations on the mitral valve. (Reproduced with permission from Kumar, Clarke (2001) *Clinical Medicine*, 5th edn. Saunders.)

Arthralgia
Chest pain
Confusion

SIGNS

Fever
Murmurs
Tachycardia
Splenomegaly
Clubbing – rare, except in prolonged illness
Oedema
Neurological deficit due to abscess or cerebral
    embolization
Embolic features and immune-complex
    deposition: splinter haemorrhages, petechiae,
    Janeway lesions, Roth spots and Osler's nodes

INVESTIGATIONS
FBC
Hb ↓ (normochromic, normocytic)
WCC ↑
Platelets normal

U + Es
Urea and creatinine may be ↑

LFTs
Albumin ↓
Immunoglobulins ↑
Otherwise usually normal

Table 1.1 Organisms grown in endocarditis

	Native value (%)	Prosthetic value (%)
Streptococcus species	55	45
Staphylococcus aureus	7	11
Gram-negative bacilli	5	1
Coagulase-negative staphylococci	4	15

ESR ↑
CRP ↑
Clotting normal
False-positive VDRL
Complement levels ↓

Urine
Proteinuria and haematuria in 50%

CXR
Cardiomegaly
Pulmonary congestion
Cannonball lesions seen with right-sided
endocarditis from septic emboli

ECG
↑ PR interval if aortic root involvement

DIAGNOSIS
Duke's criteria
Major
1. Positive blood cultures – organism grown
from two separate cultures or persistent
positive cultures 12 hours apart
2. Evidence of endocardial involvement, i.e.
echocardiographic evidence of vegetation,
abscess or new dehiscence or new valve murmur

Minor
Predisposition to endocarditis
Fever > 38°C
Vascular phenomena, e.g. splinter
haemorrhages, arterial embolism, mycotic
aneurysm, intracranial haemorrhage,
splenomegaly
Positive blood cultures (non-major)
Immunological phenomena, e.g. Osler's nodes,
Roth spots, glomerulonephritis, CRP >
100 mg/L, ESR > 1.5 upper limit of normal

Diagnosis depends on 2 major, 1 major and 3
minor or 5 minor
Blood cultures mold × 3 positive in 90%
Serology for *Aspergillus*, *Candida*, Q fever,
Chlamydia, *Brucella* if appropriate
CO_2 culture for HACEK organisms if otherwise
culture-negative

Echocardiography
Transthoracic sensitive in 58–63% in native
valve endocarditis but less if prosthetic

Transoesophageal echocardiography sensitive in
90–100%

COMPLICATIONS
Embolic
Cerebral, renal, splenic, hepatic infarcts and
mycotic aneurysms if left-sided endocarditis
Pulmonary infarcts or abscesses if right-sided
endocarditis

Cardiac
Valvular failure, unstable prosthesis, fistula
formation, abscess formation, AV nodal block
and valvular obstruction if vegetation enlarges

Renal
Vasculitis leading to renal failure

TREATMENT
Antibiotic therapy
Prolonged intravenous antibiotics (usually 4–6
weeks). Frequently benzylpenicillin and
gentamicin if penicillin-sensitive *Streptococcus*.
Staphylococci usually require flucloxacillin or
vancomycin, plus gentamicin. Follow *British
National Formulary* guidelines. Doses dependent
on MIC and MBC. Length of treatment depends
on organism isolated.

If culture negative with native valve
endocarditis, give ampicillin and gentamicin. If
prosthetic valve and culture negative, add in
vancomycin.

Surgery
Uncontrolled infection/resistant infection/relapse
after therapy
Unstable prosthesis
Severe valve incompetence, especially if causing
heart failure
Perivalvular extension of infection
Large vegetations
Staphylococcus aureus infection or fungal infection
Culture-negative endocarditis with persistent
fever

Prevention
Prophylactic antibiotics prior to:
Dental work involving work below the gum line
Surgical procedures, especially if any pre-
existing infection
Cystoscopy and urinary tract instrumentation
Prostatic biopsy

Pacemaker insertion

Rigid bronchoscopy (but not flexible)

Vaginal delivery if infection present

Colonoscopy and biopsy, especially if inflammation

Oesophageal balloon dilatation, argon ablation, variceal injection (but not routine oesophagogastroduodenoscopy)

Patients who need prophylaxis are those at high and moderate risk of endocarditis:

High-risk

Prosthetic heart valves

Previous infective endocarditis

Mitral valve prolapse with mitral regurgitation or thickened MV leaflets

Complex congenital cyanotic heart disease, e.g. Fallot's

Surgically constructed systemic pulmonary shunts

Moderate-risk

Acquired valvular disease – e.g. AS, AR, MS, MR

Non-cyanotic congenital defects, e.g. ASD, VSD, bicuspid aortic valve

Hypertrophic cardiomyopathy

Aortic root replacement

QUESTION SPOTTING

Endocarditis is a multisystem disorder that has a long differential diagnosis (see SLE). Because of the serious nature of the disease, it is essential to consider it in any patient presenting with a murmur and fever. CRP is a better marker than ESR for active disease (see SLE).

Key points that may come up in questions:

1. Transoesophageal echo is much more sensitive for vegetations than transthoracic echo
2. Echocardiographic confirmation of vegetations is not always necessary for diagnosis
3. Be aware of the prophylaxis guidelines
4. Know the relative and absolute indications for surgery

RHEUMATIC FEVER

Rheumatic fever is a systemic connective tissue disease occurring approximately 3 weeks after a group A streptococcal infection. It causes inflammation of the heart, central nervous system and joints, probably due to cross-reactivity of the streptococcal M protein with cardiac and other organ tissue, which leads to an autoimmune reaction. This leads to the pathognomonic Aschoff lesion which is collagen degeneration associated with infiltration of mononuclear cells and multinucleated histiocytes. The disease typically affects 6 to 16-year-olds, who often have a genetic predisposition.

CLINICAL FEATURES
The diagnosis is clinical and defined by the Duckett Jones criteria:

Major criteria
Pancarditis (40–50%)
Endocarditis: valvulitis most frequently involving mitral and aortic valves, causing valvular insufficiency and scarring. Murmurs are common, including a non-specific mid-systolic murmur, the Carey Coombes murmur (mid-diastolic murmur of thickened mitral valves). Nodules may form on the valve leaflets
Myocarditis: causes cardiac failure, conduction defects and arrhythmias
Pericarditis: pericardial effusion, friction rub and chest pains

Polyarthritis (60–80%)
Typically an asymmetrical, large-joint migratory polyarthritis. The arthritis tends to be more prominent than carditis in adults and vice versa in children

Chorea (5–20%)
Sydenham's chorea, St Vitus' dance
May be the only clinical finding. May include emotional lability and explosive speech

Erythema marginatum (< 5%)
Subcutaneous nodules (< 5%)

Minor criteria
Arthralgia
Fever
↑ ESR/CRP
↑ PR interval

Previous rheumatic fever
Leukocytosis
Two minor, or one major plus two minor, criteria are necessary for diagnosis. Plus supporting evidence of preceding group A streptococcal infection by throat swab culture, ↑ ASOT or other streptococcal antibody test.

INVESTIGATIONS
FBC
Hb ↓ (MCV normal)
WCC ↑ though variable. Neutrophilia
Platelets normal
ESR ↑

U + Es
Usually normal

LFTs
Albumin normal or ↓
Otherwise normal

CRP ↑
CK ↑
Troponins ↑
↑ ASOT titre and levels >200 units

CXR
Cardiomegaly
Increased pulmonary vascular markings
Pulmonary oedema

ECG
PR interval ↑
Tachycardia
AV block
Non-specific QRS and T-wave changes

Echocardiogram
Cardiac dilatation
Valvular abnormalities
Pericardial effusion

DIAGNOSIS
Clinical diagnosis based on Duckett Jones criteria and echocardiographic findings

DIFFERENTIAL DIAGNOSIS
SLE
Acute juvenile arthritis or Still's disease
Infective endocarditis

Pericarditis
Viral illness with arthralgia

TREATMENT
Bedrest until inflammatory markers are normal
Penicillin for 10 days to treat streptococcal
    infection (erythromycin in penicillin
    hypersensitivity)
Aspirin (80–100 mg/kg per day) in divided doses
    for at least a month in mild carditis or arthritis.
    Prolonged course (3–6 months) may be needed
    in severe disease
Prednisolone 1–2 mg/kg per day for 1–3 months
    if severe cardiac disease
Rebound carditis and arthritis is often seen on
    weaning off steroids, and aspirin is indicated
    for this
Valve replacement if acute severe valvular
    insufficiency
Valproate may be useful for choreiform
    movements

Primary prevention
Penicillin as early as possible in streptococcal
pharyngitis

Secondary prevention
Continuous penicillin for 5 years or until 21 years
of age (whichever is longer) if no carditis. May
be needed for longer and sometimes life if
carditis

PROGNOSIS
There is a recurrence rate of 50% in patients who
have previously had the disease who then get a
group A streptococcal pharyngitis.

QUESTION SPOTTING
Watch for the Duckett Jones criteria and be
especially alerted if chorea is present. Pericarditis
is commoner than endocarditis in rheumatic
fever. A history of sore throat is another possible
clue.

Take care to differentiate rheumatic fever from
infective endocarditis. There is considerable
overlap, but chorea and erythema marginatum
point to rheumatic fever, as does pericarditic
pain. Discrete vegetations or positive blood
cultures point more towards infective
endocarditis.

ATRIAL SEPTAL DEFECTS

The true atrial septal defects are those that originate from the fossa ovalis, giving rise to ostium secundum defects. However the term is also often used to include any communication between left and right sides of the heart at atrial level. These lesions include ostium primum defects, sinus venosus defects, inferior vena cava defects and coronary sinus anomalies.

The male-to-female ratio is 1:4. Ostium primum defects tend to present in childhood. Ostium secundum defects often present in adulthood and often with atrial fibrillation.

SYMPTOMS

Usually asymptomatic in early years
Fatigue
Exertional dyspnoea
Chest infections
Palpitations

SIGNS

Irregular pulse
↑ JVP
Right ventricular heave
S1 normal or split, S2 wide fixed split
Mid-systolic ejection flow murmur
Mid-diastolic tricuspid flow murmur
Pansystolic murmur of mitral regurgitation if associated mitral valve abnormalities, including MV prolapse

INVESTIGATIONS
ECG

Primum: RVH, RBBB, right axis deviation
Secundum: RVH, RBBB, left axis deviation
Sinus venosus: RVH, RBBB, right axis deviation, left axis P waves
May have ↑ PR interval

CXR

Large RA and RV
Large PA and pulmonary markings

DIAGNOSIS
Echocardiography

Large RA, RV and PA
Mitral valve abnormalities
Direct visualization of the defect

Cardiac catheter

Useful to work out shunting with saturation measurements
Catheter may pass through defect and may identify other defects
Right-sided pressures often normal unless pulmonary hypertension

ASSOCIATIONS

Down's syndrome

DIFFERENTIAL DIAGNOSIS

VSD
PDA
Endocardial cushion defect

COMPLICATIONS

Infective endocarditis in ostium primum defects
Pulmonary hypertension (15%) as late complication
Eisenmenger's syndrome (6–9%)
Cardiac failure
Atrial arrhythmias
Paradoxical embolus

TREATMENT

Antibiotic prophylaxis for dental work.

Surgical closure if uncomplicated ASD with significant shunt (> 1.5:1). This is best performed in children aged 2–5 and has a mortality of < 1%.

Percutaneous closure now possible with deployable dumb-bell devices but these have limitations.

QUESTION SPOTTING

May be part of an Eisenmenger's complex or be the cause of infective endocarditis.

You may find an ASD is the diagnosis on cardiac catheterization data. Remember that in ASDs the ventricular saturations will be the same, whereas in VSDs the left ventricular saturations may be different from aortic saturations.

CARDIAC MYXOMAS

Tumours of mesenchymal origin, occurring in the heart. Although they tend not to be invasive, embolization is common. The cause is not clearly established, but some tumours show cytogenetic abnormalities, especially in cases of Carney's syndrome (see below). 86% are in the left atrium, and usually arise from the septal wall, and 90% are solitary. Less commonly they arise in the right atrium and rarely in the ventricles. 10% of cases are familial and probably autosomal-dominant.

SYMPTOMS
Fever
Weight loss
Exertional dyspnoea
Paroxysmal dyspnoea
Syncope
Haemoptysis
Some symptoms may vary with body position
Also arthralgia, myalgia, chest pain
Stroke

SIGNS
Irregular pulse
Clubbing
Raynaud's phenomenon
Mid-diastolic murmur of mitral stenosis which may vary with position
Pansystolic murmur of mitral regurgitation
Loud P2 and right heart failure if right-sided
Tumour 'plop'

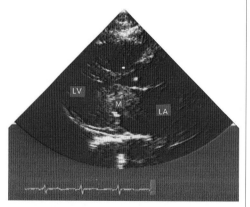

Figure 1.8 Echo showing large atrial myxoma. (Reproduced with permission from Kumar, Clarke (2001) *Clinical Medicine*, 5th edn. Saunders.)

INVESTIGATIONS
FBC
Hb ↓ (MCV normal)
WCC ↑
Platelets normal or rarely ↓
ESR ↑
Clotting normal

U + Es
Urea and creatinine ↑ if renal vasculitis or embolization

LFTs
Globulins ↑
Albumin ↓

CRP ↑

Urinalysis
Blood and protein if renal vasculitis or embolization

DIAGNOSIS
Echocardiography
Allows accurate estimation of size, position and mobility of the tumour. May be difficult to differentiate from atrial thrombus

Transoesophageal echocardiography
Often superior to transthoracic echocardiography

Cardiac catheter
Has risk of tumour embolization, but should be performed if there is suspicion of underlying coronary artery disease

ASSOCIATIONS
A few cases are as part of the syndrome myxoma or Carney's syndrome: cardiac myxoma (may be multiple, recurrent after surgery, and more often in other chambers of the heart)
Myxomas in other sites, e.g. skin
Freckled pigmentation of the skin
Endocrine tumours, e.g. pituitary, testicular, adrenal cortex

DIFFERENTIAL DIAGNOSIS
Connective tissue diseases
Infective endocarditis
Atrial thrombus

Rheumatic fever
Other occult malignancy

COMPLICATIONS

Embolization to brain, lung and peripheral vessels which may show malignant tendencies with local invasion and destruction, giving rise to myxomatous pseudoaneurysms

TREATMENT

Urgent surgical resection. Low mortality rates reported (2%)

Recurrence is in the order of 1–5% following resection (up to 22% if familial type)

QUESTION SPOTTING

Atrial myxoma may mimic connective tissue diseases but appropriate testing with ANA, ANCA or rheumatoid factor should help. If echocardiography suggests an intracardiac mass, or clinical examination suggests a new murmur, then infective endocarditis is clearly an important diagnosis to rule out. Blood cultures should be the investigation of choice in this situation.

Think of atrial myxoma in young patients with stroke-like symptoms or loss of consciousness.

RESPIRATORY DISEASE

SARCOIDOSIS

Sarcoidosis is a multisystem disorder of unknown aetiology. The hallmark of the disease is the presence of non-caseating granulomas in affected organ systems. Almost any organ system may be involved, making it the ideal MRCP topic. Afro-Caribbean and Irish people are affected more commonly. Peak age of onset 25–40 years.

CLINICAL FEATURES

May be asymptomatic and is commonly an incidental finding on a CXR. 90% have thoracic involvement

Constitutional
Fever
Malaise
Weight loss
Peripheral lymphadenopathy

Respiratory
Dry cough (> 90%)
SOB on exertion
Wheeze
Crackles occur only when fibrosis is established
Clubbing is rare
Pleural effusion (uncommon)

Skin/joints
Arthralgia (12–27%)
Acute polyarthropathy may also occur, especially at the onset of the illness
Bone pain (cysts – 5%)
Tendon and joint inflammation
Lupus pernio
Violaceous plaques
Maculopapular rash
Subcutaneous nodules
Erythema nodosum

Eyes
Painful eyes – anterior uveitis
Blurred vision (uveitis, papilloedema, chorioretinitis)
Dry eyes (lacrimitis)
Band keratopathy (from hypercalcaemia)

Neurological
Meningism (5%)
Cranial nerve palsies (especially VIIn – may be bilateral)
Thirst, polyuria (hypothalamic involvement or hypercalcaemia)
Seizures
Psychosis
Paraesthesia and focal weakness (peripheral neuropathy, transverse myelitis)

Cardiac
Sudden death (heart block, arrhythmias)
Cardiomyopathy
Ventricular aneurysm – very rare

Other
Dry mouth (parotitis)
Hepatomegaly (25%, usually asymptomatic, but may give rise to portal hypertension and varices)
Splenomegaly (25%)

INVESTIGATIONS
FBC
Usually normal
Lymphocytes may be ↓
Hb, WCC and platelets ↓ if spleen enlarged

U + Es
Usually normal

LFTs
Calcium – may be ↑
Bilirubin, ALP mildly ↑ if liver involved
Albumin may be ↓

CRP usually normal
Immunoglobulins may be ↑
Serum ACE – ↑ in two-thirds who have active disease; false-positive rate is high and includes TB
Urinary calcium often raised due to increased vitamin D absorption from the gut

CXR
Bilateral hilar lymph nodes in 90% in acute disease
May show midzone or diffuse fibrosis. See Figure 2.1 – staging the disease is more important

High-resolution CT chest
Micronodules in a subpleural and bronchovascular distribution. Small-airway trapping due to granulomas common. Possible honeycomb lung. Possible hilar and

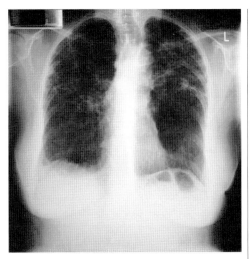

Figure 2.1 Sarcoid. This chest X-ray shows bilateral upper-lobe fibrosis secondary to sarcoid. The hila are pulled up and the lower lobes are pulled up and stretched so that tenting can be seen at the diaphragm. There are also cystic changes in the upper lobes.

mediastinal lymphadenopathy. Endobronchial disease in 55%

ECG
May show AV block or conduction delay

PFTs
Reduced FVC and TLco. FEV_1 may also be reduced due to obstructive lesions
Tuberculin test negative in two-thirds. A strongly positive test is unusual

Biopsy
Bronchoscopy
Bronchial biopsy – 41–57% positive (higher if visible abnormality)
Transbronchial biopsy – 40–90% positive
Lymphocytosis from BAL. Also seen in pneumonitis and smokers

Mediastinoscopy
90% positive yield. Useful in excluding lymphoma
Biopsy from other organ involvement, e.g. skin

DIAGNOSIS
Characteristic clinical features with radiological support (high resolution CT will also show parenchymal involvement) and preferably histological evidence of non-caseating granulomas in any tissue. Biopsy is usually obtained from bronchial or trans- bronchial biopsy. Lymphocytosis from BAL would also be useful. TB and lymphoma often need to be excluded as they can produce a similar clinical, radiological and histological picture

DIFFERENTIAL DIAGNOSIS
Sarcoid can mimic many other diseases, as its manifestations are so diverse

Lung diseases which may mimic the fibrosis of sarcoid
Interstitial lung disease
Malignancy
Infection

Differential diagnosis for BHL
Tuberculosis
Lymphoma
Metastatic Ca
Histoplasmosis
Coccidiomycosis
Berylliosis
Hypogammaglobulinaemia
Recurrent infections
Leukaemia

COMPLICATIONS
Progressive fibrosis and lung damage can lead to bronchiectasis and *Aspergillus* colonization. Fibrosis also leads to cor pulmonale
Sudden death or cardiac failure occur secondary to cardiac involvement

TREATMENT
Most patients have asymptomatic CXR changes not requiring treatment and are simply kept under surveillance

Indications for immunosuppressive therapy:
Increasing symptoms, worsening CXR and PFTs
Cardiac and neurosarcoid
Sight-threatening ocular sarcoid
Hypercalcaemia
Lupus pernio
Splenic, hepatic and renal sarcoid

Usually with high-dose steroids for 4 weeks reduced to maintenance dose around 5–15 mg of prednisolone for a few months and then slowly reduce to 5–7.5 mg for 6–12 months, which consolidates resolution

May need to consider gastric and bone protection for this group

Other drugs

Methotrexate: useful in cutaneous disease

Azathioprine: used in neurosarcoid and as a steroid-sparing agent

Antimalarials: used for skin involvement and hypercalcaemia

PROGNOSIS

Lofgren's syndrome (erythema nodosum plus BHL) – 80% enter remission

BHL alone (50%) – 80% remit within 1 year
BHL and fibrosis (25%) – 50% remit
Fibrosis alone (10%) – 25% remit
More aggressive in black populations

QUESTION SPOTTING

Sarcoidosis can be used in many different ways but often a clue is the combination of respiratory symptoms together with thirst and polyuria. Any cranial nerve lesion, especially if bilateral, should cause suspicion of sarcoid with a differential diagnosis of Lyme disease.

Questions may depict a patient with shortness of breath, a restrictive defect and a high calcium.

A defect in the *CFTR* gene located on the long arm of chromosome 7 is thought to be the cause of most cases. This gene is essential for the regulation of salt and water movement across cell membranes. The gene represents a transmembrane chloride channel, and a defect leads to an alteration in shape and thus a failure to open in response to elevated cAMP. This causes failure of excretion of chloride and so there is an increased reabsorption of sodium into the epithelial cells. With less salt there is less excretion of water and so the viscosity of mucus produced at the epithelial surface rises. The CFTR is also required for excretion of sweat and CF patients have impaired reabsorption of sodium chloride in the sweat ducts leading to excessive loss of this in sweat.

More than 800 gene defects have now been identified; the commonest is the ΔF508 mutation. This accounts for 70% of cases in the UK and USA. In southern Europe, this falls to < 50% and only 30% in Ashkenazi families. Cystic fibrosis is one of the most common hereditary diseases in Caucasians, with a carrier frequency of 1:25 and an incidence of about 1:2500 live births.

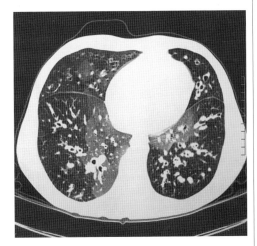

Figure 2.2 Bronchiectasis. Widespread airway enlargement with air trapping. Patches of lung tissue show higher attenuation. These are normal and reduce in size on expiration. Other areas show low attenuation which is unaltered on expiration; these are areas of alveolitis with air trapping.

CLINICAL FEATURES

Respiratory
Nasal polyps
Haemoptysis
Recurrent bronchial infections, especially with
    *Staphylococcus aureus, Pseudomonas
    aeruginosa* or *Burkholderia cepacia*
Bronchiectasis from recurrent infections
Spontaneous pneumothorax
Cor pulmonale
Allergic bronchopulmonary aspergillosis
CF 'asthma'

Gastrointestinal
Abdominal pain from:
Pancreatic inflammation and failure leading to
    steatorrhoea and *impaired glucose tolerance*.
    Pancreatitis (acute and chronic) occurs in 15%
    of CF adults and the acute form is less severe
    than the non-CF form.
Small-bowel obstruction (meconium ileus-
    equivalent)
Reflux
Biliary cirrhosis and portal hypertension from
    chronic cholestatic liver disease
Gallstones
Pericholangitis
Periportal hepatic fibrosis

Other
Male infertility
Secondary amenorrhoea
Amyloid
Arthropathy
Finger clubbing in chronic suppurative lung
    disease

Infants may present with:
Meconium ileus
Failure to thrive
Oedema from hypoalbuminaemia

INVESTIGATIONS
FBC
Hb normal
WCC ↑ if infection
Platelets normal or ↓ if splenomegaly

U + Es
Normal

LFTs

Usually abnormal
Albumin ↓
Bilirubin often ↑
AST often ↑
ALP often ↑

Ca may be normal or ↓
Amylase ↓
Glucose ↑ (impaired glucose tolerance)
Immunoglobulins normal
Vitamin A, D and E levels can be reduced
Faecal elastase is useful in screening for exocrine
pancreatic dysfunction

CXR

Pneumonia
Bronchiectasis
Pneumothorax
Fibrosis

High-resolution CT chest

Will show bronchiectasis (Fig. 2.2)

DIAGNOSIS

High sweat sodium and chloride concentration of
over 60 mmol/L; chloride usually more than
sodium
Genetic screening for known common CF
mutations should be considered

DIFFERENTIAL DIAGNOSIS

Coeliac disease (may coexist with cystic
fibrosis). Look for evidence of villous atrophy
Congenital pancreatic hypoplasia
Crohn's disease/ulcerative colitis

Causes of bronchiectasis

Postinfectious: measles, rubella, tuberculosis
Allergic bronchopulmonary aspergillosis
Gamma-globulin deficiencies
Ciliary immotility, e.g. Kartagener's syndrome
Neuropathic causes such as Chagas disease and
the Riley–Day syndrome which cause
autonomic disturbance leading to
hypersecretion of mucus
Bronchial obstruction with tumour or foreign
body
Idiopathic

TREATMENT

CF patients are best managed by a
multidisciplinary team, including
physiotherapist, specialist nurse, dietician,
psychologist and physician
Gene therapy is not yet possible

Chest

Regular physiotherapy (postural drainage, active
cycle techniques and forced expiratory
techniques)
Antibiotics are given in acute exacerbations
(intravenously if *Pseudomans*) and
prophylactically (orally or via nebulizer).
Mucolytics such as DNase also play a role, as
do bronchodilators for those with ariflow
obstruction
Advanced lung disease requires oxygen and
diuretics in view of cor pulmonale, and
non-invasive ventilation. Lung or heart–lung
transplantation in suitable cases

GI

Pancreatic enzyme replacement. Fat-soluble
vitamins (ADEK); ursodeoxycholic acid in liver
impairment and some require liver
transplantation.

Other

Treating CF-related diabetes with insulin
(different from types 1 and 2): ketoacidosis
unusual. Treatment of osteoporosis, arthritis,
sinusitis, vasculitis, fertility and offering genetic
counselling.

PROGNOSIS

Median survival is now over 30 years.

QUESTION SPOTTING

Think of CF in the young patient with
malabsorption or recurrent infections. Exclude
hypogammaglobulinaemia, which may present
with recurrent respiratory infections and
diarrhoea. You may be required to interpret the
results of a pancreatic test.

BRONCHIAL CARCINOMA

Carcinoma of the bronchus accounts for approximately 20% of all cancers and 27% of cancer deaths. Incidence is rising in women.

Cigarette smoking is thought to be responsible for 90% of lung cancers. Passive smoking may cause as much as 5%. Other factors implicated include asbestos, arsenic, chromium, iron oxide, petrol products, tar, coal, silicon, radiation and other causes of alveolitis such as cryptogenic fibrosing alveolitis and systemic sclerosis.

TYPES
Pragmatically, lung carcinoma is divided into two types:

Non-small-cell lung cancer
75–80% of all lung cancers
Squamous is the commonest; it usually presents as a mass on a chest film but may cavitate and look similar to a lung abscess or indeed rarely present as multiple cavitating lesions. Hypercalcaemia is often found.
Adenocarcinoma is not necessarily smoking-related and can present in areas of scarring or fibrosis. Should consider adenocarcinoma at other sites if the secondary lesion has caused pleural infiltration or effusion.
Alveolar cell carcinoma is rare and can be associated with fluffy CXR appearance and copious sputum production (bronchorrhoea).

Small-cell lung cancer
20–25% of all lung cancers
Often disseminated at the time of diagnosis due to haematogenous spread and frequently metastasizes to the liver, bone, brain and adrenals. SIADH can be associated; surgery usually inappropriate, but chemo- and radiosensitive.

SYMPTOMS
Weight loss
Anorexia
Lethargy
Cough (40%). Sputum production, especially if bronchial obstruction leads to recurrent pneumonia
Chest pain (20%) from pleural involvement or nerve invasion

Pancoast syndrome is pain in shoulder and inner aspect of arm from lower brachial plexus involvement (especially the T1 nerve root) and associated Horner's syndrome
Haemoptysis, particularly if the carcinoma is proximal and endobronchial
Dyspnoea if collapse, bronchial obstruction or lymphangitis
Dysphagia if mediastinal spread
Hoarseness or 'bovine' cough if recurrent laryngeal nerve involvement
Symptoms of metastatic spread
Neuro: focal neurological deficit, seizures, personality change
Bones: pain, pathological fractures
Liver: jaundice, abdominal pain
Skin: nodules

Symptoms of non-metastatic disease
Symptoms of hypercalcaemia
Paraneoplastic syndromes

SIGNS
Often normal
Lymphadenopathy, e.g. supraclavicular nodes, especially in squamous cell carcinoma
Signs of pneumonia – collapse, consolidation
Stridor
Monophonic unilateral wheeze
Hoarse voice
Dull lung base from phrenic nerve palsy
Pleural effusion
Superior vena cava obstruction
Clubbing ± hypertrophic pulmonary osteoarthropathy

PARANEOPLASTIC SYNDROMES
Endocrine (10%)
SIADH (especially small-cell)
Ectopic ACTH secretion (especially small-cell)
Hypercalcaemia secondary to PTHrP secretion (especially squamous cell lung carcinoma)
Carcinoid-like syndrome
Gynaecomastia
Thyrotoxicosis
Hypoglycaemia
Addison's disease (due to adrenal replacement with metastases)

Neurological

Polyneuropathy

Myelopathy (leading to motor neurone-like
disease)

Encephalopathy, including cerebellar
degeneration

Myasthenia (Eaton–Lambert syndrome)

Polymyopathy

Skin

Dermatomyositis

Acanthosis nigricans

Herpes zoster

Erythema gyratum repens

Vascular

Thrombophlebitis migrans

Non-bacterial thrombotic endocarditis

Disseminated intravascular coagulation

Thrombotic thrombocytopenic purpura

Anaemia (normocytic, microcytic, haemolytic)

Other

Clubbing (30%), especially in adenocarcinoma
and squamous cell carcinoma

Hypertrophic pulmonary osteoarthropathy (3%).
May be associated with gynaecomastia
(especially squamous cell and
adenocarcinoma)

Eosinophilia

INVESTIGATIONS
FBC

Hb ↓ or normal

WCC normal or ↑ if coexistent infection

Platelets normal

U + Es

Na normal or ↓ if SIADH

K normal or ↓↓ if ectopic ACTH

Urea and creatinine normal

LFTs

Albumin ↓

Deranged if liver metastases

Clotting normal

Ca ↑ if PTHrP secretion

CXR – 90% sensitive at presentation

Hilar enlargement (unilateral or bilateral)

Peripheral opacity, especially with
adenocarcinoma or alveolar cell carcinoma

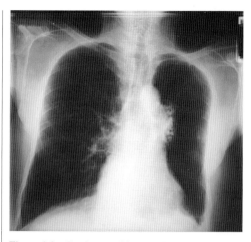

Figure 2.3   Carcinoma of lung. This chest radiograph
shows a left hilar mass. There is loss of lung volume in
the left hemithorax from previous lobectomy and there
are pathological rib fractures on the left side.

Collapse

Effusion

Rib destruction

Pericardial effusion

Lymphangitis carcinomatosa

See CXR (Figure 2.3)

DIAGNOSIS

Consider lung malignancy in those who develop
new symptoms and signs, particularly respiratory
and constitutional, such as weight loss, and those
who are at risk (e.g. smokers, asbestos exposure,
fibrosing alveolitis). All require CXR and usually
go on to have CT chest staging, bronchoscopy for
staging and tissue diagnosis, which help
determine treatment options, usually decided in
multidisciplinary meetings.

Bronchoscopy and biopsy/bronchial brushings
(80% within reach of scope, particularly if
presenting with bronchitic symptoms or
stridor)

Sputum cytology

Percutaneous needle biopsy (CT guidance or at
mediastinoscopy)

Biopsy of possible metastases (lymph node, liver
or bone marrow)

CT scan of chest (and head/abdomen for staging)

Liver ultrasound scan

Bone scan

PET imaging technique where metabolically active tissue such as tumours take up more of a radiolabelled FDG molecule. Useful in staging by detecting regional and mediastinal lymph node spread

DIFFERENTIAL DIAGNOSIS
For haemoptysis

Infection, including tuberculosis

Pulmonary embolus

Bronchiectasis

Goodpasture's syndrome

Wegener's granulomatosis

Microscopic polyarteritis

Allergic bronchopulmonary aspergillosis

Idiopathic pulmonary haemosiderosis

Trauma

Benign tumours

Hereditary haemorrhagic telangiectasia (Osler–Weber–Rendu)

For round lesions on a CXR

Carcinoma

Secondary tumours

Lung abscess

Encysted interlobar effusion

Hydatid cyst

AV malformation

Bronchial carcinoid

Aspergilloma

Rheumatoid nodule

Hamartoma

Bronchogenic cyst

For cavitating lesions on a CXR

Infection – *Staphylococcus aureus*, tuberculosis, *Klebsiella*, *Pneumocystis carinii*, hydatid, amoebic, fungal

Tumour, especially squamous cell

Infarcts

Wegener's granulomatosis

Rheumatoid nodules

TREATMENT
Surgical

85% not resectable

Careful staging essential

Contraindications to surgery

Metastases

Mediastinal organ invasion

Malignant pleural effusion

Contralateral mediastinal nodes

$FEV_1 < 1.5$ L (lobectomy), < 2.0 L (pneumoenectomy)

Severe cardiac/other condition

Radiotherapy

Radical, especially in conjunction with chemotherapy

Palliative for SVC obstruction, haemoptysis, chest pain or metastatic pain and major airway obstruction

Watch for radiation pneumonitis (early) and radiation fibrosis (late)

Combined chemotherapy

Useful in small-cell carcinoma

Other

Interventional bronchoscopy techniques for palliating airflow obstruction (photodynamic therapy, brachytherpay and laser therapy)

Steroids

Demeclocycline for SIADH

Palliative care

PROGNOSIS

NSCLC: 50% 2-year survival without spread and 10% with treatment

SCLC: 3 months median survival if no treatment; 15 months with treatment

Only 6% 5-year survival. Best results are for well-differentiated squamous cell carcinoma

QUESTION SPOTTING

Remember rare presentations of common conditions. Bronchial carcinoma is commoner than Goodpasture's syndrome as a cause of haemoptysis! Abnormal blood tests may be caused by metastatic or paraneoplastic phenomena.

COMMUNITY-ACQUIRED PNEUMONIA

A common disease associated with significant morbidity and mortality. It is the commonest infectious cause of death and up to 40% with CAP require hospital admission in the UK. Mortality is significant, currently estimated at 5–10% but up to 50% in those admitted to the intensive care unit. There are a number of ways a pathogen breaches host defences and gains entry into the bronchial tree below the larynx. These include microaspiration (occurs in nearly 50% of healthy individuals during sleep), direct or haematogenous spread, inhalation and activation of dormant infection. This section will cover general and specific features of some of the commoner pathogens involved, including atypical organisms such as *Mycoplasma pneumoniae* and *Legionella pneumophila*. The organisms are not identified in up to 15–20% of cases and the proportion of cases infected with more than one organism is not known.

RISK FACTORS
Aspiration – usually anaerobes and Gram-negative organisms
Immunosuppression
Alcoholism
Diabetes
COPD – bacterial pneumonia is common in this group; common organisms are *Haemophilus influenzae* and *Moraxella catarrhalis*
Institutionalization – a common risk factor for elderly nursing-home residents

ORGANISMS CAUSING CAP
Streptococcus (pneumococcal) *pneumoniae* – Most frequent organism, particularly in the winter season
Legionella pneumophila – 50% are travel-related; epidemics occur in relation to water-containing systems
Staphylococcus aureus – common in the winter season and 40% of patients have coexisting influenza infection
Mycoplasma pneumoniae – epidemics in the community
Chlamydia psittaci – uncommon, usually acquired from birds but human-to-human spread can occur

Coxiella burnetii (Q fever) – occur in epidemics in relation to animal source (uncommon)

CLINICAL FEATURES
Fever
Cough
Sputum
Breathlessness
Chest pain (pleuritic)
Elderly patients can present non-specifically with confusion or reduced mobility
High temperature or hypothermia
Tachypnoea
Tachycardia
Localizing chest signs – crackles, bronchial breath sounds, dullness, reduced air entry (present in the vast majority of CAP cases)

Specific clinical features
Streptococcus pneumoniae – high fever with pleuritic chest pain; common in the elderly and those with comorbidity including cardiovascular disease, diabetes, COPD and those with a history of alcohol excess
Legionella pneumophila – younger age group, smokers; more severe infection, including ITU admission, is more common. Evidence of multisystem disease with neurological symptoms and deranged liver and muscle enzymes
Mycoplasma pneumoniae – more common extrapulmonary involvement such as haemolysis, skin and joint problems. Younger age group
Chlamydia psittaci – longer duration of symptoms and dry cough
Klebsiella pneumoniae – leukopenia and thrombocytopenia
Streptococcus milleri – dental or abdominal abscess source

INVESTIGATIONS
FBC
Hb – may be low in *Mycoplasma* pneumonia due to haemolysis
WCC (neutrophilia)>15 indicates bacterial infection. >20 or < 4 indicates severe infection

U + Es
Raised urea in severe infection

Creatinine may be raised if dehydrated or severe sepsis

Sodium – may be low; not just in atypical pneumonia

LFTs

Deranged liver enzymes with bacteraemia and right-lower-lobe pneumonia

CRP

More sensitive than WCC or temperature

Can be useful in assessing response to treatment

Cultures

Blood cultures

Ideally before antibiotic therapy but *should not delay it*!

Sputum culture and sensitivity

Pleural fluid

Microscopy, culture and sensitivity. Also to rule out empyema and should be sent for cytology in those at risk of malignancy

Serological testing

Paired samples at onset and in 7–10 days should be sent, particularly in severe illness

Specific investigations

Mycoplasma pneumonia – complement fixation test (CFT) is the gold-standard serological test.

Legionnaire's disease – urinary antigen can be obtained early and is sensitive and specific. Direct immunofluorescence (DIF) tests for *Legionella pneumophila* and culture of sputum, BAL and endotracheal aspirate are also good tests. Serology tests in the form of PCR and antibody testing are also available

Chlamydia – Detected by DIF

Influenza A and B, adenoviruses and RSV

Specific serological tests

TREATMENT

Oxygen

Low threshold for intravenous fluids with urine output monitoring are essential

Nutritional support in prolonged illness

Most hospitals have protocols to treat CAP empirically with antibiotics. The clinical scenario and severity of the disease occasionally prompt modification or additional antibiotic cover with intravenous administration in severe disease. Penicillins with clavulanic acid and third-generation cephlosporins cover most organisms. Macrolides are also commonly prescribed empirically to cover atypical organisms. *Pseudomonas* is usually covered with ciprofloxacin or ceftazidime and *Staphylococcus aureus* is covered with flucloxacillin or with vancomycin if MRSA is suspected.

COMPLICATIONS

CRP falls by $> 50\%$ in 4 days for those who respond to treatment. If it doesn't, then consider the following reasons for treatment failures and complications:

Slow response in the elderly, those with local (e.g. bronchial carcinoma) and systemic (e.g. myeloma) impaired immunity

Incorrect diagnosis (e.g. pneumonitis, pulmonary embolism or pulmonary oedema)

Inappropriate or incorrect antibiotic therapy (e.g. tuberculosis, fungal or resistant organism)

Secondary complications such as parapneumonic effusion, empyema and abscess formation

PROGNOSIS

Can be assessed using the acronym CURB65.

C = confusion

U = urea > 7 mmol/L

R = respiratory rate ≥ 30 breaths/min

B = blood pressure systolic ≤ 90 mmHg $\pm$ diastolic ≤ 60 mmHg

65 = 65 years or over

The British Thoracic Society has shown good evidence that this risk score severity assessment correlates with the following mortality figures:

4 factors – mortality 83%

3 factors – mortality 33%

2 factors – mortality 23%

1 factors – mortality 8%

No factors – mortality 2.4%

QUESTION SPOTTING

Legionella and *Mycoplasma* are often favourite organisms in the MRCP CAP case.

Consider *Legionella* in:

Foreign travel – especially if air conditioning in old or Third-World hotel
Non-lobar pneumonia
Diarrhoeal prodrome
Failure to respond to penicillins
Deranged LFTs or low sodium (although not confined to atypical pneumonias)

Mycoplasma may present as:

Chest infection plus anaemia
Chest infection plus rashes
Chest infection that does not respond to amoxycillin
Chest infection with multisystem involvement in a patient who is otherwise not particularly unwell
Note that this combination can occur in any type of pneumonia

PNEUMOCYSTIS PNEUMONIA

Pneumocystis carinii pneumonia (PCP) is the clinical syndrome from infection with the fungus *P. jiroveci* (previously *P. carinii*). Infection is common and usually asymptomatic, but can be life-threatening in the immunocompromised host. Cell-mediated immunity is required to prevent clinical disease. It is one of the most common diseases to occur in HIV-infected patients and is one of the AIDS-defining diseases.

It usually remains confined to the lungs where it causes pneumonitis, rarely becoming disseminated. The organism may remain dormant for years; however, PCP is thought to follow new infection in the immunocompromised host rather than reactivation of latent infection. There are recognized risk groups other than HIV-infected individuals; these include those on chemotherapy treatment such as fludarabine and those receiving corticosteroids, especially ones with haematological malignancy.

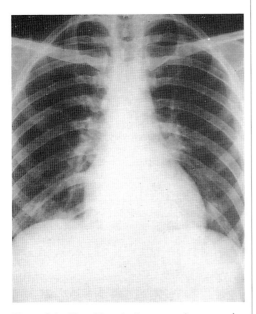

Figure 2.4 Chest X-ray in *Pneumocystis* pneumonia. Note remarkably normal appearance despite significant symptoms and hypoxia. (Reproduced with permission from Forbes, Jackson (2003) *Colour Atlas and Text of Clinical Medicine*, 3rd edn. Mosby.)

SYMPTOMS
Triad of:

Fever
Shortness of breath
Cough – persistent and usually non-productive

Disease may be preceded by upper respiratory tract infection or diarrhoea, and may run a subacute course.

SIGNS
Fever
Tachypnoea
Cyanosis
Crackles in the chest are rare

INVESTIGATIONS
FBC
Hb normal
WCC not useful as may be ↓ or ↑
Platelets normal

U + Es
Normal

LFTs
Normal
Lactate dehydrogenase is typically raised but is a non-specific finding.

ABGs
May be normal at rest, but desaturation occurs on exertion

CXR
The typical appearance is of diffuse alveolar shadowing, starting at the hila and spreading laterally. The apices and bases are spared until late in the disease. Other recognized features include local infiltrate, nodule, cavity or pneumothorax. The radiograph appearance lags behind the clinical disease and may be normal. (Fig. 2.4)

High-resolution CT chest
This demonstrates bilateral ground-glass pattern. Not routinely used in the diagnosis of PCP but useful in cases where there is a high index of suspicion with normal CXR (approximately 10%).

DIAGNOSIS

Induced sputum in an appropriate negative-pressure room. This has around 60% diagnostic yield in HIV-infected individuals but less in other immunocompromised groups who have lower organism burden. Bronchoscopy and BAL are superior to induced sputum. Silver staining or immunofluorescence has a specifity of nearly 100% and sensitivity of > 80% (lower in non-HIV-infected individuals, reflecting a lower pathogen load). Transbronchial biopsy also has a high sensitivity but is reserved for those who have a non-diagnostic BAL in view of the increased risk of complications.

DIFFERENTIAL DIAGNOSIS

CMV
TB
Other bacterial, viral or fungal infection, e.g. *Cryptococcus*, histoplasmosis, aspergillosis
Pneumonitis secondary to drugs, especially cytotoxic drugs, e.g. methotrexate

TREATMENT

Oxygen
HIV testing if no other cause for immunocompromise
Intravenous high-dose co-trimoxazole. Treatment can switch to oral once the patient is responding
Alternative treatment is pentamidine, but this has a high rate of side-effects
Steroids may have a useful role in reducing mortality in patients with respiratory failure
Prophylaxis is required following the acute attack as the organism is never eliminated. Oral co-trimoxazole is effective; oral dapsone and pyrimethamine are also useful. Inhaled pentamidine can also be used for prophylaxis
Primary prevention should be given to HIV-infected patients with CD4 count < 200/mm^3
Secondary prophylaxis is also recommended

PROGNOSIS

100% mortality without treatment
5–15% mortality with treatment (higher rates in cancer patients and > 50% mortality in mechanically ventilated HIV-infected patients)

QUESTION SPOTTING

Watch out for PCP in unwell patients with shortness of breath but no respiratory signs and a normal chest X-ray. 'Young man' in a question should make you consider HIV infection, and look for other features suggestive of HIV infection such as weight loss and *Candida* infection. Normal oxygen saturations at rest do not exclude the diagnosis.

ALPHA-1-ANTITRYPSIN DEFICIENCY

α_1-Antitrypsin (α1AT) is an inhibitor of neutrophil elastase. One in 10 of the population carries a mutation – the M allele produces a normal amount of protein, Z produces 15% and S produces 40% of normal. Homozygotes for the Z mutation occur at a rate of 1 per 2500 population. Unopposed neutrophil elastase activity leads to accelerated lung damage, especially in smokers, with consequent emphysema. The Z mutation also accumulates in hepatocytes, leading to hepatocyte death and cirrhosis. Heterozygotes for Z produce less severe disease, but may result in cirrhosis.

SYMPTOMS
Progressive SOB, wheeze
Weight loss
Late onset
Jaundice, abdominal swelling
Ankle oedema (cor pulmonale and cirrhosis)

SIGNS
Wheeze, reduced breath sounds
Hyperexpanded chest
Signs of cor pulmonale (late)
Jaundice
Spider naevi
Palmar erythema
Ascites
Encephalopathy (late)

INVESTIGATIONS
FBC
Hb ↑ in severe lung disease
WCC normal
Platelets usually normal

U + Es
Normal

LFTs
May all be elevated
INR raised in cirrhosis

ECG may reflect cor pulmonale (RVH, p pulmonale)
CXR shows basal emphysematous changes
PFTs show reduced FEV_1/FVC ratio. Increased residual volume and reduced TLco

DIAGNOSIS
Liver biopsy shows diastase-resistant PAS-positive inclusions in hepatocytes, together with evidence of cirrhosis. α1AT mutations are detected by isoelectric focusing on gel electrophoresis.

ASSOCIATIONS
Bronchiectasis
Glomerulonephritis
Panniculitis
Inflammatory bowel disease
Wegener's granulomatosis

TREATMENT
Avoid smoking (including passive) as this accelerates disease
Avoid pyrexia in infants (high temperatures are thought to encourage deposition of Z protein in the liver, contributing to the infantile hepatitis and liver dysfunction seen in ZZ homozygotes)
Transplantation in advanced respiratory failure
Genetic councelling and screening siblings are important

PROGNOSIS
10% of infants who are ZZ homozygotes become jaundiced during the first year of life. 10–15% of these develop juvenile cirrhosis; the rest appear to recover at least partially
50% of adults with ZZ will eventually develop cirrhosis. Hepatocellular carcinoma may develop as a result
In ZZ disease, emphysema typically becomes apparent at age around 50, but non-smokers are usually asymptomatic. Suspect in young patients with COPD and those who smoke

QUESTION SPOTTING
The combination of emphysema and liver dysfunction is usually a pointer to α1AT deficiency. Watch out for emphysema in a young person, especially if a non-smoker.

ALLERGIC BRONCHOPULMONARY ASPERGILLOSIS

Allergic bronchopulmonary aspergillosis (ABPA) is usually caused by the fungus *Aspergillus fumigatus* and rarely causes disease in immunocompetent non-atopic people. However, *Aspergillus* may also cause a wide array of clinical syndromes which include aspergilloma (a fungus ball within a pre-existing cavity) and invasive aspergillosis (immunosuppressed individuals are particularly at risk). ABPA is caused by the inhalation and trapping of spores in the viscid secretions of atopic and cystic fibrosis patients.

ABPA affects up to 20% of patients with asthma. Men and women are equally affected. Most patients are less than 35 years old at presentation.

SYMPTOMS
Low-grade fever
Cough productive of brown mucus plugs
Wheezing
Increasing shortness of breath
Pleuritic chest pain
Haemoptysis
'Recurrent pneumonia'

SIGNS
Diffuse wheeze
Prolonged expiratory phase
Crackles are only heard when pulmonary
   infiltrates are present
Finger clubbing may occur if fibrosis is present

INVESTIGATIONS
FBC
Hb normal
WCC normal or ↑ but eosinophils ↑↑ ($> 1.0 \times 10^9$/L)
Platelets normal

U + Es
Normal

LFTs
Usually normal

Total protein may be ↑
IgE ↑
ESR ↑
Sputum samples show fungal hyphae on
   microscopy (not a specific test)

Positive *Aspergillus* skin test and/or *Aspergillus*-
   specific IgE RAST

CXR
Transient patchy infiltrates with or without
   collapse or consolidation. More common in
   upper lobes. Bronchiectasis of proximal
   airways may be seen. Fibrosis with
   honeycombing also occurs later on
High-resolution CT may show bronchiectasis,
   fibrosis and infiltrates. Lung function tests
   show a reversible obstructive defect
Bronchoscopy and lavage show positive culture
   to *Aspergillus fumigatus*, numerous hyphae,
   mononuclear cells and eosinophils

DIAGNOSIS
Diagnosis requires a positive skinprick test (beware
high false-positive rate), increased total IgE with
increased IgE and IgG to *Aspergillus* species
(serum precipitins) and radiological evidence of
ABPA with the appropriate clinical features

DIFFERENTIAL DIAGNOSIS
Churg–Strauss syndrome
Tuberculosis
Sarcoid
Parasitic infestation
Extrinsic allergic alveolitis
Eosinophilic pneumonia
Bacterial infection
Invasive pulmonary aspergillosis

COMPLICATIONS
Bronchiectasis secondary to immune complex
   deposition
Upper-lobe fibrosis and honeycomb lung
Cor pulmonale (rare)
Haemoptysis (rare)

TREATMENT
Oral corticosteroids (prednisolone 30–40 mg) for
2 weeks initially and then tapered to control
symptoms

PROGNOSIS
Remission is usual after steroids, but
exacerbations are common, and may occur up to

7 years after the acute stage. Progression to steroid dependence (to control asthma or ABPA or both) is not uncommon, and this may eventually lead to pulmonary fibrosis, cor pulmonale and death, though this is rare.

QUESTION SPOTTING

The typical patient will be young and will have asthma or cystic fibrosis. The most common scenario will be abnormalities on a chest X-ray in the absence of extra clinical features, or an exacerbation of shortness of breath with other features such as mucus production and fever. Remember to work out eosinophil counts if part of a blood differential is given.

OBSTRUCTIVE SLEEP APNOEA SYNDROME

This disorder is due to upper-airway narrowing which is provoked by sleep, causing sleep fragmentation to result in significant daytime symptoms, usually manifest as excessive daytime somnolence. It affects around 0.5–1% of adult males in the UK with a 5:1 male-to-female ratio. Prevalence figures are expected to rise with the rise of the prevalence of obesity in the UK and other western countries.

SYMPTOMS
Triad of:

Hypersomnolence (measured on the Epworth Sleepiness Scale: > 9/24 is considered abnormal)
Heavy snoring and apnoeic episodes, often noticed by bed partner
Restless sleep

Other symptoms
Morning headaches secondary to CO_2 retention
Depression
Poor concentration
Nocturnal enuresis
Loss of libido

SIGNS
Obesity
Large collar size (usually > 16)
Undersized or set-back mandible
Oropharynx narrowing due to ENT cause, indicating referral

INVESTIGATIONS
FBC
Hb ↑
WCC normal
Platelets normal

U + Es
Normal

LFTs
Normal

ABGs
po_2 normal or ↓
pco_2 normal or ↑
pH may be ↑

DIAGNOSIS
Is usually based on the results of a sleep study. Often overnight pulse oximetry alone along with typical clinical features is enough to make the diagnosis. Limited polysomongraphy in addition will identify most cases, allowing trial of CPAP treatment.

DIFFERENTIAL DIAGNOSIS
Nocturnal myoclonus – repeated leg movements during sleep that disrupt sleep pattern and produce daytime somnolence
Narcolepsy – sleep attacks, cataplexy (sudden loss of muscular tone associated with emotion), sleep paralysis and hypnagogic hallucinations
Idiopathic hypersomnolence
Laryngeal obstruction from complications of rheumatoid arthritis or Shy–Drager syndrome
Poor sleep hygiene

COMPLICATIONS
Cor pulmonale
Hypertension
Polycythemia
Respiratory failure, especially if pre-existing respiratory obstruction such as asthma or chronic airway obstruction

TREATMENT
Treatment of underlying cause if acromegaly, myxoedema, enlarged tonsils or SVC obstruction
Weight loss
Avoidance of respiratory depressants, sedatives and muscle relaxants such as alcohol, strong analgesics and benzodiazepines
Continuous nasal positive airways pressure via a nasal mask at night is effective if tolerated
Tricyclic antidepressants may be effective if only mild
Surgery (uvulo-palato-pharyngoplasty) is advocated by some centres but is not proven to be effective
Tracheostomy is effective but not without its own problems. However it may be life-saving as a temporary measure whilst treating the underlying cause of the apnoea

The patient's quality of life and livelihood, such as heavy-goods vehicle driving, are key in making a treatment choice

QUESTION SPOTTING

Obstructive sleep apnoea may masquerade as a cause of daytime confusion, loss of concentration or depression. Do not confuse with narcolepsy, which has a different clinical pattern. Medical history of acromegaly, hypothyroidism and hypertension with daytime somnolence should also give you a clue.

If shown nocturnal oxygenation chart, this should be an easy-to-spot diagnosis.

Hypersensitivity pneumonitis (HP) (also known as extrinsic allergic alveolitis) is a hypersensitivity reaction to inhaled dusts, which may be inorganic but are usually organic. Examples include fungal spores from mouldy hay (farmer's lung), avian proteins (pigeon fancier's lung) and sugar (bagassosis). An acute illness may occur, mediated by a type III hypersensitivity reaction, and a chronic inflammatory disease process also occurs, leading to granuloma formation and lung fibrosis.

Many asymptomatic exposures to the antigen may occur before the onset of an acute episode. Often the disease is divided into acute and chronic forms based on the time course of presentation. The acute phase is more reversible than the chronic phase but overlap of the two phases is also recognized and is referred to as subacute. Prevalence is not accurately known but it is estimated that 8% of budgerigar and pigeon keepers and 5% of farmers may develop HP. Less common in smokers, for unknown reasons.

ACUTE ILLNESS
Symptoms – onset 4–8 h after exposure to antigen
Dry cough
Flu-like illness

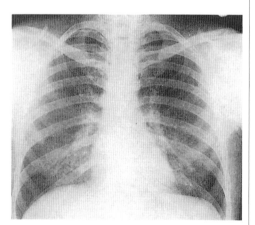

Figure 2.5 Chest X-ray of acute phase of hypersensitivity pneumonitis. Note obliteration of lung markings. (Reproduced with permission from Forbes, Jackson (2003) *Colour Atlas and Text of Clinical Medicine*, 3rd edn. Mosby.)

Breathlessness
Fever
Myalgia
Wheeze is uncommon

Signs
Fever
Bibasal crackles

CHRONIC ILLNESS
Symptoms
Cough
Insidious breathlessness
Fatigue
Weight loss
May be history of acute episodes

Signs
Crackles may be absent
Clubbing is uncommon until late in disease
Signs of right heart failure occur in advanced disease

INVESTIGATIONS
FBC
Hb normal
WCC neutrophilia (in acute illness only)
No eosinophilia
Platelets normal

U + Es
Normal

LFTs
Normal

Calcium normal
Immunoglobulins normal
Serum precipitins (IgG) are often positive, indicating exposure

CXR (Fig. 2.5)
Shows bibasal alveolar shadowing in acute illness. May be normal.
Reticulonodular shadowing in chronic illness; often in upper and middle zones.
Lymphadenopathy is not a feature

High-resolution CT chest
Diffuse well-defined centrilobular nodules, ground-glass change, increased lucency from air trapping. Can mimic usual interstitial pneumonia

PFTs

Show reduced TLco and FVC in acute and chronic disease. Occasionally FEV_1 may be disproportionately reduced

Bronchoscopy

BAL usually shows lymphocytosis but this is non-specific. Transbronchial biopsy can provide a tissue diagnosis; however surgical lung biopsy is superior.

DIAGNOSIS

History of antigen exposure, typical clinical features such as onset of symptoms within 4–8 hours after exposure, recurrent episodes, weight loss and crackles on examination in combination with HRCT findings are useful in making the diagnosis. Absence of serum precipitins is very unusual but has been described. In cases where the diagnosis is uncertain, a lung biopsy to show characteristic histological features would be useful.

DIFFERENTIAL DIAGNOSIS

Usual interstitial pneumonia (UIP)
Cryptogenic organizing pneumonia (COP)
Sarcoidosis
Tuberculosis
Atypical pneumonia
Pneumoconioses
Pulmonary vasculitis
Pulmonary alveolar proteinosis

TREATMENT

Avoidance of the triggering antigen is the mainstay of treatment. If difficult, for example in farmers, measures to reduce exposure such as facemasks should be put in place. Steroids can curtail an acute attack; they may have a role in attenuating chronic disease, but once fibrotic changes occur, the course of the chronic disease tends to be irreversible.

PROGNOSIS

Acute attacks usually resolve in 12–48 hours, leaving no residual lung damage. Chronic disease may progress to end-stage lung fibrosis with cor pulmonale.

QUESTION SPOTTING

A person with pets, birds or an interesting-looking environmental history or occupation (not just farmers!), who presents with an acute respiratory illness, may have HP. Note that the presence of precipitins does not necessarily mean that the diagnosis is HP.

The presence of a restrictive defect with impaired gas transfer suggests lung fibrosis; the short story may suggest a diagnosis.

CHRONIC OBSTRUCTIVE PULMONARY DISEASE

This is a chronic progressive disorder of airways obstruction which lacks reversibility. The term COPD includes chronic bronchitis and emphysema. Asthma is a separate disease entity and the vast majority of patients have one or the other, rather than both.

Age > 35 years, smoking history, chronic dyspnoea, sputum production and lack of diurnal variation in FEV_1 favour a diagnosis of COPD. Chronic bronchitis is classically defined as sputum production on most days for 3 months of 2 successive years and symptoms improve in > 90% if they stop smoking. Emphysema is more of a histological diagnosis, described as enlargement in air spaces distal to the terminal bronchioles with associated destruction of the alveolar wall.

Prevalence of COPD is very high – estimated at 1.5 million in the UK, with 25 000 deaths per year in England and Wales.

SYMPTOMS
Cough
Sputum
Dyspnoea
Wheeze

SIGNS
Tachypnoea
Hyperinflation
Use of accessory muscles of respiration
Reduced cricosternal distance (< 3 cm)
Reduced expansion symmetrically
Resonant or hyperresonant percussion note with quiet breath sounds, especially over large bullae
Cyanosis
Rhonchi/wheeze
Signs indicating right-sided heart failure (cor pulmonale)
COPD is not a cause of clubbing

'Pink puffers and blue bloaters' are terms that are going out of fashion. Essentially, they are disease states at two ends of a spectrum. The former group may go on to develop type 1 respiratory failure, and are often breathless but not cyanosed. The latter group rely on their hypoxic drive and are cyanosed but not necessarily breathless during their baseline respiratory status. They should receive supplemental oxygen with care.

INVESTIGATIONS
FBC
Raised Hb
Raised Hct
Raised WCC (often due to current high-dose oral steroid therapy)

U + Es
Usually normal

LFTs
Usually normal
If deranged and young patient, consider $\alpha1AT$ deficiency

CXR
Hyperinflation (> 6 anterior or > 10 posterior ribs above the diaphragm in the mid-clavicular line), flattening of the hemidiaphragms, prominent pulmonary vessels, paucity of lung vascular markings in the periphery and bullae. Useful tool in exacerbations.

ECG
Right atrial and ventricular hypertrophy

ABG
Reduced po_2 ± raised pco_2. (Normal pH and raised bicarbonate in stable disease states)

PFTs
Obstructive with air trapping with FEV_1 < 80% predicted and FEV_1:FVC ratio < 70%. Raised TLC and RV with reduced DLCO in emphysema. Rarely, spirometry and static lung volumes can be normal despite gross emphysema.

High-resolution CT chest
Sensitive in showing bullous disease and emphysema. Useful when considering bullectomy or volume reduction surgery (in upper-zone emphysema).

DIAGNOSIS
Usually the patient will present with insidious breathlessness on effort ± bronchitic symptoms and supporting spirometry and CXR findings.

Exacerbations usually occur in those who have been diagnosed previously.

Severity of COPD

Mild = FEV_1 60–80% predicted
Moderate = FEV_1 40–59% predicted
Severe = FEV_1 <40% predicted

TREATMENT
Non-pharmacological

Smoking cessation
Exercise
Dietary modification (low BMI and obesity)
Influenza and pneumococcal vaccinations
Pulmonary rehabilitation and palliative care in
more advanced disease

Pharmacological

Mild: PRN inhaled antimuscarinic
Moderate: regular antimuscarinic ± long-acting
beta-agonist ± inhaled corticosteroid (FEV_1
< 50% > 2 exacerbations per year)
Severe: combination of long-acting beta-agonist
and steroid with regular antimuscarinic or long-
acting antimuscarinic. Regular nebulized therapy
may play a role. Consider theophylline with
blood level monitoring and long-term oxygen
therapy (LTOT). This is > 15 hours/day of low-
flow oxygen delivered from a concentrator for
those who have advanced stable disease with a
po_2 < 7.3 kPa (< 8 kPa in cor pulmonale) and
who are not exposed to cigarette smoke

Other

Mucolytics
Sublingual small-dose benzodiazepine in anxiety
Antidepressants

COMPLICATIONS
Exacerbations

A common reason for acute hospital admission,
often secondary to one or a combination of the
following factors:

Infection
Tumour
Anxiety
Pneumothorax
Sedatives
Pulmonary embolism
Acute coronary syndrome

Other complications

Respiratory failure
Cor pulmonale
Bronchiectasis secondary to recurrent infections
Depression

QUESTION SPOTTING

Look for obstructive defect on spirometry with
classical 'scalloping effect' on the flow/volume
loop in a patient with a significant smoking
history.

HISTIOCYTOSIS X (LANGERHANS-CELL HISTIOCYTOSIS)

Histiocytosis X, or pulmonary Langerhans-cell histiocytosis (LCH) is a rare condition commonly affecting adults aged 20–40 years, characterized by infiltration of the lung with histiocytes (Langerhans cells). This condition overlaps with other conditions that have similar pathological findings but diverse clinical features. These range from local disease involving a single organ (e.g. eosinophilic granulomas of bone) to systemic diseases affecting multiple organs, such as Hand–Schueller–Christian syndrome. Chest physicians are more likely to see the isolated form of the disease; however, pulmonary manifestations also occur in systemic disease.

Patients are usually heavy smokers and it is speculated that this might be the antigen stimulus for activating Langerhans cells. These cells arrange into granulomata and are located in bronchiolar walls and from there invade adjacent structures. This explains the initial appearance of nodules on CT scan which then goes on to become cystic.

CLINICAL FEATURES

Exertional breathlessness

Cough

Chest pain from rib lesions

Systemic symptoms of fever and weight loss are less common

Pneumothorax is a recognized complication in 10%

Asymptomatic in 25% and examination is usually normal

INVESTIGATIONS

FBC

Usually normal. No eosinophilia

U + Es

Usually normal

LFTs

Usually normal

Serum ACE

May be elevated

CXR

Normal or shows diffuse reticulonodular shadowing, sometimes with cystic changes in the upper and middle lobes

HRCT

Diffuse centrilobular nodules (± cavitation) and variable wall thickness cysts. The lesions are of different age and interspersed with normal lung, with upper- and middle-lobe predominance. Purely nodular or purely cystic appearances may occur

PFTs

Obstructive, restrictive or mixed patterns have been observed. Gas transfer is usually reduced, sometimes with preserved lung volumes

DIAGNOSIS

High-resolution CT sometimes shows a distinctive pattern of mid- to upper-zone nodules and cysts. This pattern may be sufficient to make the diagnosis. If the pattern is less specific, biopsy is needed

Surgical lung biopsy is preferred over transbronchial biopsy

Extrathoracic tissue (e.g. from bone) in systemic disease is occasionally diagnostic. Tissue should be stained for Langerhans cells

Bronchoalvolar lavage may also be diagnostic: > 5% Langerhans cells make the diagnosis, but the test is insensitive

DIFFERENTIAL DIAGNOSIS

On HRCT: emphysema cysts lack walls

Lymphangioleiomyomatosis: where cysts are present they are distributed uniformly

ASSOCIATIONS

Pulmonary hypertension

Manifestations of systemic LCH (diabetes insipidus, skin disease, lytic bony lesions)

Lymphoma

Lung cancer is more common, probably related to smoking history

TREATMENT

Spontaneous improvement is common but
relapse may occur

Smoking cessation is the mainstay of treatment

Corticosteroids have been used in
systemic disease but this treatment lacks
evidence base

Lung transplantation should be considered in
those with advanced respiratory failure or
pulmonary hypertension

PROGNOSIS

Variable but median survival is 12 years from
diagnosis

QUESTION SPOTTING

Suspect this diagnosis in young adult smokers
with cystic changes on CXR or HRCT or with
those who develop recurrent pneumothoraces

LYMPHANGIOLEIOMYOMATOSIS

Lymphangioleiomyomatosis (LAM) is a rare condition affecting women in their 30s. It is characterized by abnormal proliferation of smooth-muscle cells in a hormone-dependent manner and therefore can also occur in postmenopausal women on oestrogen replacement. Lung, airways, blood vessels and lymphatics are progressively involved in the disease process, eventually leading to cyst formation from airway and lymphatic obstruction. The cause of this disease is unknown and the incidence is estimated at 1 in 1.1 million.

ASSOCIATIONS
40% of adult females with tuberous sclerosis develop pulmonary changes identical to LAM

SYMPTOMS
Recurrent pneumothorax (65%)
Dyspnoea (40%)
Cough (20%)
Haemoptysis (14%)
Chylothorax (10%)
Chest pain

SIGNS
Often no signs
Crepitations
Pleural effusion
Palpable abdominal masses

Other organs affected
Kidney: angiomyolipoma in 50% of cases. Can cause flank pain and bleeding into the renal tract
Abdomen: lymphadenopathy, usually asymptomatic in 30% of patients
Skin: cutaneous swellings likely due to localized oedema

INVESTIGATIONS
FBC
Usually normal

U + Es
Usually normal

LFTs
Usually normal

CA-125 levels may be elevated

PFTs
Normal or predominantly obstructive pattern. Restriction a lot less common. Gas transfer reduced

CXR
Normal
Hyperinflation with septal lines (obstructed lymphatics) and reticular shadowing

High-resolution CT chest
Multiple cysts of varying size throughout the lung, usually thin-walled and < 1 cm in size. Normal adjoining lung parenchyma. Pleural effusions may be present

DIAGNOSIS
Is usually on clinical picture plus high-resolution CT findings. Occasionally, lung biopsy may be required

DIFFERENTIAL DIAGNOSIS
Causes of preserved lung volumes with reduced transfer factor:

Tuberous sclerosis
Langerhans cell histiocytosis
Neurofibromatosis

Lymphoma
Tuberculosis
Asthma/COPD
Other interstitial lung disease

TREATMENT
Should be aimed at those who are symptomatic or declining
Diet: low-fat diet with medium-chain triglycerides supplements prevents chylothorax recurrence. No strong evidence for this
Bronchodilators – useful for airflow obstruction
Hormone manipulation has been beneficial in slowing decline in PFTs but again, there have been no large studies
Smoking cessation

PROGNOSIS
Variable but may slowly progress to respiratory failure. 70% are alive at 10 years, 25% at 20 years

QUESTION SPOTTING

Consider this diagnosis in young and middle-aged women with decline in respiratory function (especially in pregnancy) or if they develop recurrent pneumothoraces.

Commonly associated with tuberous sclerosis and angiomyoleiomas or other retroperitoneal tumours.

GASTROENTEROLOGY AND HEPATOLOGY

PRIMARY BILIARY CIRRHOSIS

An autoimmune disease of unknown aetiology. PBC is characterized by granulomatous destruction of small intrahepatic bile ducts, leading to slowly progressive cholestasis and eventual cirrhosis. 90% of patients are female, with a peak age of onset of 40–60 years.

SYMPTOMS

PBC is often asymptomatic at presentation

Early
Pruritus (usually first symptom)
Tiredness

Late
Jaundice
Haematemesis
Abdominal discomfort
Steatorrhoea

SIGNS
Hepatomegaly
Scratch marks
Other signs of chronic liver disease; spider naevi are often absent
Xanthelasma
Splenomegaly, clubbing, jaundice, ascites and oedema are all late findings

INVESTIGATIONS
FBC
Usually normal but all counts reduced in hypersplenism

U + Es
Usually normal

LFTs
ALP ↑, usually markedly
ALT slightly ↑
Bilirubin ↑ later in disease
GGT ↑
Albumin ↓ in cirrhosis

Cholesterol ↑
INR ↑ in decompensating cirrhosis
IgM often ↑
Immune complexes normal
Serum ACE may be ↑ but is not specific for PBC

Antinuclear antibody may be positive, and many other antibodies may be found, including anti-SSA (Ro), anticentromere, antithyroid and anti-AChR antibodies.

DIAGNOSIS
Antimitochondrial antibody is positive in 95%
Specificity of the M2 subtype is 98%; this antibody is found at low titre in autoimmune hepatitis
Liver biopsy shows granulomas and small bile duct destruction, progressing to piecemeal necrosis and cirrhosis

ASSOCIATIONS
Gallstones
Almost any autoimmune process can be associated:

Sicca syndrome (75%)
Thyroiditis (20%)
Rheumatoid arthritis
SLE
Dermatomyositis
Scleroderma/CREST
Autoimmune thrombocytopenia
Addison's disease
Fibrosing alveolitis
IgA deficiency
Membranous glomerulonephritis
Ulcerative colitis
Transverse myelitis
Renal tubular acidosis
Coeliac disease
Lichen planus
Graves disease
Myasthenia gravis

DIFFERENTIAL DIAGNOSIS
Chronic viral hepatitis
Alcoholic liver disease
Primary sclerosing cholangitis
Autoimmune hepatitis
Sarcoidosis
Drug reactions
Note that overlap syndromes with sclerosing cholangitis and autoimmune hepatitis also occur

COMPLICATIONS
Portal hypertension leading to varices
Hepatic encephalopathy
Ascites
Oedema
Renal tubular acidosis
Osteoporosis
Hypercholesterolaemia
Osteomalacia (long-standing severe disease only)

TREATMENT
Cholestyramine relieves pruritus. Osteoporosis should be treated with calcium, vitamin D and bisphosphonates
Liver transplantation: 85–90% survival at 1 year. Recurrence is rare. Consider when bilirubin > 100 mmol/L
Ursodeoxycholic acid is somewhat controversial, but may prolong the interval before death or liver transplant
Methotrexate may also be of value, but ciclosporin, colchicine and steroids do not appear to improve prognosis, although they may improve symptoms

PROGNOSIS
Asymptomatic patients: 10–16-year median survival
Symptomatic patients: 7-year median survival

QUESTION SPOTTING
PBC must be on the differential of any grey case involving a woman with liver disease. Other features to look for are:

Pruritus in a middle-aged woman
Elevated ALP and hepatomegaly without a very high bilirubin
Liver disease with a number of other autoimmune conditions, especially hypothyroidism, dry eyes or scleroderma
Raised cholesterol and elevated IgM are other possible clues

AUTOIMMUNE HEPATITIS

An autoimmune disease of unknown aetiology. It may have either a chronic or acute, fulminant course. Histology shows piecemeal necrosis in zone 1 of the hepatic parenchyma, with a lymphocytic infiltrate. There is a link with the HLA B8/DR3 and HLA DR4 haplotypes

SYMPTOMS
Tiredness
Anorexia
Nausea
Jaundice, RUQ tenderness and abdominal distension may occur in acute or subacute illness

SIGNS
Palmar erythema
Spider naevi
Hepatomegaly
Splenomegaly
Moon face, abdominal striae and central obesity may be evident even without steroid treatment

INVESTIGATIONS
FBC
Hb ↓
MCV normal
WCC usually normal – ↓ in hypersplenism
Platelets usually normal – ↓ in hypersplenism

U + Es
Normal

LFTs
Bilirubin ↑ in 25–50% at presentation
ALT ↑ 2–20 times normal
ALP slightly ↑
Albumin low
INR ↑ in advanced disease

ESR ↑
IgG ↑ in 90%
IgA, IgM usually normal

Antibodies
ANA positive in 40–70% – may be antibodies against dsDNA
Anti-smooth-muscle antibodies positive in 60%
Anti-LKM-1 antibodies may also be positive
Anti-mitochondrial antibodies occasionally positive at low titre

DIAGNOSIS
Liver biopsy shows lymphocyte infiltration, piecemeal necrosis and fibrosis as the disease progresses. The biliary tree is relatively spared.

Presence of features of hepatitis, anti-smooth-muscle antibodies and typical histology usually clinch the diagnosis. A prompt response to immunosuppression is almost always seen; lack of response in patients taking adequate doses of steroids suggests a different diagnosis.

Disease is classified into three types by antibody profile:

Type 1: ANA and anti-smooth-muscle antibodies
Type 2: anti-LKM-1 antibodies
Type 3: anti-soluble liver antigen/liver pancreas antigens

ASSOCIATIONS
Other autoimmune conditions are present in 60% of cases of autoimmune hepatitis

Sicca syndrome (35%)
Renal tubular acidosis (24%)
Peripheral neuropathy (10%)
Hashimoto's thyroiditis (7%)
Ulcerative colitis (4%)
Rheumatoid arthritis (2%)
Thrombocytopenia/haemolytic anaemia
Mixed connective tissue disease
Diabetes mellitus
Diabetes insipidus
Graves disease
Pulmonary fibrosis
Coeliac disease
Myasthenia gravis
Polymyositis
Glomerulonephritis

DIFFERENTIAL DIAGNOSIS
Acute disease
Hepatitis A, B, C, E infection
EBV/CMV hepatitis

Wilson's disease
Drug toxicity

Chronic disease
Chronic hepatitis B/C
Primary biliary cirrhosis (PBC)
Primary sclerosing cholangitis
Wilson's disease
α_1-antitrypsin deficiency
Alcohol abuse

COMPLICATIONS
Cirrhosis with other features of liver failure
Varices with associated bleeding may occur
Hepatocellular carcinoma
Hypersplenism
Hepatic encephalopathy may complicate acute or
   end-stage disease

TREATMENT
Steroids, with azathioprine as a steroid-sparing
agent once in remission. Mycophenolate,
cyclophosphamide or ciclosporin can be used in
patients failing to respond to azathioprine.

Relapse occurs within 3 years in > 80% of
patients who discontinue immunosuppression.

Patients with no histological evidence of
inflammation at 3 years can have a trial without
immunosuppressants, but most patients will
require long-term immunosuppression.

Liver transplantation is successful for end-
stage disease. Recurrent disease can occur in the
transplanted liver.

PROGNOSIS
> 95% 10-year survival if no cirrhosis present
65% 10-year survival if cirrhosis present

QUESTION SPOTTING
Acute or chronic liver disease, especially in a
young woman, should lead to consideration of
autoimmune hepatitis.

Pointers to the diagnosis are:

Negative viral serology
Markedly raised ALT/AST
High immunoglobulin levels (or large difference
   between total protein and albumin)
Presence of anti-smooth-muscle antibodies
No history of drugs or alcohol

HEREDITARY HAEMOCHROMATOSIS

Hereditary condition leading to inappropriately high absorption of iron by the gut mucosa with increased transfer of iron to plasma. This leads to excessive total body iron and deposition of iron in cells of the liver, heart, pancreas, joints, skin, gonads and other endocrine organs. This in turn causes tissue damage, fibrosis and functional failure. The deposition in parenchymal cells of the liver contrasts with normal individuals who tend to deposit iron in the bone marrow. Liver damage is fibrotic. Hepatitis suggests viral infection or alcohol abuse.

The *HFE* gene is located on chromosome 6p21, closely linked with HLA A3. There is a lesser linkage with HLA B14. 80–90% of patients have a single mutation at site 282. Heterozygotes have increased iron absorption without the disease (25% have abnormal iron studies). The precise mechanism whereby the mutation leads to increased iron absorption remains unclear.

Women are protected by menstruation and so present clinically later than men, who typically present aged 40–50.

SYMPTOMS

Often asymptomatic
Weakness
Lethargy
Abdominal pain
Arthralgia
Loss of libido and impotence
Symptoms of cardiac failure
Symptoms of diabetes such as thirst and polyuria

SIGNS

Hepatomegaly
Splenomegaly
Loss of body hair
Gynaecomastia
Testicular atrophy
Skin pigmentation – 'bronze'
Arthritis
Signs of diabetes mellitus

INVESTIGATIONS
FBC
Normal

U + Es
Normal
Glucose normal or ↑

LFTs
AST ↑
ALP ↑
Bilirubin ↑
Albumin normal

Iron ↑
Ferritin ↑
TIBC ↓
Fasting transferrin saturation ↑
(iron ÷ TIBC × 100%)
Testosterone ↓
Urine iron excretion ↑ after desferrioxamine
Joint X-rays show cartilage calcification
Dual-energy CT scan (which requires modifications to the CT scanner for the test) has high correlation for iron overload, but is less sensitive for lower levels

DIAGNOSIS

Raised ferritin (> 300 ng/mL) is suggestive but not sensitive or specific for the disease
Transferrin saturation > 55% for men or > 50% for women is sensitive and specific for iron overload – this forms the first line of investigation
Positive genotyping is found in > 90% of UK patients and is used to confirm the diagnosis
If clinical suspicion is high but tests are inconclusive:
Liver biopsy may be indicated if signs of liver disease and iron overload but negative genotyping – it can be used to determine whether cirrhosis is present together with the degree of iron overload
A trial of phlebotomy may be used – the ability to maintain haemoglobin levels after 4 g of iron removed (20 × 450 mL phlebotomies) confirms iron overload

DIFFERENTIAL DIAGNOSIS

Chronic liver disease, e.g. alcoholic cirrhosis, chronic viral hepatitis, post portocaval shunt
Parenteral iron overdose (intravenous iron, transfusions, haemodialysis)

Ineffective erythropoiesis, e.g. thalassaemia major, sideroblastic anaemia treated by blood transfusion

Porphyria cutanea tarda

Congenital atransferrinaemia

Neonatal iron overload

African iron overload (inherited, non-HLA-linked)

COMPLICATIONS

Cirrhosis of the liver – later in women

Cardiac – restrictive cardiomyopathy, arrhythmias and cardiac failure

Diabetes mellitus

Hepatocellular carcinoma (200 $\times$ risk) – 30% of patients with cirrhosis will develop this

Rarely, cholangiocarcinoma

Chondrocalcinosis and degenerative joint disease

Infertility in men

Patients are also at greater risk of certain infections, especially, hepatitis B and C, *Listeria* and *Yersinia*

TREATMENT

Weekly phlebotomy of 500 mL of blood until erythrocytosis is iron-dependent (i.e. haemoglobin or haematocrit does not recover by the next phlebotomy). Monitor the transferrin saturation and ferritin. Continue phlebotomy until transferrin saturation is < 50% or ferritin < 50 ng/mL. Then bleed 500 mL blood every 2–3 months

Avoid alcohol and vitamin C, which can increase iron absorption

Liver transplant may be considered but results are poor, with only 50–60% survival rates

First-degree relatives should be offered biochemical and genetic screening – start phlebotomy if the disease is confirmed

PROGNOSIS

Normal prognosis if no cirrhosis and compliant with phlebotomy treatment

QUESTION SPOTTING

The typical patient will be a male in his 40s who presents with cirrhotic liver disease, who will have incidental findings of diabetes. These two findings should immediately alert you to the possibility of haemochromatosis.

Also consider the diagnosis if there is a combination of some of the following:

Cardiac failure
Arthralgia
Skin pigmentation
Gonadal failure
Chondrocalcinosis

WILSON'S DISEASE (HEPATOLENTICULAR DEGENERATION)

An autosomal-recessive disease caused by mutations of the *ATP7B* gene on chromosome 13. This leads to failure of hepatocyte excretion of copper into the bile. Copper accumulates in the liver and, when saturated, in other organs, notably the brain, cornea and lens, kidney, red blood cells, bones and skin.

Onset is usually between 6 and 40 years of age and the clinical picture can be very variable.

SYMPTOMS
Tremor
Small handwriting
Dysarthria
Personality changes
Behaviour disturbance, including depression
    and psychosis
Abdominal discomfort
Swelling of abdomen or ankles
Tiredness

SIGNS
Hepatic
Jaundice
Ascites
Hepatomegaly
Often asymptomatic

Central nervous system
Tremor
Dysarthria
Drooling
Chorea
Dystonic spasms or posturing
Akinesia
Rigidity
Seizures
Impaired cognition – late
Hearing, vision and sensation are not usually
    affected
Reflexes are usually normal, as are the plantar
    responses

Ocular
Kayser–Fleischer rings – present in 60% of cases;
    almost always in neurological disease
Sunflower cataracts

Renal
Renal tubular acidosis (usually proximal) with osteomalacia/rickets

Haematological
Haemolytic anaemia (10%). This is typically non-spherocytic and Coombs-negative.

Skin
Copper deposition leads to bluish tinging, and blue lunulae in the nailbeds

Other features
Osteoarthritis of the spine (Scheuermann's disease)

Polyarthritis
Hypermobile joints
Chondromalacia patellae

INVESTIGATIONS
FBC
Normal

U + Es
Normal

LFTs
Bilirubin ↑
AST ↑
ALP ↑
Albumin ↓
Clotting prolonged if severe liver disease

Bicarbonate ↓ if RTA
Caeruloplasmin ↓ or normal
Total copper ↓ (or normal)
Free copper ↑↑
Autoantibodies (e.g. anti-smooth-muscle
    antibody) may be positive
IgG may be elevated

Urinalysis
Glucose +
Protein +
Amino acids +
↑ Urinary 24-hour copper (may be raised in
    other chronic liver disease and in proteinuria)
CT/MRI brain scans show cerebral atrophy and
    degeneration of basal ganglia

DIAGNOSIS

Liver biopsy shows ↑↑ copper levels (> 250 μg/g dry weight). An alternative test is to measure 24-hour copper excretion whilst giving d-penicillamine; the diagnostic threshold is > 25 μmol/24 hours

DIFFERENTIAL DIAGNOSIS

Acute liver failure

Paracetamol overdose/other drug toxicity
Mushroom poisoning
Autoimmune hepatitis
Viral hepatitis
Liver ischaemia

Chronic disease

Haemochromatosis
Viral or autoimmune liver disease
Parkinsonian syndromes
Multiple sclerosis
Drug side-effects
Cerebral tumour

COMPLICATIONS

Cirrhosis
Portal hypertension with splenomegaly, varices and ascites
Pigment gallstones from haemolysis
Hepatocellular carcinoma – rare, in contrast to haemochromatosis
May present as fulminant hepatic failure
Cardiac arrhythmias
Renal tubular acidosis
Haemolytic anaemia

TREATMENT

Penicillamine for life
Trientine may be used if penicillamine-intolerant
Some clinicians advise potassium sulphide or zinc as additional therapy, as they reduce copper absorption in the gut
A low-copper diet is also advised, as is abstinence from alcohol
Some worsening in symptoms may be seen early on in treatment and response is rare before 6–12 months. Treatment may be reduced once copper levels are normalized but should be continued for life. Neurological damage does not usually reverse with treatment
Liver transplant is useful in young patients with severe disease, especially as it corrects the metabolic defect, so that treatment may be stopped
Relatives of patients with Wilson's disease should be screened

PROGNOSIS

Death occurs in 5–14 years without treatment

QUESTION SPOTTING

Consider the diagnosis if:

Fulminant liver failure occurs in a young patient where there is no obvious cause
A young patient has odd neurological symptoms and deranged LFTs – especially if tremor, dysarthria or chorea is present

Chronic inflammatory disease invariably affecting the rectum which can spread in a confluent manner to involve the whole colon (pancolitis). Mucosa can return to normal when the inflammation subsides but there is usually some residual glandular distortion.

The cause of ulcerative colitis (and Crohn's disease) is not known, and it is possible that the two diseases represent manifestations of the same disease, but different environmental factors determine which disease phenotype occurs. Ulcerative colitis, for instance, is less likely in smokers, unlike Crohn's disease. However the pathogens implicated in Crohn's disease (*Mycobacterium* and viruses) have not been found in ulcerative colitis. Likewise xANCA (antigen is lactoferrin) is raised in ulcerative colitis but not in Crohn's disease. A number of genetic associations, including with MHC and IL-1 gene variants, have been proposed.

SYMPTOMS

Bloody diarrhoea with mucus
Urgency of defecation and tenesmus
Lower abdominal pain
Weight loss
Fever
Malaise
Nausea
Anorexia
Arthritis

SIGNS

May be none
Anaemia
Tachycardia
Fever
Mouth ulcers
Abdominal tenderness
Finger clubbing – rare

INVESTIGATIONS

FBC

Hb ↓ (MCV normal or ↓ if chronic blood loss)
WBC ↑
Platelets normal or ↑

U + Es

Normal

LFTs

Albumin ↓
Bilirubin, ALT and ALP may all be elevated – see differential diagnosis

ESR and CRP ↑

Stool analysis

Negative for pathogens
Positive for blood

AXR

May show colonic dilatation
Sacroiliitis
Ankylosing spondylitis

Barium studies

Not used for diagnosis nowadays. Double-contrast study will show abnormal mucosal pattern and ulceration if present. Plain abdominal radiography should precede barium study to exclude toxic dilatation. Long-standing disease may show the 'lead pipe' sign – a smooth, straight descending colon and sigmoid colon (Fig. 3.1).

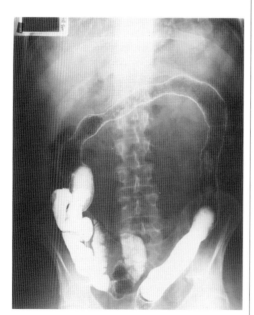

Figure 3.1 Barium enema showing shortened, featureless 'lead pipe' descending colon in long-standing ulcerative colitis.

DIAGNOSIS

Is by colonoscopy and biopsy. Mucosa shows erythema and reduced vascular pattern. Ulcers tend to occur late. Pseudopolyps and mucosal bridging may occur. Colonoscopy also allows the extent of the disease to be mapped.

Rectal biopsy

DIFFERENTIAL DIAGNOSIS

See Crohn's disease

Differential diagnosis of abnormal LFTs in inflammatory bowel disease

Acute colitis: acute-phase response and fatty change
Pericholangitis: mostly benign. Usually in pancolitis and resolves with colectomy
Viral hepatitis: may be transfusion-related
Gallstones
Autoimmune cholangiopathy: similar to autoimmune chronic active hepatitis and responds to steroids
Primary sclerosing cholangitis (70% of patients with PSC have UC)
Drug-induced
Hepatic granulomas
Liver abscess
Amyloid

COMPLICATIONS

Carcinoma 5–10% after 20 years of disease. May be multifocal and often mucinous in type
Abscess formation
Acute toxic bowel rare but commoner than Crohn's
Perforation rare but commoner than Crohn's
Haemorrhage rare but commoner than Crohn's
Fistulae (external, rectovaginal) – very rare, unlike Crohn's
Stricture formation – very rare, unlike Crohn's

TREATMENT

General medical measures: fluid and electrolyte replacement, blood transfusion as required
Oral steroids and topical steroids via rectal enemas (only in the acute attack)

Oral aminosalicylate (effective in acute attack and also to maintain remission)
Topical mesalazine enemas if refractory to oral aminosalicylate and topical steroids
Azathioprine and 6-mercaptopurine are effective steroid-sparing agents in maintaining remission in those patients not controlled by aminosalicylates. Ciclosporin is also used to control severe active inflammation not responding to other measures
Metronidazole has no proven use in ulcerative colitis, and elemental feeding does not reduce disease activity in ulcerative colitis (see Crohn's disease)

Surgery

Absolute indications
Uncontrolled haemorrhage
Perforation
Carcinoma

Relative indications
Severe colitis ± toxic megacolon not responding to maximal medical therapy
Severe intractable symptoms
Intolerable side-effects from disease-modifying medications
Intolerable extracolonic manifestations, e.g. pyoderma gangrenosum, haemolytic anaemia or arthritis, but note the course of primary sclerosing cholangitis is independent of disease activity and colectomy
Operation may either be a proctocolectomy with ileostomy or total colectomy with ileoanal anastomosis and pouch formation

QUESTION SPOTTING

Either ulcerative colitis or Crohn's disease may be presented and differentiation may be made by clues in the history or the investigation results and by the extraenteric manifestations. Watch for sclerosing cholangitis in UC and gallstones/oxalate renal stones in Crohn's. Either may give a history of arthritis, eye problems or a rash, which may be confused with one of the connective tissue disorders.

Questions may revolve around the management of an acute attack of UC and indications for surgery. In long-standing UC, watch for the development of colonic carcinoma.

Chronic inflammatory disease affecting any part of the gut with special predisposition for the terminal ileum, colon and anorectum.

The cause of Crohn's disease is still not known. A single aetiological factor has not been found and most now believe that the disease is due to poorly regulated immune and inflammatory processes within the gut wall. The initial response is likely to be caused by a bacterial or other environmental stimulus, but genetically susceptible individuals then suffer from an overexpression of both local immune reactions and systemic inflammatory cell infiltrate. These continue, unchecked by the normal counterinflammatory mechanisms.

A possible association is with a low-residue, high-refined-sugar diet, and a clear link with smoking has been established.

Genetic studies have demonstrated that several genes give rise to increased susceptibility to inflammatory bowel disease, and family members with predisposing genotype are as likely to get Crohn's disease as ulcerative colitis. However, the phenotype may be determined by environmental factors, especially smoking.

SYMPTOMS
Diarrhoea
Abdominal pain

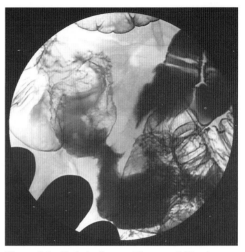

Figure 3.3 Crohn's disease. The second film shows a double-contrast barium study. There are more typical 'rose thorn' ulcers. The barium refluxes back into the ileum, which is also abnormal.

Weight loss
Fever
Rectal bleeding, especially in colonic disease
Perianal disease
Obstructive symptoms of colic and vomiting, especially in ileal disease.
Tiredness and shortness of breath if anaemic
Bone pain secondary to osteomalacia if malabsorption of vitamin D
Excessive bleeding if malabsorption of vitamin K (rare)

SIGNS
May be normal
Anaemia
Mouth ulcers
Glossitis
Clubbing of nails
Abdominal tenderness
Palpable abdominal mass, particularly right iliac fossa
Anal fissures, fistulae and skin tags

INVESTIGATIONS
FBC
Hb ↓ (mixed deficiencies can cause MCV ↓ or ↑)
WCC ↑ (neutrophilia)

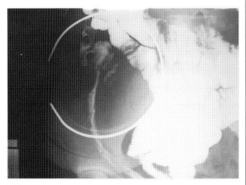

Figure 3.2 Crohn's disease. The first X-ray is a barium followthrough. The round marker is a compression disc which pushes bowel away from the area of interest. This film shows collapsed severe Crohn's disease of the terminal ileum with the classical string sign. There are multiple 'rose thorn' ulcers and ulcerated pits. This film also demonstrates area of normal bowel between areas of disease – so-called skip lesions. This is typical of Crohn's disease.

Platelets ↑

B_{12} and folate may be low

Ferritin is best marker of iron stores but may be ↑ in acute phase

U + Es

Na normal

K ↓ due to diarrhoea

Urea and creatinine normal

LFTs

Bilirubin, AST and ALP ↑ (especially a mild ↓ in AST and ALP) (see also UC)

Albumin ↓ in active disease (due to negative acute-phase reaction and protein-losing enteropathy)

Calcium ↓ in severe small-bowel disease

Mg^{2+}, Zn^{2+} and selenium may be ↓

AXR may show evidence of intestinal obstruction, sacroiliitis or ankylosing spondylitis

Ultrasound of the abdomen may demonstrate an inflammatory RIF mass and bowel oedema

DIAGNOSIS

Colonoscopy with terminal ileal or colonic biopsy can sometimes be used to diagnose the disease. Rectal sparing often occurs, even in Crohn's colitis. Resected surgical specimens are another source of tissue diagnosis.

In the early stages, aphthous ulcers have normal mucosa around them (unlike ulcerative colitis, which shows erythema and reduced vascular pattern) and later cobblestoning, fissuring ulcers and oedema are seen. Ulcers tend to be linear and become confluent: ulcerative colitis typically shows inflamed diffuse granular friable dark red mucosa and ulcers only occur in severe disease. Pseudopolyps and mucosal bridges occur in both.

Radiological diagnosis

Barium meal with follow-through or infusion (Figure 3.4) which may show thickened valvulae coniventes, small aphthous ulcers, 'rose thorn' ulcers, cobblestoning, fissures and wall thickening.

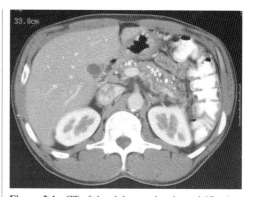

Figure 3.4 CT of the abdomen showing calcification in pancreas due to chronic pancreatitis. (Reproduced with permission from Kumar, Clarke (2001) *Clinical Medicine*, 5th edn. Saunders.)

DIFFERENTIAL DIAGNOSIS

Ulcerative colitis

Infective colitis, including TB, *Shigella*, *Campylobacter*, *Escherichia coli*, amoebiasis and pseudomembranous colitis

Vasculitis, including SLE and PAN

Ischaemic colitis

Colonic carcinoma

Collagenous and lymphocytic colitis

Irritable-bowel syndrome

Solitary rectal ulcer syndrome

Radiation colitis

Neutropenic colitis

Diverticulitis

Eosinophilic gastroenteritis

Small-bowel lymphoma

Alpha-chain disease

Amyloid

Behçet's disease

COMPLICATIONS

Acute toxic bowel, perforation, haemorrhage (rare)

Strictures of small or large bowel

Malabsorption (due to inflammation and bowel resection) – causing vitamin deficiencies, steatorrhoea, and, if severe, short-bowel syndrome

Fistulae (enterocolic, gastrocolic or from bowel to bladder or vagina. Can cause pneumaturia or faeces in either urine or vaginal discharge)

Involvement of ureters (right > left) may cause sterile pyuria, urinary tract infection or ureteric stricture

Carcinoma (3–5%) in colonic disease. Small-bowel carcinoma has also been documented, although this is rare

TREATMENT

Stop smoking (this will significantly reduce relapse rate)

Diet

Elemental diet is as effective as steroids in acute disease. However it is poorly tolerated, and polymeric diet may have a better compliance. TPN is used if preoperative or severely ill

Low fibre is used if strictures are present

Low fat is used in steatorrhoea

Vitamin supplements if deficient

Drugs

Loperamide helps diarrhoea in inactive disease

Steroids in active disease

5-aminosalicylic acid – not very effective except at high doses in active disease affecting the colon

Azathioprine or 6-mercaptopurine for at least 2 years to be effective

Methotrexate is effective but has a high incidence of side effects

Antibiotics are useful if bacterial overgrowth supervenes and causes malabsorption

Cholestyramine if diarrhoea is due to bile salt malabsorption

Rectal hydrocortisone enemas if proctitis present

TNF antagonists (e.g. infliximab) are licensed for refractory disease and for fistulating disease

Surgery

70–80% require an operation

Minimal resection margins are recommended

Bypass operations and pouch surgery are contraindicated

Fistulae should be determined anatomically with sinograms and only excised after antibiotic treatment, control of active disease

and nutrition correction. Infliximab is now licensed for treatment of fistulating disease and is usually tried first

Colostomy may be useful to defunction bowel for 12–18 months

Indications

Failure of medical management

Strictures causing obstruction

Fistulae

Abscess or perforation

Extraenteric manifestations and frequencies in Crohn's and ulcerative colitis (Table 3.1)

Other

Psoas abscess

Amyloidosis

QUESTION SPOTTING

See under ulcerative colitis.

Table 3.1

	Crohn's	UC
Hepatobiliary		
Chronic active hepatitis	2–3%	Rare
Cirrhosis	5%	20%
Fatty liver	6%	Common
Pericholangitis	20%	25%
Primary sclerosing cholangitis	Very rare	5–12%
Cholelithiasis	30%	5% (normal incidence in population)
Renal		
Oxalate stones		Not seen
Ureteric obstruction		Not seen
Rheumatological		
Enteropathic arthritis	6–12%	10%
Ankylosing spondylitis	2–6%	2–6%
Sacroiliitis	15–18%	15–18%
Osteoporosis	3–10%	3–10%
Ocular		
Uveitis or iritis		
Episcleritis		
Conjunctivitis		
Dermatological		
Erythema nodosum	5–10%	2%
Pyoderma gangrenosum	0.5%	3%
Aphthous ulceration	20%	Uncommon
Perianal skin tags	Common	Rare
Nutrition deficiency diseases	Common	Rare

BUDD–CHIARI SYNDROME

Obstruction of the larger hepatic veins. This may occur acutely or in a more chronic form.

CAUSES
Unknown in 30%
Thrombosis due to hypercoagulable state – polycythaemia vera, paroxysmal nocturnal haemoglobinuria and antithrombin III, protein C or protein S deficiencies, pregnancy or oral contraceptive pill use
Malignancy – particularly hepatic, renal and adrenal carcinomas
Congenital venous web – rare outside Japan
Hepatic infection, e.g. hydatid cysts
Radiotherapy
Trauma

SYMPTOMS
Nausea and vomiting – acute
Upper abdominal pain – acute
May be few symptoms if chronic – non-specific malaise and abdominal fullness

SIGNS
Tender hepatomegaly
Ascites
Jaundice – chronic
Splenomegaly – chronic
Peripheral oedema only occurs if inferior vena cava involved
Hepatojugular reflex usually absent

INVESTIGATIONS
FBC
Normal

U + Es
Normal

LFTs
Variable
AST ↑
ALP ↑
Bilirubin ↑
Albumin ↓

Ca normal
Clotting may be abnormal

Ascites
Protein > 25 g/L initially but falls in chronic phase

DIAGNOSIS
Liver ultrasound with Doppler to examine flow in the hepatic vein
Abdominal CT or MRI can also be used to demonstrate hepatic vein occlusion
Liver biopsy shows centrilobular congestion with fibrosis

DIFFERENTIAL DIAGNOSIS
Cirrhosis from other causes
Veno-occlusive disease – rare disease caused by widespread non-thrombotic obliteration of the central hepatic veins. Pyrrolizidine alkaloids (from the plants used to make tea), cytotoxic drugs and hepatic irradiation are the most common causes. Clinically very similar to Budd–Chiari syndrome
Right-sided cardiac failure
Constrictive pericarditis
Inferior vena cava obstruction

TREATMENT
Treat the underlying cause if identified
Ascites should be treated with diuretics, sodium and water restriction and paracentesis. The ascites may prove difficult to treat and portal venous shunting by transjugular intrahepatic portasystemic stent shunting (TIPSS) or peritoneal-systemic shunting (the LeVeen procedure)
Side-to-side portocaval or splenorenal anastomosis may be useful to decompress the liver
Surgery for congenital webs
Rarely thrombolytics such as streptokinase may be tried with subsequent anticoagulation
Liver transplantation is becoming more common

PROGNOSIS
Generally poor. 30–60% die within 1 year.
Survivors may develop cirrhosis

QUESTION SPOTTING

May present with the picture of cirrhosis, but with no obvious underlying cause except that the patient may have some reason for a hypercoagulable state – if you suspect the diagnosis, look for an underlying cause, e.g. antiphospholipid syndrome, polycythaemia rubra vera. Also consider if a picture of acute hepatitis occurs with ascites.

COELIAC DISEASE

An autoimmune disease with hypersensitivity to the gliadin fraction of gluten and related products in wheat, rye and barley, characterized by destruction of the normal small-bowel mucosal architecture.

Mucosal destruction of the proximal bowel leads to malabsorption of fat, protein and carbohydrate, along with low vitamin A, D, E and K levels, low iron and folate.

There is high prevalence in Ireland and in Punjabi immigrants. There is often a family history.

SYMPTOMS

Many cases are asymptomatic, with anaemia or other disturbances picked up on routine screening tests
Abdominal bloating and discomfort
Diarrhoea and steatorrhoea
Weight loss
Weakness
Anaemic symptoms (tiredness, breathlessness)
Bone pain
Paraesthesia and tetany if hypocalcaemia
Bruising (from vitamin K coagulopathy – rare)

SIGNS

Anaemia, particularly in pregnancy
Proximal muscle weakness (vitamin D malabsorption)
Mouth ulcers and stomatitis
Clubbing (rare)
Associated rash of dermatitis herpetiformis

INVESTIGATIONS

FBC
Hb $\downarrow$
WCC and platelets $\downarrow$ (folate/B_{12} deficiency)
MCV $\downarrow$ if Fe-deficient, $\uparrow$ if folate/B_{12}-deficient. May be normal if mixed deficiency or mild disease

U + Es
Usually normal
K $\downarrow$ in diarrhoea

LFTs
Bilirubin normal
ALP may be $\uparrow$ in osteomalacia, or from liver/bowel source

Albumin often $\downarrow$
Fe often $\downarrow$
TIBC often $\uparrow$
Red cell folate usually $\downarrow$
B_{12} may be $\downarrow$
Calcium $\downarrow$ or low normal
Phosphate $\downarrow$
IgA often raised, with low IgM levels
INR may be elevated (vitamin K malabsorption)

Blood film
Dimorphic picture if mixed iron deficiency – microcytes, macrocytes, hypersegmented neutrophils
Features of hyposplenism – target cells, Howell–Jolly bodies, etc.
Barium studies show dilated bowel, smooth outline with prominent (oedematous) valvulae conniventes

DIAGNOSIS

Duodenal biopsy via endoscopy. Histology shows atrophy of villi with crypt hypertrophy. Plasma cells and lymphocytes are seen invading the lamina propria
Antigliadin and antiendomysial antibodies – 90% sensitivity. May be negative in individuals with IgA deficiency (10% of coeliacs). Tissue transglutaminase antibodies are a new specific and sensitive test
Symptoms improve on a gluten-free diet

ASSOCIATIONS

Dermatitis herpetiformis (gluten-sensitive rash)
IDDM
Thyroid disease
Addison's disease
Fibrosing alveolitis
SLE
Polyarteritis
Inflammatory bowel disease
Temporal lobe epilepsy
10% also have IgA deficiency (compared with 0.5% of the general population)

DIFFERENTIAL DIAGNOSIS

Other causes of malabsorption, including:
Crohn's disease
Giardia infection

Postinfectious malabsorption
Whipple's disease
Radiation enteritis
Bacterial overgrowth
Amyloidosis
Lymphoma
Common variable immunodeficiency
Cow's milk intolerance

COMPLICATIONS
Osteoporosis
Osteomalacia
Splenic atrophy
GI lymphoma
Ulcerative jejunoileitis
Oesophageal carcinoma
Pharyngeal carcinoma
B_{12} deficiency (associated pernicious anaemia or bacterial overgrowth)

TREATMENT
Gluten-free diet. Vitamin supplementation may be necessary for 3–4 months until the mucosa regenerates. Corticosteroids may be given acutely for severe disease.

QUESTION SPOTTING
Consider coeliac disease in any patient with generalized malabsorption – look for steatorrhoea, weight loss, low calcium, anaemia. Also consider in anyone with iron deficiency and no obvious source for the blood loss.

Often, the difficulty is to distinguish between coeliac disease and the other causes of malabsorption listed above. Look out for:

Recurrent anaemia
A long history, perhaps of poor growth in
    childhood
No prior history of GI infection
Villous atrophy on small-bowel biopsy
Lack of strictures or small-bowel surgery
Presence of a rash (dermatitis herpetiformis)
Family history
At-risk groups

CHRONIC PANCREATITIS

Unlike acute pancreatitis, the chronic inflammation in this disease leads to progressive and irreversible structural damage with permanent impairment of endocrine and exocrine function. The pancreatic acini are destroyed by the chronic fibrotic process. The pancreatic ducts become dilated and irregular, and protein plugs and calcification may appear. Clinical evidence of pancreatic exocrine insufficiency occurs after loss of > 90% of function. Deficiencies of fat-soluble vitamins (A, D, E and K) are possible, but very rare, in comparison with malabsorption such as coeliac disease. Pancreatic endocrine insufficiency occurs and, although glucose intolerance is common, overt diabetes mellitus occurs very late in the disease. Patients are also glucagon-deficient (unlike idiopathic insulin-dependent diabetes), and so are at more risk of treatment-related hypoglycaemia.

CAUSES

Alcohol (70–80%)

Idiopathic (10–20%) – bimodal distribution, men = women, some patients found to have a mutation in the cystic fibrosis gene without having cystic fibrosis

Patients with overt cystic fibrosis

Other causes (5–10%) include:

Hyperlipidaemia – especially hypertriglyceridaemia

Hereditary – rare, autosomal-dominant

Tropical – rare in UK, but common in parts of Africa and Asia. Affects children who are malnourished and cassava fruit has been implicated. Abdominal pain is less frequent

Obstructive

Chronic hypercalcaemia, e.g. hyperparathyroidism – occurs in 10–15% of these patients if untreated

Haemochromatosis

Trauma

Postsurgical

Pancreas divisum – failure of fusion of the two embryonic parts to the pancreas. Only a small proportion progress to chronic pancreatitis

Gastrinoma

Alpha-1-antitrypsin deficiency

Deficiencies of amylase, lipase, trypsinogen or enterokinase

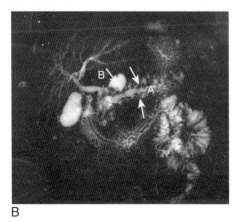

A

B

Figure 3.5 Imaging in chronic pancreatitis. (A) CT scan showing a grossly dilated and irregular duct with calcified stone (arrow A). Note the calcification in the head of the gland (arrow B). (B) MRCP of the same patient showing marked ductal dilation with abnormal dilated side branches (arrows A). A small cyst is also present (arrow B). (Reproduced with permission from Boon, Colledge, Walker et al. (2006) *Davidson's Principles and Practice of Medicine*, 20th edn. Churchill Livingstone.)

CLINICAL FEATURES

Abdominal pain – highly variable pattern

Anorexia

Weight loss – often due to fear of eating

Nausea and vomiting

Mild fever common

Steatorrhoea with bloating, abdominal cramps and flatus

Skin nodules

Disseminated fat necrosis – rare

INVESTIGATIONS

FBC
Normal

U + Es
Normal

LFTs
Raised if concurrent liver disease or cholestasis, but otherwise normal

Amylase ↑ or normal later in the disease. No prognostic value

Lipase may be ↑ or normal

Glucose raised (if diabetes supervenes)

72-hours faecal fat collection > 20 g/24 hours (normal < 7 g/24 hours)

Pancreatic exocrine function tests (e.g. pancreolauryl test) show pancreatic insufficiency

AXR
Shows pancreatic intraductal calcification in 30% (especially alcohol-induced)

Ultrasound
Abdominal ultrasound may show focal or diffuse enlargement, ductal irregularity dilatation and pseudocysts (sensitivity 60–70%).

DIAGNOSIS
Abdominal CT has specificity of 90%

MRCP is also useful to confirm the diagnosis – this is a non-invasive alternative to ERCP for defining ductal abnormalities

Endoscopic ultrasound is increasing in use. Can also perform fine-needle aspiration by this method, and look for complications such as pseudocysts

DIFFERENTIAL DIAGNOSIS
Pancreatic malignancy is the major differential

Coeliac disease

Crohn's disease

Also consider:

Other malignancy

Other causes of malabsorption, e.g. bacterial overgrowth

Gallstones

Peptic ulcer disease

Irritable-bowel syndrome

Endometriosis

COMPLICATIONS
Pancreatic pseudocyst formation. Cause of 5–10% of deaths with chronic pancreatitis due to complications of mechanical obstruction, erosion into blood vessels and infection. If small they require no treatment, but if larger may require percutaneous aspiration or surgery

Abscess formation

Gastrointestinal bleeding

Mechanical obstruction to duodenum – pain after eating and early satiety

Mechanical obstruction to common bile duct – pain and jaundice with abnormal liver function tests

Pancreatic fistulae with ascites or a pleural effusion (these exudates have very high amylase levels)

Splenic vein thrombosis with portal hypertension – may require splenectomy

Pseudoaneurysm formation involving the splenic artery – treat with coil embolization if possible

TREATMENT
Stop alcohol – improves prognosis, but may not affect pain

Pain control – beware problems of addiction to opiates

Intravenous vitamin supplementation

Oral pancreatic enzyme supplements – this often improves pain by diminishing the stimulation of cholecystokinin

Diet, oral hypoglycaemics and insulin may be required in the treatment of diabetes

Coeliac plexus nerve block may be considered, but side-effects include postural hypotension, diarrhoea and paraparesis

Surgery is controversial. It has been used for pancreatic resection and ductal drainage procedures. Surgery may also be indicated for drainage of larger pancreatic pseudocysts

Endoscopic treatments include sphincterotomy, pancreatic duct stent placement, stone extraction and pseudocyst drainage

QUESTION SPOTTING

The question is unlikely to include all three of alcohol abuse, abdominal pain and raised amylase. A question with abdominal pain, weight loss and nausea/vomiting is likely to raise the suspicion of abdominal malignancy, but chronic pancreatitis should also be considered. Consider the diagnosis whenever malabsorption is the presenting feature, and look out for calcification of the pancreas on abdominal films or CT. Other clues include raised glucose.

Colorectal cancer is the third commonest internal cancer in the UK. Two-thirds of tumours are found distal to the splenic flexure, and 2–3% of tumours have additional metachronous colonic tumours at the time of diagnosis. Colorectal cancers usually arise from dysplastic polyps; the incidence is much higher in patients with familial adenomatous polyposis and hereditary non-polyposis colon cancer (HNPCC) syndrome. Low levels of dietary fibre and high levels of meat appear to increase the risk of bowel cancer.

Oesophageal cancer has historically been due to squamous cell carcinoma, but the incidence of this is declining, whereas the incidence of adenocarcinoma is rising. Tobacco and alcohol are risk factors for squamous cell carcinoma; Barrett's oesophagus is an important risk factor for adenocarcinoma.

Stomach cancer (adenocarcinoma) is less common than 50 years ago in western countries but remains very common in East Asia. Smoked and preserved foods, as well as cigarette smoking, may play a role. *Helicobacter pylori* has also been implicated as a risk factor. There is a link with blood group A, pernicious anaemia and previous partial gastrectomy. Stomach cancers are found in the middle and lower parts of the stomach in 80% of cases, and may appear as polyps, ulcers or diffuse thickening of the stomach wall.

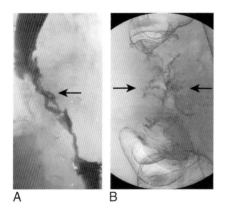

A   B

Figure 3.6 Barium studies showing (A) oesophageal cancer and (B) colon cancer. (Reproduced with permission from Boon, Colledge, Walker et al. (2006) *Davidson's Principles and Practice of Medicine*, 20th edn. Churchill Livingstone.)

SYMPTOMS
Weight loss
Tiredness
Breathlessness
Abdominal pain
Anorexia

Upper GI
Indigestion
Dysphagia – initially to solids
Nausea, vomiting
Cough
Haematemesis, melaena
Hoarse voice

Lower GI
Constipation
Diarrhoea
Blood in stool
Mucus in stool
Abdominal swelling

SIGNS
Anaemia
Lymphadenopathy (especially in left supraclavicular fossa)
Jaundice (if advanced liver metastases)
Cachexia
Hepatomegaly
Ascites
Palpable masses
Abdominal distension (if obstruction)
Abdominal tenderness
Ankle oedema (due to low protein, IVC compression or DVT)

INVESTIGATIONS
FBC
Hb – often low
MCV – often low
WCC – usually normal
Plts – usually normal

U + Es
Normal

LFTs
Elevated if liver metastases – ALP may be elevated if bony metastases

INR
Usually normal

Calcium
May be elevated if bony metastases present

ECG
Usually normal

CXR
May show pulmonary metastases, bony metastases

AXR
Usually normal. May show large stomach air bubble if gastric outlet obstruction; dilated bowel if bowel obstruction

DIAGNOSIS
Is by endoscopy. Upper GI endoscopy with biopsy diagnoses oesophageal and stomach cancer; endoscopic ultrasound helps to delineate the extent of local spread and any nodes. Colonoscopy and biopsy is the gold standard for diagnosing colorectal cancer; flexible sigmoidoscopy and barium enema can be used in patients unable to tolerate a full colonoscopy.

CT and MRI have a supplementary role to play in staging the cancer by ascertaining the degree of local and distant spread.

DIFFERENTIAL DIAGNOSIS
Other causes of GI bleeding – peptic ulcer, oesophagitis/ulceration; angiodysplasia, diverticular disease, varices

Other malignancy, e.g. lung, breast, pancreas, lymphoma

Chronic infection, e.g. tuberculosis, Whipple's disease

Chronic inflammatory disorders, e.g. Crohn's disease, diverticulitis

ASSOCIATIONS
Colorectal cancer
Familial adenomatous polyposis (including Gardner's syndrome)

HNPCC – diagnosed in families where 3 or more cases occur, at least 2 of which are in first-degree relatives with one diagnosed at age < 50 years

Peutz–Jeghers syndrome

COMPLICATIONS
GI bleeding (lower or upper)
Ascites
Liver and other metastases
Perforation with peritonitis
Intestinal obstruction
Malnutrition
Local invasion (e.g. pericardium, lung, aorta; bladder, vagina, coeliac plexus)
Paraneoplastic effects (e.g. acanthosis nigricans)

TREATMENT
Surgical
Stomach cancer
Gastrectomy (partial or total)

Adjuvant chemo- plus radiotherapy may reduce recurrence; adjuvant chemotherapy alone has little effect

Gastrojejunostomy is used as a palliative procedure to bypass gastric outlet obstruction

Palliative chemo- and radiotherapy may provide some symptomatic improvement

Oesophageal cancer
Oesophagectomy – via abdominal or thoracic approach

Neoadjuvant radio- and chemotherapy in combination appears to improve survival; postoperative chemo- and radiotherapy do not

Palliative manoeuvres (usually for dysphagia) include stenting of the stricture, photodynamic laser ablation of cancerous tissue at endoscopy and external beam radiotherapy

Colorectal cancer
Surgical excision (hemicolectomy); cancers within a few centimetres of the anal margin require abdominoperineal resection (with loss of the anus and consequent permanent stoma). Total mesorectal excision is the surgical technique usually employed now to ensure clearance of rectal tumours. Surgery is also used palliatively to bypass intestinal obstruction, and excision of solitary hepatic metastases may also be carried out to prolong life.

Radiotherapy
Reduces local recurrence after surgery in rectal cancer. Also useful for local recurrence in a palliative setting.

Chemotherapy

Adjuvant chemotherapy improves outcome in Dukes C colorectal cancer, and combination chemotherapy may improve symptoms and prolong life in metastatic disease.

As with all cancers, palliative care remains an important treatment modality for most patients.

PROGNOSIS

Oesophageal cancer

For patients fit enough to undergo surgery, 5-year survival is approximately 20%

Overall survival is 5–10% at 5 years

Stomach cancer

90% of cancers have either metastasized or invaded lymph nodes at diagnosis. 5-year survival is 5–15%

Colorectal cancer

Dependent on staging:

Dukes A (confined to mucosa) – 90% 5-year survival

Dukes B (submucosal invasion; no nodal spread) – 70% 5-year survival

Dukes C (regional node involvement) – 30–50% 5-year survival

Dukes D (distant spread) – < 10% 5-year survival

QUESTION SPOTTING

Consider the diagnosis in anyone with weight loss and anaemia, or change in bowel habit and weight loss. Questions may centre around management decisions or how best to investigate patients, especially patients with comorbid disease.

ALCOHOLIC LIVER DISEASE

Liver dysfunction caused by excessive ingestion of alcohol. Changes progress through fatty infiltration and chronic inflammation to fibrosis and cirrhosis. 20% of heavy drinkers will develop cirrhosis; the amount of alcohol required to do so varies widely from person to person. Heavy drinking may also precipitate alcoholic hepatitis – an acute inflammatory condition with neutrophilic infiltration of the liver.

SYMPTOMS
Nausea, vomiting
Ankle swelling
Increasing abdominal girth
Fatigue

SIGNS
Most signs are not specific for alcohol-induced chronic liver disease:

Alcohol on breath
Asterixis
Parotid enlargement
Gynaecomastia
Spider naevi
Jaundice
Loss of hair
Small testes
Hepatomegaly (not if cirrhotic)
Splenomegaly
Ascites
Ankle oedema

INVESTIGATIONS
FBC
Hb – low if GI bleeding
MCV – usually elevated
WCC – may be low
Plts – often low

U + Es
Na – low if decompensated disease
K – often low
Urea – often low
Creatinine – usually normal

LFTs
Bilirubin – may be elevated
ALT – normal or elevated
ALP – may be elevated

GGT – usually elevated

Amylase – usually normal
Glucose – normal or low
Magnesium – often low
Phosphate – often low
Calcium – usually normal
INR – elevated if established liver damage or severe jaundice
Ultrasound – may show fatty change of the liver, hepatomegaly or a small nodular liver if cirrhotic. May also show splenomegaly and ascites

DIAGNOSIS
Is usually based on evidence of liver disease (deranged LFTs, signs of chronic liver disease) plus a history of heavy alcohol intake. Biopsy is only very rarely required when the suspicion of an alternative diagnosis is high.

DIFFERENTIAL DIAGNOSIS
Other causes of chronic liver disease, especially:

Hepatitis B/C
Primary biliary cirrhosis
Acute alcoholic hepatitis – consider paracetamol overdose (usually very high ALT, bilirubin relatively low)
Acute hepatitis B infection
Amanita poisoning

COMPLICATIONS
GI bleeding from varices (oesophageal, gastric, rectal)
Hepatic encephalopathy
Spontaneous bacterial peritonitis if ascites present
Malnutrition; low magnesium and phosphate
Hepatorenal syndrome
Bleeding at other sites due to coagulopathy
Hepatocellular carcinoma (in long-standing cirrhosis)

TREATMENT
Alcohol abstinence is the most important treatment
Vitamin B complex to protect against neurological damage

Antibiotic prophylaxis if ascites is present

Decompensations may require drainage of ascites with replacement of albumin; spironolactone; vitamin B-complex administration and treatment of any precipitating factors (e.g. infection, GI bleeding). Nutritional support is often needed

Spontaneous bacterial peritonitis is diagnosed on microscopy and culture of ascites; treat with broad-spectrum antibiotics with ongoing antibiotic prophylaxis

Varices are managed by fluid resuscitation and transfusion; give terlipressin as a holding measure and carry out emergency endoscopy as soon as possible. Sequential banding or sclerotherapy via endoscopy is used to obliterate the varices; propranolol also reduces rebleeding by reducing portal pressures. Refractory cases may require shunting (TIPSS or rarely surgical shunt)

Encephalopathy is treated by removing precipitants (e.g. drugs), fluid and nutritional support and bowel decontamination (give lactulose with or without antibiotics)

Hepatorenal syndrome is treated by close attention to fluid balance (often with the help of a CVP line). Terlipressin and albumin may help to reverse the syndrome

End-stage cirrhosis may require liver transplant; not all patients are psychologically suitable to receive a transplant

PROGNOSIS

Dependent on the grade of cirrhosis. Abstinence can improve survival to 90% at 5 years; survival is less than 50% at 5 years with continued drinking. Spontaneous bacterial peritonitis is associated with a particularly poor outcome in the medium term, as is hepatorenal failure.

QUESTION SPOTTING

The diagnosis is usually obvious; you are more likely to be asked about management of decompensations of liver disease, e.g. variceal bleeding, liver failure. Detoxification from alcohol is often a complicating factor. Also look out for alcoholic hepatitis as a differential; the bilirubin is usually very high, the ALT only moderately elevated and nausea, vomiting and RUQ pain often occur with a fever and high WCC.

NEPHROLOGY

4

HAEMOLYTIC–URAEMIC SYNDROME (HUS) AND THROMBOTIC THROMBOCYTOPENIC PURPURA (TTP)

This is a syndrome comprising microangiopathic haemolysis, renal failure and thrombocytopenia, thought to be due to endothelial cell dysfunction. A variety of insults may trigger the syndrome:

WITH DIARRHOEAL PRODROME
Escherichia coli O157, *Shigella*, *Yersinia* spp. (all produce Shiga toxin)

WITHOUT DIARRHOEAL PRODROME
Viral or pneumococcal URTI
HIV
Idiopathic; may be familial
Pregnancy/postpartum
Malignant hypertension
Renal transplant
Other glomerulonephritis
SLE
Scleroderma
Drugs, including OCP, ciclosporin, Mitomycin C, 5-fluorouracil, ticlopidine
Diarrohea and upper respiratory tract infection are the commonest trigger factors of HUS
HUS is commonly associated with renal problems
HUS is commoner than TTP and occurs more often in children,with median age of 6 months to 4 years. TTP occurs at any age but peaks at 35 years

SYMPTOMS
Bloody diarrhoea 1 week prior to onset
Tiredness, SOB (due to anaemia)
Nausea, vomiting, itching (due to uraemia)
Occasionally macroscopic haematuria
Neurological deficits are uncommon in HUS, but are common in TTP and include:
Seizures
Psychosis
Focal deficits; may be transient or permanent
Hallucinations

SIGNS
Pale (anaemia)
If onset is insidious, may see raised BP, hypertensive retinopathy

Asterixis (uraemia)
Fever
Purpuric rash
Jaundice (haemolysis)

INVESTIGATIONS
FBC
Hb ↓
WCC ↑
Platelets ↓

U + Es
Na may be ↓ in ARF
K usually ↑
Urea and creatinine ↑

LFTs
Bilirubin ↑
Albumin ↓

Haptoglobins ↓ or absent
Reticulocytes ↑
Coombs test negative (the anaemia is not immunologically mediated)
Urate ↑
LDH ↑
INR and APTT normal
Fibrin degradation products usually ↑

Blood film shows schistocytes and spherocytes
Blood cultures are negative in *E. coli* disease

CT of the brain may show areas of infarction, or less commonly haemorrhage, in TTP

ADAMTS13 levels. This is a von Willebrand factor-cleaving protease which is normal in HUS and depressed in TTP – an assay for the future that may help distinguish between the two diseases and allocate those who would benefit from plasma exchange (TTP)

DIAGNOSIS
The diagnosis of these conditions is based on clinical findings coupled with lab findings. Clinical features, the blood film appearance noted above, along with an Hb less than 8 g/dL and moderate thrombocytopenia with normal coagulation would suggest HUS. Markedly elevated LDH along with neurological manifestations is more common in TTP.

DIFFERENTIAL DIAGNOSIS

Vasculitis

Malignant hypertension

Carcinomatosis

Septicaemia with DIC (clotting is abnormal)

Ischaemic colitis or ulcerative colitis

Haemorrhagic fevers, including dengue

Malaria

Snake bite

SBE, especially on prosthetic valves

HELLP syndrome (pregnancy) and pre-eclampsia

Evans syndrome (ITP + autoimmune haemolytic
    anaemia)

AV malformations

COMPLICATIONS

Bowel perforation/infarction may occur

GI bleeding

Pancreatitis (DM rare)

Acute coronary ischaemia

Myocarditis occurs rarely

TREATMENT
HUS

Supportive treatment includes correcting
    hypovolaemia, hyperkalaemia and anaemia.
    Dialysis is often necessary

Steroids are widely used but have not been
    proven to affect outcome

Plasma exchange is also used, but its efficacy is
    unclear at present and is reserved for severe
    cases

Likewise, the benefit of using heparin or
    prostacyclins is also unproven

TTP

Plasma exchange against FFP is the treatment of
choice; this has been shown to reduce mortality.
Some patients appear to improve on steroids; use
of steroids may reduce the chance of relapse.
Platelet transfusion is contraindicated as it can
worsen the disease

PROGNOSIS
HUS

Mortality rate is 5–15%. The outlook is worse for
older children and adults. More than 80% of
children recover with supportive care.

TTP

Untreated, has a mortality nearing 100%. Early
diagnosis and treating with plasma exchange
have changed this grim prognosis to a lot more
promising 90% survival rate. 30% will relapse
over a 10-year period.

QUESTION SPOTTING

A 'classic' presentation involves a diarrhoeal
prodrome, followed by:

Renal failure

Microangiopathic haemolytic anaemia

Thrombocytopenia

Normal clotting

In such a case, the major differential diagnosis is
TTP, which more commonly has neurological
manifestations, and less commonly produces
renal failure. The diseases are thought to be two
ends of a spectrum of microthrombotic disease,
however.

HUS may occur without an obvious prodrome,
and may have an insidious onset.

RENAL TRANSPLANT FAILURE

Renal transplants may fail for the same reasons as native kidneys, or for reasons specific to transplanted kidneys. Causes include:

PRERENAL
Sepsis
Dehydration
Haemorrhage
Myocardial failure

INTRINSIC RENAL FAILURE
Arterial thrombosis
Venous thrombosis
Acute tubular necrosis
Infection
Rejection (hyperacute, acute or chronic)
Ciclosporin A toxicity
Relapse of original renal disease, especially focal segmental glomerulosclerosis, but also membranous, IgA, mesangiocapillary and anti-GBM disease
Renal artery stenosis
New glomerulonephritis, including CMV infection

POSTRENAL
Bladder outflow obstruction
Ureteric obstruction (e.g. from a lymphocoele, ureteric stenosis, clot in ureter)

CLINICAL FEATURES
Arterial thrombosis
Abrupt loss of graft function (anuria, biochemical derangement)
Often no other signs, but may be hypertensive if subtotal thrombosis
Occurs in first few days after transplant

Venous thrombosis
Occurs days to weeks after transplant
Loss of function (oliguria/anuria)
Painful, swollen graft
May have swollen ipsilateral leg
Graft occasionally ruptures, leading to haemorrhagic shock

Ureteric obstruction
Reduced graft function (oliguria/anuria)
Graft may slowly increase in size
Ipsilateral leg may swell (iliac vein compression)

Ciclosporin A toxicity
Reduced graft function
Improves when drug dose is reduced
Usually hypertensive (but this is often the case when ciclosporin A dose is in the therapeutic range)

Hyperacute rejection
Occurs within minutes of graft being perfused
Graft fails to work at all

Acute rejection
Most often occurs in first 3–6 months after transplant
Fever
Painful, swollen graft
Reduced function (oliguria/anuria)
Features may be less dramatic when taking ciclosporin

Chronic rejection
Usually asymptomatic; may present with symptoms of uraemia. There is usually no pain, swelling or fever

Infection
Painful, swollen graft
Fever, rigors
Dysuria and frequency
Reduced graft function

INVESTIGATIONS
FBC
Hb ↓ in chronic failure
WCC ↑ in sepsis, acute rejection. This response may be attenuated by azathioprine
Platelets usually normal

U + Es
Na may be ↓ in acute failure
K may be ↑
Urea and creatinine are ↑ in any form of transplant failure. It is important to know the baseline level however

LFTs

Usually normal, but may be mildly ↑ (from azathioprine)

Calcium low or normal

ESR, CRP are raised in sepsis, acute rejection and recurrent vasculitis

Coagulation screen usually normal

PO_4 raised in transplant failure, especially if chronic

Urinalysis

Blood and protein in arterial or venous thrombosis, infection, acute rejection or some forms of vasculitis

Protein only in chronic rejection or some forms of recurrent renal disease. Mild proteinuria also occurs in ciclosporin A toxicity

Early acute rejection may show decreased urinary Na, increased urinary creatinine, proteinuria and so-called 'activated cells' in the urine sediment

DIAGNOSIS

Acute rejection is characterized by rising creatinine, fever and graft pain. Chronic rejection presents with gradual rise in creatinine and proteinuria. The following tests help identify the underlying cause:

Renal US with Doppler flow; this will diagnose obstruction to urine outflow, arterial and venous thrombosis and lymphocoele

MSU for infection

Ciclosporin A levels for potential toxicity

Renal biopsy: can show acute or chronic rejection, or recurrent glomerulonephritis/other renal disease. Acute rejection produces interstitial oedema, with a lymphocytic infiltrate and evidence of vascular injury

DIFFERENTIAL DIAGNOSIS

For a slow rise in urea or creatinine:

Recurrence of original renal disease
Ciclosporin A toxicity
Chronic rejection

Also consider other nephrotoxic drugs, e.g. antibiotics, diuretics, ACE inhibitors

Fever, pain, swelling and rising creatinine:

Acute rejection
Sepsis, including UTI

Prerenal causes

Venous thrombosis

TREATMENT

Acute rejection: high-dose methylprednisolone and in resistant cases antithymocyte globulin or monoclonal OKT3 antibody can be used

Prerenal failure; ensure good fluid loading and treat the cause

Recurrence of original renal disease: may need increased immunosuppression

Ciclosporin A toxicity: reduce dose

UTI: treat with antibiotics

Chronic rejection: no useful therapy at present

QUESTION SPOTTING

You will usually be told that a transplant is present; if not, the iliac fossa mass is the clue

Transplant failure is evidenced by a rising creatinine, which may be accompanied by oliguria or anuria

Remember that transplant failure may not be due to rejection

Remember that other opportunistic infections affect immunosuppressed transplant patients (e.g. TB, PCP, *Candida*, CMV)

AMYLOIDOSIS

Deposition of fibrillar amyloid protein in target organs, which can include almost any organ in the body. Several types of amyloid are recognized, including AL (derived from Ig light chains), AA (derived from amyloid protein A, an acute-phase reactant), and ATTR, derived from a mutant transthyretin protein.

CAUSES OF AMYLOIDOSIS
AL amyloid
Myeloma
Waldenström's macroglobulinaemia
Non-Hodgkin's lymphoma
Other monoclonal gammopathies

AA amyloid
Any long-standing infection or inflammation, including:
Tuberculosis
Bronchiectasis
Osteomyelitis
Infected ulcers or burns
Whipple's disease
Leprosy
Rheumatoid arthritis
Behçet's disease
Adult Still's disease
Ankylosing spondylitis
Reiter's disease
Crohn's disease (rare in UC)
Familial Mediterranean fever
Renal cell carcinoma
Hodgkin's disease
Renal dialysis

CLINICAL FEATURES (AL AMYLOID)
Skin
Purpura, easy bruising. Amyloid plaques

Cardiac
Restrictive cardiomyopathy – tiredness, SOB, nausea. Right-sided signs more prominent
Conduction problems/heart block

Renal
Nephrotic syndrome, chronic renal failure: oedema, pruritus, anaemia
Usually normotensive
Kidneys enlarged and may be palpable

Hepatic/GI
Hepatomegaly
Diarrhoea, constipation, early satiety, dysphagia
Malabsorption

Lung
Usually asymptomatic, but lung function changes seen

Neurological
Sensory neuropathy: distal > proximal. Motor neuropathy is rare, as is CNS involvement
Prominent autonomic features, especially postural hypotension

Other
Hyposplenism in 24%. Splenomegaly in 5%
Lymphadenopathy is usually absent
Macroglossia (20%)
Nail dystrophy
Shoulder-pad sign, polyarthropathy
Hypothyroidism (20%). Hypoadrenalism

Differences for AA amyloid
Cardiac involvement is rare
No macroglossia
Splenomegaly is more common
Gut involvement is usually asymptomatic

Differences with ATTR amyloid
Neurological dysfunction common
No macroglossia
Renal disease is mild
Cardiomyopathy less prominent, but conduction system problems are common

INVESTIGATIONS
FBC
Hb ↓ in renal failure
WCC normal
Platelets normal

U + Es
Na ↓ in hypoadrenalism
Urea, creatinine ↑ (renal impairment)

LFTs
Bilirubin usually normal
ALT usually normal
ALP ↓
Albumin ↓

ESR, CRP reflect underlying disease

Clotting occasionally deranged (due to binding of clotting factors to amyloid or severe liver disease)

Immunoglobulins may show monoclonal band in AL amyloid

TFTs may show low T_4, raised TSH (if thyroid involved)

Blood film may show Howell–Jolly bodies (hyposplenism)

Urine shows proteinuria. May show Bence–Jones proteins (AL)

ECG: may show poor R-wave progression, conduction delays/block

Echo: may show diastolic ventricular impairment (restrictive), bright echo pattern to myocardium

PFTs show reduced Kco

Chest X-ray may show pleural effusions and reticulonodular shadowing

DIAGNOSIS

Rectal, fat or target organ biopsy. All have 70–80% sensitivity. Amyloid stains red with Congo red, and shows apple-green birefringence under polarized light

Diagnosis of AL amyloid

Monoclonal Ig or Bence–Jones protein in 90%
Monoclonal plasma cells on bone marrow biopsy

Diagnosis of ATTR amyloid

Isoelectric focusing of plasma to identify mutant transthyretin protein

TREATMENT

Avoid calcium channel blockers and digoxin if cardiac involvement (may worsen condition)

Restrictive cardiomyopathy may require warfarin

Colchicine is effective in FMF amyloid

Chemotherapy can prolong life in AL amyloid, but is poorly tolerated if cardiac involvement is present

Liver transplant is the treatment of choice for ATTR amyloid

PROGNOSIS

1–2 years for AL amyloid. Median survival 6 months if cardiac involvement

Up to 15-year survival from diagnosis in ATTR amyloid

Prognosis is dependent on the underlying disease in AA amyloid

QUESTION SPOTTING

The combination of hepatomegaly with or without splenomegaly plus renal impairment is a strong pointer to amyloidosis. Mention of a large tongue should also make one consider the diagnosis, as should autonomic neuropathy.

Proteinuria and renal impairment in a patient with an underlying inflammatory disorder should prompt consideration of amyloid.

Renal cell adenocarcinoma (hypernephroma) is usually derived from proximal tubular epithelial cells. Bilateral tumours occur in 1%. 25% present with metastases, usually to bone, lung or liver.

SYMPTOMS

Haematuria (65%)
Loin pain (20–40%)
Weight loss
Anorexia
Fevers/sweats (20%)
Left-sided scrotal swelling (2% of males due to obstruction of testicular vein)

SIGNS

Fever
Mass in flank (6–50%)
Hypertension (12%)
Left-sided varicocoele

INVESTIGATIONS

FBC

Hb ↑ in 4% (erythropoietin production). ↓ in 35% (reduced erythropoietin)
WCC usually normal
Platelets usually normal; ↑ in 11%

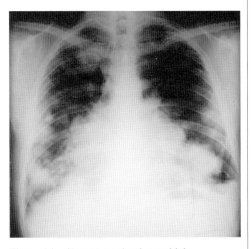

Figure 4.1 Chest X-ray showing multiple 'cannonball' metastases from renal cell carcinoma.

U + Es

Usually normal

LFTs

May be ↑ if liver metastases. ALP may be ↑ if bony metastases or if reactive hepatitis present. Bilirubin usually normal

Calcium may be ↑
ESR often ↑ (40%)
Urine often shows haematuria. Does not usually contain malignant cells

Chest X-ray may show 'cannonball' metastases (Fig. 4.1)

Contrast-enhanced CT

This has largely replaced ultrasound and excretory urography in staging and differentiating benign from malignant renal tumours
MRI is helpful in assessing vena caval involvement

DIAGNOSIS

A large proportion of patients are diagnosed incidentally. A combination of flank pain, haematuria and flank mass occurs in 10% of patients and indicates advanced disease. Diagnosis is on cross-sectional imaging; biopsy is not usually required.

DIFFERENTIAL DIAGNOSIS

Other causes of haematuria
Other causes of a PUO
Rarer mesenchymal renal tumours
Xanthogranulomatous pyelonephritis
Renal cysts

COMPLICATIONS

Amyloidosis (3–5%)
Reactive hepatitis (4%) with hepatomegaly

TREATMENT

The treatment options of renal cell carcinoma are surgery, radiation, chemotherapy, hormonal therapy, immunotherapy or a combination of these. Metastatic tumours occasionally disappear after the primary is excised.

Chemo-, hormonal and immunotherapy options have been limited in positively influencing the outlook of the disease.

Radical nephrectomy for limited-stage disease.

PROGNOSIS

50% 10-year survival for tumours confined to one kidney

5% 10-year survival for metastatic disease

QUESTION SPOTTING

May present as a non-specific illness involving weight loss, fever, raised ESR; there is usually another clue to the diagnosis, e.g. haematuria or raised Hb ± raised calcium.

You are unlikely to be told about a mass in the flank!

RENAL TUBULAR ACIDOSIS (RTA)

Failure of the kidney to create acid urine by either distal tubular failure to exchange Na^+ for H^+ leading to excess bicarbonate in the filtrate or proximal tubule failure to excrete hydrogen ions. An important cause of normal anion gap acidosis.

There are four types:

TYPE I – DISTAL RTA

Distal RTA is the most common type. The disease presents at any age.

CAUSES

Congenital

Autosomal-dominant, recessive and sex-linked have all been documented

Acquired

Autoimmune ($\uparrow$ immunoglobulin), e.g. Sjögren's syndrome, chronic active hepatitis, cryoglobulinaemia

Nephrocalcinosis, e.g. hyperparathyroidism, excess vitamin D, medullary sponge kidney

Drugs, e.g. amphotericin, lithium, analgesics

Renal disease, e.g. transplanted kidney, obstructive uropathy, chronic pyelonephritis, sickle-cell disease

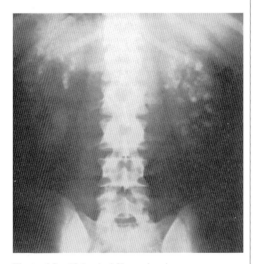

Figure 4.2 Abdominal X-ray showing nephrocalcinosis in a patient with renal tubular acidosis. (Reproduced with permission from Souhami, Moxham (2002) *Textbook of Medicine*, 4th edn. Churchill Livingstone.)

SYMPTOMS

Anorexia

Fatigue

Renal colic from stones

Polyuria and polydipsia

Bone pain and weakness (due to osteomalacia caused by calcium loss in the urine and calcium from bone buffering excess H^+)

Constipation

Recurrent urinary tract infections secondary to renal stones

Renal failure

INVESTIGATIONS

FBC

Normal

U + Es

Na normal

K $\downarrow$

Urea and creatinine normal

Cl $\uparrow$

pH $\downarrow$

$HCO^{3-} < 21$ mmol/L

Urinalysis

Urinary pH never < 5.5

Urine ammonia $\downarrow$

Urine calcium $\uparrow$ and urine citrate $\downarrow$, which leads to the formation of renal stones in the presence of an alkaline urine

TREATMENT

Treatment of underlying condition if possible

Sodium bicarbonate supplements

Potassium supplements

Citrate supplements

Thiazide diuretics may reduce plasma volume and thus increase proximal bicarbonate reabsorption

Vitamin D if osteomalacia

TYPE II – PROXIMAL RTA
CAUSES
Congenital

Hereditary – autosomal-dominant

Cystinosis

Wilson's disease

Galactosaemia

Von Gierke's disease
Lowe's syndrome
Hereditary fructose intolerance

Acquired

Autoimmune with ↑ immunoglobulins, e.g.
  Sjögren's syndrome
Drugs, e.g. acetazolamide, lead, tetracyclines
Dysproteinaemic states, e.g. myeloma
Others, e.g. hyperparathyroidism, amyloid,
  nephrotic syndrome

Type II RTA is less common than type I. It most
  commonly occurs as part of a generalized
  proximal tubular defect that results in
  glycosuria, aminoaciduria, phosphaturia and
  renal tubular acidosis – the Fanconi syndrome
The defect is a failure to secrete H^+ from the
  proximal tubule. This means that too much
  bicarbonate is left in the filtrate for the distal
  tubule to reabsorb. As the plasma bicarbonate
  falls, so the filtered bicarbonate load falls until
  the distal tubule is able to reabsorb all the
  bicarbonate and homeostasis is restored (at a
  plasma bicarbonate level of approximately 12–
  15 mmol/L). Because of the failure of the $Na^+/$
  H^+ pump in the proximal tubule, there is Na^+
  wasting, causing polyuria and hypotension. This
  stimulates aldosterone secretion and the resulting
  Na^+/K^+ exchange causes hypokalaemia
Renal calculi are not a feature. Rickets/osteomalacia
  are seen, but only as a failure of vitamin D
  metabolism, which is often part of the Fanconi
  syndrome and not due to calcium buffering

SYMPTOMS

Polyuria and polydipsia
Muscle weakness – rare. Caused by
  hypokalaemic myopathy
Bone pain from osteomalacia – rare

INVESTIGATIONS
FBC

Normal

U + Es

Na normal
K ↓
Urea and creatinine normal

Cl ↑
pH normal or ↓
Bicarbonate ↓
Ca may be ↓

Urinalysis

Urinary calcium normal
Glucose +
Protein +
Aminoaciduria +
pH normal

TREATMENT

Treatment of underlying condition
  if possible.
Sodium bicarbonate supplements – huge
  doses may be required to overcome
  the 'leak'
Potassium citrate as required

TYPE III RTA

A combination of type I and type II and
incredibly rare, so will not be covered here

TYPE IV – HYPORENINAEMIC HYPOALDOSTERONISM

Probably the commonest of the renal tubular
acidoses. Patients are acidotic and have
hyperkalaemia

CAUSES

Chronic tubulointerstitial disease, e.g. reflux
  nephropathy
Diabetes mellitus leading to a failure of
  renin production
Primary adrenal disease, e.g. Addison's disease
Hereditary inborn errors of steroid synthesis –
  rare

The defect is caused by either hypoaldosteronism
or renal resistance to the effects of aldosterone.
This reduces the capacity of the distal nephron to
secrete H^+. Hyperkalaemia is directly due to loss
of aldosterone action. This causes suppression of
renal production of NH_4^+ which exacerbates
the acidosis. The condition is more commonly

seen in patients on prostaglandin inhibitors such as NSAIDs as renin production is partly dependent on prostaglandin synthesis.

SYMPTOMS
Polyuria and polydipsia
Loin pain if reflux nephropathy

INVESTIGATIONS
FBC
Normal

U + Es
Na normal ($\downarrow$ if Addison's)
K $\uparrow$
Urea and creatinine normal
pH $\downarrow$
Bicarb $\downarrow$
Ca normal

TREATMENT
If significant acidosis or hyperkalaemia, treat with fludrocortisone

QUESTION SPOTTING
May present with non-specific symptoms of polyuria and polydipsia, along with renal stones or osteomalacia. These features should alert you to the possibility of renal tubular acidosis

This disorder is ideal for data interpretation-type questions. If given enough information in the question, always work out the anion gap:

Anion gap = $(Na + K) - (Cl + HCO_3)$.

Normal range = 10–18 mmol/L

If the anion gap is high in the presence of an acidosis, this means that there is an increased amount of an unmeasured anion, such as lactic acid or exogenous acid

If the anion gap is normal in the presence of an acidosis, this means that HCl is being retained or HCO_3 is being lost

There are a number of causes for each type:

Normal anion gap acidosis
GI bicarbonate loss by ileostomy or by diarrhoea, e.g. cholera diarrhoea
Renal tubular acidosis types I, II, IV
Cystectomy with implantation of ureters
Acetazolamide therapy
Pancreatic loss of HCO_3 via a pancreatic fistula
Ammonium chloride ingestion
Increased catabolism of lysine or arginine

High anion gap acidosis
Ketoacidosis
Insulin deficiency
Excess alcohol ingestion
Starvation

Lactic acidosis
Type A – poor tissue perfusion, often with hypoxia occurs in shock (septic, hypovolaemic or cardiogenic), postseizure, severe hypoxia and carbon monoxide poisoning
Type B – reduced hepatic metabolism of lactic acid that may occur in diabetic ketoacidosis, metformin excess, haematological malignancies, hepatic failure and alcohol excess
Exogenous acids
Salicylate overdose
Ethylene glycol or methanol ingestion

BARTTER'S SYNDROME AND RELATED DISORDERS

Bartter's syndrome is caused by a defect in one of three ion channels in the thick ascending loop of Henle; the Na/K/2Cl channel (site of action of loop diuretics) is the prototypical mutant site. A closely related disorder, Gitelman's syndrome, is caused by mutations in the thiazide-sensitive Na/Cl transporter in the distal convoluted tubule. Both these conditions may be mimicked by diuretic abuse or by rare autoimmune disorders affecting the afore-mentioned transporters. Bartter's and Gitelman's syndromes are autosomal-recessive conditions.

SYMPTOMS
Polyhydramnios in utero (Bartter's only)
Weakness
Muscle cramps
Polyuria

SIGNS
BP is usually normal with no postural drop

INVESTIGATIONS
FBC
Usually normal

U + Es
Na usually normal
K invariably ↓
Urea and creatinine usually normal

LFTs
Usually normal
ESR usually normal unless other autoimmune disorders
Bicarbonate usually ↑ (metabolic alkalosis)
Plasma renin ↑
Plasma aldosterone ↑

Urine
Urinary Na ↑
Urinary K ↑
Urinary Cl ↑
Urinary protein < 300 mg/24 hours
Urine microscopy normal

DIAGNOSIS
1. Exclude diuretic abuse by repeated urine sampling for diuretics

2. Bartter's syndrome typically shows hypercalciuria plus raised urinary prostaglandins. It is usually evident at birth or in early childhood
3. Gitelman's syndrome typically shows hypocalciuria, hypomagnesaemia plus raised urinary prostaglandins. It may not present until adulthood
4. Immune-related K^+-losing interstitial nephritis; suspect if other autoimmune phenomena present and urinary prostaglandins normal

Renal biopsy (not often needed):
Hyperplasia of the juxtaglomerular apparatus (JGA) is evident with Bartter's and Gitelman's syndromes

COMPLICATIONS
Nephrocalcinosis due to chronic hypercalciuria

TREATMENT
Bartter's and Gitelman's: NSAIDs, K^+ supplements.

PROGNOSIS
In many cases good, and individuals usually lead normal lives

QUESTION SPOTTING
Good data interpretation cases. For all the above diagnoses, the clue is a hypokalaemic alkalosis with a normal blood pressure. A normal blood pressure argues against Cushing's or Conn's, and there is usually no history of vomiting, diarrhoea, fistulae or other drug ingestion
The urine values show Na and K wasting with normal creatinine, pointing to a renal tubular problem.
Bartter's: tend to be young (< 10 years), with high urinary calcium
Gitelman's: tend to be adults, with low urinary calcium
Diuretic abuse: suspect if a member of nursing staff, or job is allied to medicine, or a relative on diuretics
Autoimmune: suspect if other features of autoimmune disease (e.g. rash, arthropathy)

GOODPASTURE'S SYNDROME

An autoimmune disease which is characterized by deposition of antibodies against the glomerular basement membrane (anti-GBM antibodies) in various tissues, typically the lungs and kidneys. Due to different specificities of these antibodies, the disease may present in a variety of ways, and may not always present with the most typical features of haemoptysis and glomerulonephritis.

The incidence is bimodal with peaks at age 30 (more men) and 60 (more women). The disease more typically presents in spring and this may be related to associated infection. Inhalation of hydrocarbons is also thought to trigger the disease.

SYMPTOMS
Cough
Shortness of breath
Pulmonary haemorrhage – variable and more common in smokers
Haematuria (often microscopic)

SIGNS
Rare
Hypertension is not usually a feature
Note that systemic features of fever, rash, myalgia, malaise, headaches, joint pains and weight loss are not common but may occur. Chest pain and pleurisy are rare; compare with pulmonary embolism.

INVESTIGATIONS
FBC
Hb ↓ (MCV ↓ with prolonged haemoptysis due to iron deficiency)
WCC normal or ↑
Platelets normal or ↑

U + Es
Na normal
K normal or ↑ (with renal failure)
Urea ↑ with renal impairment
Creatinine ↑ with renal impairment

LFTs
Albumin ↓
ANCA may be positive in 30%. Usually pANCA
ANA-negative

Urinalysis
Dysmorphic red cells with red cell casts very common
Proteinuria is also common, though not usually in the nephrotic range

CXR
Patchy shadows of intra-alveolar blood, typically spreading out from the hilum. May be single or multiple. Shadows resolve within 2 weeks if no further bleeding

PFTs
Increased CO transfer typical of pulmonary haemorrhage
A restrictive defect may occur with progressive disease

DIAGNOSIS
Alveolar haemorrhage with renal failure and positive anti-GBM antibodies (usually IgG but may be IgA or IgM) is sufficient to make the diagnosis. False-negative rate of 5–10%
Renal biopsy:
Linear immunofluorescence with rapidly progressive glomerulonephritis (RPGN) or crescentic glomerulonephritis. Linear staining occurs in Goodpasture's, SLE and diabetes. Anti-GBM antibodies may be demonstrated bound to renal tissue, even if absent from plasma

DIFFERENTIAL DIAGNOSIS
Renal/pulmonary syndromes may be seen in:

SLE
Wegener's granulomatosis
Systemic sclerosis
Rheumatoid arthritis
Other systemic vasculitis: PAN, Churg–Strauss, Behçet's, giant cell arteritis, cryoglobulinaemia
Infection: TB, *Legionella*
Others: TTP and HUS, malignancy with glomerulopathy

TREATMENT
Plasma exchange
Pulsed methylprednisolone and cyclophosphamide

These two therapies are the only truly effective therapies. Prednisolone is rarely effective in the acute phase but tends to be used in conjunction with cytotoxics such as cyclophosphamide or azathioprine to prevent rebound after the plasma exchange

Transplantation is now increasingly used. Goodpasture's may recur in the transplanted kidney, but this is usually a milder form (possibly due to time delay from initial onset of disease, and due to the immunosuppressive regimen)

PROGNOSIS

Generally poor despite treatment if advanced renal disease. Although anti-GBM antibody titres show poor correlation with prognosis, patients with high ANCA but low anti-GBM titres tend to do well, but show relapses which do not tend to occur in ANCA-negative patients.

QUESTION SPOTTING

The typical patient is a young white male smoker who presents with haemoptysis. Anti-GBM antibodies with renal biopsy should be diagnostic but look to exclude other conditions seen in the differential, like SLE.

You may be asked to interpret a renal biopsy in the setting of a patient with rapidly progressive glomerulonephritis. This occurs in Goodpasture's, SLE, Wegener's, cryoglobulinaemia, Henoch–Schönlein purpura, PAN, as well as the typical postinfectious and idiopathic types. Think of Goodpasture's if asked to interpret lung function tests showing a raised Kco.

RHEUMATOLOGY

5

SYSTEMIC LUPUS ERYTHEMATOSUS

SLE is a multisystem autoimmune disorder of unknown aetiology, characterized by widespread derangement of humoral and cell-mediated immunity. Failure of the apoptotic mechanism in inducing tolerance may play a role. Vasculitis, usually of small vessels, underlies many of the organ derangements. A minority of sufferers have mutations of complement components, especially C_1, C_2 and C_4. It is much commoner in women (9:1), affecting mostly younger women (often of child-bearing age). There is an association with HLA B8/DR3 and HLA DR2.

FEATURES
(% = SYMPTOMS AT ONSET
OF DISEASE)
Musculoskeletal
Arthralgia, arthritis (60%). Usually non-erosive, migratory. Effusions are uncommon. Jaccoud's arthropathy may develop
Myalgia
Myositis (10%)

Skin (60%)
Raynaud's phenomenon (25%)
Livedo reticularis
Photosensitive rashes, e.g. butterfly rash
Urticaria
Purpura
Discoid lesions (may occur alone)
Alopecia

Renal (25%)
Glomerulonephritis
Vasculopathy with hypertension

Neurological (20%)
Psychosis
Fits
Headaches
Memory impairment
Cranial nerve palsies
Aseptic meningitis
Peripheral neuropathy

Cardiac
Endocarditis (Libman–Sacks)
Pericarditis
Myocarditis

Lung (5%)
Pleuritic pain; effusions are uncommon
Pneumonitis (acute or chronic)

GI (uncommon)
Pancreatitis
Peritonitis
Mesenteric vasculitis

Other
Hepatomegaly, splenomegaly
Lymphadenopathy (non-tender) (15%)
Arterial and venous thrombosis (due to antiphospholipid syndrome)
Weight loss

INVESTIGATIONS
FBC
Hb sometimes $\downarrow$ (haemolysis, chronic disease)
MCV normal ($\uparrow$ in haemolysis)
WCC often $\downarrow$ (especially lymphocytes)
Platelets sometimes $\downarrow$
Reticulocytes $\uparrow$ in haemolysis

U + Es
Urea and creatinine $\uparrow$ in renal disease

LFTs
Bilirubin $\uparrow$ in haemolysis
ALT, ALP $\uparrow$ in active disease, especially after administration of salicylates
Haptoglobins absent in haemolysis
INR normal
APTT prolonged in antiphospholipid syndrome
ESR $\uparrow$
CRP usually normal; $\uparrow$ in serositis or concomitant disease, e.g. infection
CK $\uparrow$ in myositis
Igs $\uparrow$
Immune complexes $\uparrow$
C_3 $\downarrow$
C_4 $\downarrow$
Total complement activity $\downarrow$

Antibodies
ANA positive in 95%
dsDNA positive in 60%; high specificity for SLE
anti-Ro positive in 20–60%. Also positive in Sjögren's syndrome
anti-La positive in 15–40%. Also positive in Sjögren's syndrome
anti-Sm positive in 10–30%. High specificity for SLE
anti-RNP is a marker for mixed connective tissue disease

Rheumatoid factor positive in 25–50%

VDRL often false-positive (antiphospholipid syndrome)

Urine may show proteinuria, haematuria

CSF may show elevated protein levels and white cells in cerebral lupus

DIAGNOSIS

Four from the following must be present at some stage in the illness:

Malar (butterfly) rash

Discoid rash

Photosensitivity

Oral ulcers

Arthritis

Serositis (pleuritic, pericarditis)

Renal disease (> 500 mg proteinuria/day, cellular casts)

Neurological disorder

Haematological disorder (low Hb, WCC or platelets)

Positive ANA

Immunological disorder (LE cells, anti-dsDNA, anti-Sm or false-positive VDRL)

DIFFERENTIAL DIAGNOSIS
Autoimmune disease
Rheumatoid arthritis

Adult Still's disease

Mixed connective tissue disease

Systemic sclerosis

Polymyositis

Behçet's disease

Primary vasculitides

Primary antiphospholipid syndrome

Infections
Viral arthritis

Whipple's disease

SBE

Lyme disease

Syphilis

TB

Other
AIP

TTP/HUS

PNH

Drug reactions

Lymphoma

Sarcoidosis

Atrial myxoma

Inflammatory bowel disease

Familial Mediterranean fever

TREATMENT
Mild (skin and joints only)
NSAIDs

Hydroxychloroquine

Topical steroids

Sunblock

Moderate
Oral steroids

Azathioprine as a steroid-sparing agent

Severe (progressive renal disease, neurological disease)
Cyclophosphamide, azathioprine

Steroids

COMPLICATIONS
Infections

End-stage renal failure

Atherosclerosis

Pulmonary embolus/haemorrhage

Osteonecrosis

Permanent neurological damage

Shrinking-lung syndrome

PROGNOSIS
> 90% 5-year survival. Early deaths are usually due to renal disease and lupus itself

70% alive at 20 years. Cardiovascular disease is now a major cause of late death in SLE

QUESTION SPOTTING
SLE is the multisystem disorder par excellence. Clues to the diagnosis are:

Young female patient

Low WCC ± low platelets

Renal disease

Rashes

High ESR with relatively normal CRP

Consider SLE whenever multiple organ systems are involved in a young woman and there is no immediately obvious cause or she has unexplained spontaneous abortions or neuropsychiatric illness

Unknown mechanism, but autoimmunity is the most likely. The trigger is thought to be T-helper cell activation leading to production of proinflammatory mediators such as IL-1 and TNF-α. This in turn leads to persistent cellular activation, autoimmunity and inflammation. Tissue damage is caused by immune complex deposition and direct cell-mediated immunity. Inflammation of synovium causes thickening and effusions with joint and bone destruction.

1% of the population worldwide have rheumatoid arthritis. Male-to-female ratio 1:3. Peak incidence in 4th–5th decade, but can occur at any age. There is a family history in 5–10% of patients

Classical disease gives early-morning stiffness and pain in a few peripheral joints initially, but disease can be highly variable

PATTERN OF DISEASE
Insidious (70%)
Acute (15%)
Systemic (10%)
Palindromic (5%)

CLINICAL FEATURES
Joints
Swelling
Pain

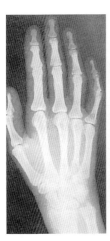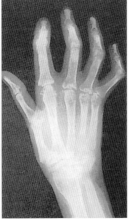

Figure 5.1   X-ray showing rheumatoid changes in hands. (Reproduced with permission from Souhami, Moxham (2002) *Textbook of Medicine*, 4th edn. Churchill Livingstone.)

Stiffness (especially if joint inactive)
Reduced joint motion
Subluxation
Joint instability
Deformity
Contractures
Classical changes in the hands and feet include:
  ulnar deviation of fingers, swan-neck
  deformities, boutonnière deformity,
  Z deformity of thumbs, clawing of toes
Tendinitis
Bursitis

Extra-articular
Systemic
Fever
Weight loss
Fatigue
Increased infection risk

Musculoskeletal
Muscle wasting

Haematological
Anaemia
Splenomegaly
Lymphadenopathy (50%)

Skin
Nodules
Fistulae
Pyoderma gangrenosum
Ulcers

Neurological
Cervical cord compression secondary to
  atlantoaxial subluxation
Mononeuritis multiplex
Compression neuropathy, especially carpal
  tunnel syndrome
Peripheral neuropathy (sensorimotor)
Stroke

Ocular
Episcleritis
Scleritis
Scleromalacia
Keratoconjunctivitis sicca (10%)

Cardiovascular – rare except for pericarditis
Pericarditis causing effusions and sometimes
  pericardial constriction
Myocarditis

Endocarditis
Conduction abnormalities
Coronary vasculitis
Aortitis, arteritis

Pulmonary
Nodules – may cavitate
Effusions – very common: exudates with ↑ white
cells, ↑ LDH, ↓ glucose, ↑ Rheumatoid factor,
↓ complement
Fibrosis
Bronchiolitis obliterans
Haemorrhage
Caplan's syndrome

Other
Amyloidosis

INVESTIGATIONS
FBC
Hb ↓ (MCV normal, ↑ or ↓; sulfasalazine causes
↑ MCV)
WBC ↑ – if leukopenia and thrombocytopenia,
think of Felty's syndrome
Eosinophilia may occur
Platelets ↑
Hb may be ↓ due to:

1. Iron-deficiency anaemia from NSAIDs
2. Folate deficiency (↑ cell turnover)
3. B_{12} deficiency due to pernicious anaemia
4. Chronic disease
5. Haemolytic anaemia
6. Aplastic anaemia secondary to drug therapy

U + Es
Na normal
K normal
Urea and creatinine ↑ if renal involvement or
drug toxicity (NSAIDs, penicillamine, gold,
ciclosporin A)

LFTs
May be raised with sulfasalazine or methotrexate

ESR ↑ may stay high, even when disease not
active
CRP ↑
Complement C_3 and C_4 ↓
Rheumatoid factor often positive (75%)
ANA may be positive (30%)
Cryoglobulins may be present

X-rays (Fig. 5.1)
Periarticular osteoporosis
Loss of joint space
Erosions
Subluxation and ankylosis
Joint aspiration
Yellow, cloudy, 2000–10 000 cells/mm^3;
predominantly neutrophils

DIAGNOSIS
At least four of the following criteria should
be met for at least 6 weeks:

Morning stiffness > 1 hour
Arthritis of three or more joint areas
At least one of wrist, MCP or PIP involved
Symmetrical joint involvement
Presence of rheumatoid nodules
Positive rheumatoid factor
Erosive changes or periarticular osteoporosis on
hand X-rays

DIFFERENTIAL DIAGNOSIS
Infective arthritis
Rheumatic fever
SLE
Adult Still's disease
Sero-negative arthritis such as psoriatic arthritis,
ankylosing spondylitis, etc.
Polymyalgia rheumatica
Osteoarthritis

COMPLICATIONS
Amyloid
Lymphoma
Other malignancy
Cardiovascular disease
Infections

TREATMENT
Symptom relief
Suppression of disease process
Bedrest and physiotherapy
Rest splints
Simple analgesics, e.g. paracetamol, codeine,
tramadol
Non-steroidal anti-inflammatory drugs (NSAIDs)

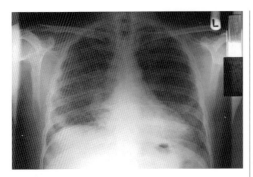

Figure 5.2 Fibrosing alveolitis secondary to rheumatoid arthritis. This chest X-ray shows small lung volume for maximal inspiration. There is widespread reticular nodular shadowing in the mid and lower zones with a peripheral distribution. These appearances are typical for any fibrosing alveolitis, including cryptogenic, drug-induced and that secondary to connective tissue diseases.

Disease-modifying drugs – used in combination from an early stage (e.g. methotrexate + sulfasalazine). Failure to obtain remission should prompt a change in therapy

Methotrexate

Sulfasalazine

Leflunomide

Hydroxychloroquine

Penicillamine

Gold

Dapsone (note: slow acetylators prone to haemolytic anaemia)

Systemic steroids – in severe exacerbation or severe extra-articular manifestations, e.g. scleritis.

Intra-articular steroids – used as an adjunct to DMARD therapy

Immunomodulation with azathioprine, cyclophosphamide, cyclosporin A, but only in severe disease where other therapies failed.

TNF blockers (infliximab, etanercept) – can be used in patients with highly active disease (>5 joints active) who have failed to respond to at least two other DMARDs including methotrexate.

Surgery for tendon repairs, synovectomy, soft tissue decompression, arthroplasty, joint replacement, arthrodesis.

Modification of cardiovascular risk factors (BP reduction, cholesterol reduction, DM, smoking)

PROGNOSIS

Variable. Worse if: high RF titre, insidious onset, continuous active disease without remission, nodules, erosions, extra-articular disease.

QUESTION SPOTTING

Ideal for these questions. Multiple extra-articular manifestations make it easy to confuse with SLE, rheumatic fever. Look for classical pattern of small joint changes, but also consider as a cause of unexplained anaemia with multisystem symptoms.

SYSTEMIC SCLEROSIS

An autoimmune disease of unknown aetiology which results in vascular damage and fibrosis in a number of organ systems. Various forms are recognized, including CREST syndrome, systemic sclerosis and morphea. All forms are more common in women (3:1) and peak age of onset is 30–50. CREST (limited cutaneous scleroderma) consists of:

Calcinosis
Raynaud's phenomenon
Oesophageal dysmotility
Sclerodactyly (usually limited to distal limbs)
Telangiectasia

CLINICAL FEATURES
Skin
Raynaud's phenomenon
Nailfold capillary abnormalities
Itching and oedema of skin
Thickened, waxy skin
Hyperpigmented or hypopigmented areas
Telangiectasia
Calcium deposits in skin

GI tract
Dysphagia
Dry mouth (sicca syndrome)
Restricted mouth opening
Nausea, anorexia (gastric paresis)
Malabsorption
Constipation ± diarrhoea (hypomotility)
Pseudo-obstruction

Musculoskeletal
Arthritis
Tendinitis
Myositis

Renal
Hypertensive renal crisis with renal failure
Lung
Fibrosing alveolitis
Pulmonary vessel disease, leading to pulmonary hypertension

Cardiac
Cor pulmonale
Myocardial fibrosis: arrhythmias, heart block

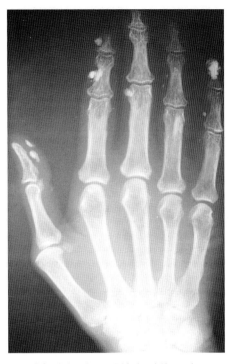

Figure 5.3 Scleroderma. This hand X-ray shows finger pulp calcinosis which is almost exclusive to scleroderma. There is also some evidence of tuft erosion to the terminal phalanx.

Other
Impotence
Trigeminal neuralgia
Carpal tunnel syndrome
Sensorimotor neuropathy
Autonomic neuropathy
Dry eyes
Gut and pulmonary involvement may progress over a period of years

INVESTIGATIONS
FBC
Hb may be ↓
MCV normal
WCC usually normal
Platelets usually normal

U + Es

Urea and creatinine ↑ in renal disease
Calcium normal

LFTs

Abnormal in PBC
Bilirubin ↑ in haemolysis

TFTs may show hypothyroidism
CK ↑ in myositis
ESR often ↓
Cold agglutinins may be present
Blood film may show fragmented RBCs in
hypertensive renal crises

Antibodies

ANA positive in 80–90%
Rheumatoid factor positive in 30–40%
Anticentromere is specific for limited cutaneous
disease; 60% sensitivity
Scl-70 is specific for diffuse systemic sclerosis;
40% sensitivity
Antimitochondrial antibody positive in 10–15%;
increased chance of developing PBC
A number of other antibodies (anti-RNP, anti-
PM-Scl) may also be detected

X-rays

Hand X-rays show resorption of phalangeal tufts,
calcinosis
Chest X-ray may show basal fibrosis

PFTs

Reduced FVC
Restrictive pattern
Low Kco
ECG may show evidence of heart block or
conduction delay. LVH if hypertensive renal
disease has been present for some time

DIAGNOSIS

Is on clinical grounds – sclerodactyly of some
degree should be present; presence of Scl-70 or
anticentromere antibody is useful confirmation.

ASSOCIATIONS

Primary biliary cirrhosis in 3% of patients with
limited cutaneous scleroderma
Thyroid disease (especially hypothyroidism) in
20–40%

DIFFERENTIAL DIAGNOSIS

Sarcoidosis
Myxoedema
Chronic graft-versus-host disease
Overlap connective tissue disease
Porphyrias
Acromegaly
Amyloidosis
Mycosis fungoides
Also consider other causes of microangiopathy
and other causes of pulmonary/renal
syndromes (e.g. Wegener's, Goodpasture's,
SLE)

TREATMENT

Raynaud's: hand care, hand warmers and calcium
channel blockers. Prostacyclin infusions,
bosentan, prazosin and losartan can also be
used for severe Raynaud's
Sclerodactyly: methotrexate has been used, as
has cyclophosphamide, but benefit is small
Dysmotility/gastro-oesophageal reflux: proton
pump inhibitors, prokinetic agents (e.g.
metoclopramide)
Bowel dysmotility: aperients, loperamide
Hypertensive crises/renal disease: ACE inhibitors
(even once dialysis-dependent)
Pulmonary fibrosis: cyclophosphamide, although
rigorous evidence of benefit is lacking
Pulmonary artery hypertension: iloprost or
bosentan. Both improve symptoms and
exercise capacity; iloprost and maybe
bosentan improve survival. Oxygen is also of
benefit
Surgery may help calcium deposits, and digital
sympathectomy may aid pregangrenous digits
Monitoring of patients for complications is
important (regular U + Es, echo, PFTs)

PROGNOSIS

5-year survival for diffuse disease is 40–75%.
Pulmonary hypertension and macrovascular
disease are now the leading causes of death;
the advent of ACE inhibitors and dialysis
has reduced the mortality from renal
crises.

QUESTION SPOTTING

Perhaps more likely to present as a complication in a patient known to have systemic sclerosis, e.g.

Renal hypertensive crisis
Lung fibrosis/right-sided heart failure
PBC
Malabsorption

WEGENER'S GRANULOMATOSIS

Vasculitis affecting small arteries in which granulomas are a feature (compare with polyarteritis nodosa).

The classical triad is:

Upper respiratory tract granulomas
Lower respiratory tract granulomas
Necrotizing focal glomerulonephritis

Peak incidence is in the fifth decade and more common in men. There is also a limited form with pure pulmonary disease and no damaging renal vasculitis.

CLINICAL FEATURES
General
Malaise
Arthralgia
Fever

Upper respiratory
Rhinitis
Epistaxis
Sinusitis
Serous otitis media
Nasal destruction leading to collapsed nasal bridge
Ulcers in palate, pharynx and sinuses

Lower respiratory
Note that there is often paucity of clinical signs despite florid radiographical changes

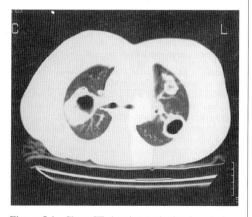

Figure 5.4 Chest CT showing cavitating lung lesion typical of Wegener's granulomatosis. (Reproduced with permission from Souhami, Moxham (2002) *Textbook of Medicine*, 4th edn. Churchill Livingstone.)

Cough
Haemoptysis
Chest pain
Dyspnoea
Bronchial obstruction causing atelectasis
Pleural involvement causing pleural effusions and pneumothorax

Renal
Glomerulonephritis – ranges from insidious to fulminant

Skin
Vasculitic rash – maculopapular or bullous. May become necrotic
Nailfold infarcts

Nervous system
Peripheral neuropathy, including mononeuritis multiplex
Intracerebral granulomas

Eyes
Episcleritis
Scleritis
Uveitis
Retinal vasculitis
Optic neuritis
Optic pseudotumour causing proptosis

Cardiovascular
Pericarditis
Coronary arteritis

INVESTIGATIONS
FBC
Hb ↓ (MCV normal)
WCC ↑ (neutrophilia – no eosinophilia)
Platelets ↑

U + Es
Na normal
K normal (unless acute renal failure)
Urea and creatinine ↑

LFTs
Albumin ↓
Otherwise normal

CRP ↑
ESR ↑

cANCA-positive (70–90%) (cytoplasmic ANCA against proteinase-3)

pANCA-positive (5–10%) (perinuclear ANCA against myeloperoxidase)

Rheumatoid factor occasionally positive

ANA occasionally positive

Anti-GBM antibodies negative

Anti-smooth-muscle antibodies occasionally positive

IgA ↑ or normal

IgG and IgM normal

Urinalysis

Blood + and red cell casts

Protein +

Chest X-ray

Typically multiple nodules (which may cavitate) throughout both lung fields (see lung cancer for differential). Nodules may reach several centimetres in size, but rapidly resolve or evolve

Evidence of pleural involvement with pleural effusions or rarely pneumothorax. Bronchial obstruction may be seen as localized atelectasis

DIAGNOSIS

Two of:

Red cell casts or microscopic haematuria

Granulomatous vasculitis on biopsy

Cavities, nodules or fixed opacifications on chest X-ray

Oral ulcers or nasal discharge (with or without blood)

An alternative diagnostic criterion is: typical involvement of upper airway, lung or kidney with positive biopsy or positive cANCA

Lung biopsy (preferred)

Typical features include giant cells at the centre of a necrotic nodule with generalized arterial and venous inflammation. Upper-airway histology is less specific

Renal biopsy (less useful)

Focal necrotizing glomerulonephritis with frequent crescent formation which is indistinguishable from Goodpasture's syndrome and Henoch–Schönlein syndrome

DIFFERENTIAL DIAGNOSIS

See polyarteritis nodosa. Also consider other causes of granuloma formation – sarcoidosis, tuberculosis

Pulmonary–renal syndromes

Goodpasture's disease

Henoch–Schönlein syndrome

Churg–Strauss

Rheumatoid arthritis

SLE

Microscopic polyarteritis

TREATMENT

Induction of remission: high-dose steroids with cyclophosphamide (IV if acute renal failure or life-threatening lung disease) for 3–6 months

Possible to switch to low-dose azathioprine or methotrexate with low-dose prednisolone for maintenance treatment (at least a year). May be needed long-term if relapses occur

Refractory cases may be helped by intravenous gamma-globulin or rituximab. Co-trimoxazole may reduce the rate of relapses. Limited (upper-airway) disease may be treated with steroids plus methotrexate

PROGNOSIS

80% 5-year survival if treated. 90% dead at 1 year untreated

QUESTION SPOTTING

An atypical history may be misleading and Wegener's may be difficult to distinguish from other forms of vasculitis. A raised WBC and platelets argue against SLE, and a positive cANCA (if given) will help the diagnosis. Churg–Strauss syndrome and microscopic polyarteritis may be positive for either pANCA or cANCA, but Churg–Strauss patients will be atopic, and microscopic polyarteritis does not involve the upper airway and the lung lesions do not cavitate.

The typical triad of upper and lower respiratory involvement and renal involvement should point to the diagnosis.

POLYARTERITIS NODOSA

A necrotizing vasculitis of unknown aetiology, affecting medium to small-sized arteries and leading to occlusion and aneurysm formation. It is associated with a number of other diseases, including hepatitis B and HIV infection. Granuloma formation is not a feature of the disease. The disease typically affects middle-aged/elderly men.

CLINICAL FEATURES

General
Fever
Tachycardia
Weight loss

Skin (50%)
Digital gangrene
Purpura
Livedo reticularis

Musculoskeletal
Myalgia (50%)
Arthralgia (50%)
Arthritis (20%)

Gastrointestinal (30%)
GI bleeding
Acute abdomen, e.g. RIF or RUQ pain
Mesenteric infarction

Cardiac
Hypertension (25%)
Pericarditis
Myocardial infarction
Chronic heart failure

Renal
Chronic or acute renal failure
Glomerulonephritis (uncommon)

Hepatic
Hepatitis (uncommon)
Hepatic necrosis (uncommon)

Neurological
Mononeuritis multiplex (50–70%)
Stroke, myelitis (less common)

Other
Pneumonitis (uncommon)
Retinal haemorrhage (uncommon)

INVESTIGATIONS

FBC
Hb ↓
MCV normal
WCC ↑
Platelets sometimes ↑

U + Es
Urea and creatinine often ↑

LFTs
ALP may be ↑ in liver involvement
Albumin ↓
Clotting usually normal

ESR ↑
CRP ↑
C_3, C_4 may be ↓
Total complement activity is ↓
Immune complexes often present
Rheumatoid factor occasionally positive
ANA negative
pANCA usually negative (see below)
Urine shows proteinuria and haematuria

DIAGNOSIS
Diagnosis is usually on clinical features (particularly weight loss, renal impairment, livedo, testicular pain, myalgia, hypertension, neuropathy) plus demonstration of:

1. Aneurysms in medium-sized vessels at angiography and/or
2. Necrotizing vasculitis in medium-sized arteries on biopsy of an affected organ

In most cases of 'classical' PAN, pANCA is negative; however, it may be positive (10%) if small vessels are also involved. The presence of hepatitis B surface antigen also contributes to the diagnostic criteria for PAN.

DIFFERENTIAL DIAGNOSIS
Other primary vasculitides, e.g.

Wegener's granulomatosis
Microscopic polyarteritis
SLE
Rheumatoid arthritis
Buerger's disease

Ergotism
SBE
Atrial myxoma
Cryoglobulinaemia
Cholesterol embolism
TTP
Systemic sepsis
Malignancy

TREATMENT

High-dose corticosteroids, with additional
cyclophosphamide or methotrexate, especially
if any evidence of small-vessel involvement or
in case of relapse
Hepatitis B-associated PAN is treated with
plasmapheresis and antivirals (vidarabine,
interferon) in addition to steroids

PROGNOSIS

80% 5-year survival with treatment. 15% 5-year
survival without treatment. Mesenteric infarction,
renal failure and cardiovascular disease are
common causes of death.

QUESTION SPOTTING

Any organ dysfunction plus hypertension may be
due to PAN, especially if there is evidence of
glomerulonephritis or recurrent GI symptoms.
Catastrophic events (due to infarction) are
common in PAN.

PAN is typically ANA- and ANCA-negative;
these are the clues to differentiate it from other
vasculitides.

Watch for risk factors for hepatitis B, or
evidence of chronic liver disease.

PAGET'S DISEASE OF BONE

An increase in bone osteoclast activity, which leads to increased osteoblast activity. Bone turnover is thus increased, with areas of bone thickening and resorption. This weakens the bone, leading to fractures. The aetiology is unclear, but viral inclusion bodies have been found in osteoclasts. Prevalence in the UK is 3–9%, rising with age.

SYMPTOMS
Deafness
Bone pain
Bone deformity
Joint pain
Numbness/paraesthesia

SIGNS
Bony deformity
Warm bones
Reduced hearing acuity
Reduced sensation
Dermatomal from nerve root entrapment
Cord compression (rare)
Signs of cardiac failure (rare)

INVESTIGATIONS
FBC
Normal

U + Es
Normal

LFTs
ALP $\uparrow$ (bone isoenzyme)
GGT normal

Calcium normal unless immobile
ESR normal
Acid phosphatase may be $\uparrow$
PSA normal
PO_4 normal
PTH normal
Vitamin D normal
Urinary hydroxyproline $\uparrow$

X-rays
Expanded bone, coarse trabeculae
Areas of sclerosis and porosis
Axial skeleton most often affected
Periarticular calcification
Microfractures on convex surface of deformed bone
See hip and skull X-rays for typical examples (Figures 5.5 and 5.6)
Bone scan shows greatly increased uptake in affected areas

DIAGNOSIS
A typical X-ray appearance, especially in the context of warm, deformed bones. Raised bony ALP with normal calcium, PO_4 and vitamin D is

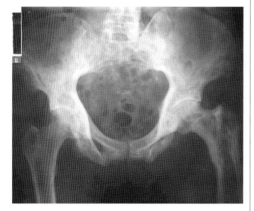

Figure 5.5 Paget's disease of bone. This pelvic X-ray shows very typical features of Paget's disease of bone. There is diffuse and severe sclerosis with coarse trabeculation and bony expansion. The disease is also apparent in the proximal femurs.

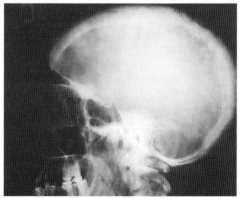

Figure 5.6 Paget's disease of bone. The skull X-ray also shows typical features of Paget's disease of bone.

likely to be due to Paget's. Bone scan may give further evidence in doubtful cases.

DIFFERENTIAL DIAGNOSIS

Metastatic malignancy (especially prostate)
Osteomalacia
Differential diagnosis of isolated raised ALP:
Paget's disease of bone
Primary biliary cirrhosis
Hepatic metastatic malignancy
Hepatic abscess/drug reaction

COMPLICATIONS

Increased risk of fracture
Osteoarthritis (especially of knee)
Osteogenic sarcoma (< 1%)
High-output cardiac failure in very extensive
  disease
Cord compression
Nerve root entrapment
Cranial nerve palsies

TREATMENT

Bisphosphonates are the treatment of choice; IV pamidronate is used if pressure symptoms are present, otherwise oral bisphosphonates can be used. Calcium and vitamin D may be needed to prevent secondary hyperparathyroidism.
Calcitonin may be used as an adjunct to control pain in the short term.

QUESTION SPOTTING

Most likely to present as non-specific aches and pains in an older person – perhaps with reduced mobility. A raised ALP is usually seen with other bone markers normal and a normal GGT.
Beware: a slightly raised calcium may occur if the patient has been immobile due to the disease. May rarely occur as part of a cord compression scenario or a cause of deafness.

BEHÇET'S DISEASE

Behçet's disease is a multisystem vasculitic disease of unknown aetiology. It is thought to have an autoimmune basis, but infective triggers may also play a role. It is most common in peoples living along the old silk route (especially Iran and Turkey), and is also common in the Japanese population. There is an association with HLA B5 and B51. Prevalence by sex varies depending on the geographical area; the disease tends to affect younger adults.

CLINICAL FEATURES
Mouth ulcers
Dysuria
Dyspareunia (from genital ulcers)
Epididymitis

Skin lesions (75%)
Erythema nodosum
Acne
Papulopustular lesions

Eye lesions (50%)
Anterior uveitis (bilateral in 90%)
Posterior uveitis
Choroidoretinitis
Keratitis
Conjunctivitis

Neurological (5–20%)
TIAs/stroke-like deficits
Myelitis
Meningoencephalitis
Seizures
Psychosis
Sudden deafness
Pseudobulbar palsy
Cranial nerve palsies

Arthritis (50%)
May follow any pattern, including sacroiliitis.
Usually non-erosive

GI tract
Diarrhoea
Rectal, intestinal and stomach ulcers

Cardiac (5–10%)
MI, myocardial ischaemia
Granulomatous endocarditis
Arrhythmias
Pericarditis

Rarer associations
Myositis
DVT, IVC/SVC thrombosis
Budd–Chiari syndrome
Arterial occlusion and aneurysms
Renal vein thrombosis
Glomerulonephritis
Pulmonary vasculitis
Amyloidosis (2%)
Lymphadenopathy

INVESTIGATIONS
FBC
Hb may be $\downarrow$
WCC mildly $\uparrow$ or normal
Platelets usually normal

U + Es
Usually normal

LFTs
Usually normal

ESR $\uparrow$
CRP $\uparrow$
C_3/C_4 normal or $\uparrow$
Immune complexes show modest $\uparrow$ in 50%
Rheumatoid factor negative
ANA negative
IgA often $\uparrow$
IgM, IgG levels are variable
Antiphospholipid antibodies: occasionally positive, more often in retinal vein/artery occlusion

CSF: may show elevated protein, WCC and immunoglobulins

DIAGNOSIS
Diagnostic criteria
Oral ulceration three times in 1 year plus two of:

Recurrent genital ulceration
Uveitis or retinal vasculitis
Skin lesions as described above
Positive pathergy test
Pathergy test: a sterile needle is used to produce a subcutaneous lesion, and the result read after 48 hours. Presence of an erythematous papule > 2 mm in diameter is considered a positive test

The test is not specific; positive results are also seen in CML and spondyloarthropathies.
The test is more likely to be positive in active disease and in certain populations

DIFFERENTIAL DIAGNOSIS
Rheumatoid arthritis
Reiter's syndrome
Stevens–Johnson syndrome
Crohn's disease
Ulcerative colitis
Neurological lesions may mimic MS
HIV infection

TREATMENT
Eyes, skin: topical steroids
Colchicine may be useful for joint involvement and erythema nodosum
Systemic steroids may be needed for internal disease; azathioprine is also effective
Thalidomide is useful for difficult-to-treat ulcers, and ciclosporin can be used for resistant uveitis

Severe vasculitis (renal, CNS) may require cyclophosphamide or chlorambucil in addition to high-dose steroids
Other therapies that are occasionally used include TNF-blockers, interferon-alpha and sulfasalazine (for bowel involvement)

PROGNOSIS
Disease runs a relapsing/remitting course.
Prognosis is good unless neurological, pulmonary or vascular problems supervene – mortality rate in such cases is 20–50% at 5 years.

QUESTION SPOTTING
A clue to the diagnosis is often Turkish or Japanese origin of the patient. A combination of oral ulcers, genital ulcers and iritis suggests the diagnosis; if neurological symptoms are also present, the diagnosis becomes very likely (neurological symptoms should not occur in Crohn's or Reiter's).

POLYMYOSITIS AND DERMATOMYOSITIS

Polymyositis is a connective tissue disease that causes inflammation and necrosis of muscle fibres. When accompanied by a rash it is known as dermatomyositis. It affects women more than men. It may run an acute course or a more chronic course.

There are five categories of disease:

1. Adult polymyositis
2. Adult dermatomyositis
3. Dermatomyositis or polymyositis with malignancy
4. Childhood dermatomyositis
5. Polymyositis as part of other connective tissue disease

CLINICAL FEATURES
Muscles
Proximal muscle weakness, especially affecting shoulder and pelvic girdles
Muscle tenderness or pain in approximately 50%
Muscle wasting (occurs later than the weakness)
Pharyngeal and respiratory muscle involvement may cause dysphagia, dysphonia and respiratory failure

Skin
'Heliotrope' rash (25%)
Gottron's papules (violet, scaly rash on knuckles)
Rash on elbows, knees (30–50%)
Cutaneous and muscular calcification
Loss of skin elasticity may give appearances similar to systemic sclerosis
Nailfold changes
Periungual erythema
Cuticular hypertrophy
Infarcts

Cardiac
Often asymptomatic
Heart block
Arrhythmias
Myocardial infarction
Pericarditis

Other
Fever
Weight loss
Mild arthralgia or inflammatory polyarthritis affecting the small joints of the hands
Raynaud's syndrome in 30%

Renal involvement is rare except if myoglobinuria causes renal impairment
Pulmonary fibrosis (particularly associated with the Jo-1 antibody)

INVESTIGATIONS
FBC
Hb ↓ (MCV normal)
WCC ↑ if severe with neutrophilia
Platelets normal or ↑

U + Es
Na normal
K normal
Urea and creatinine ↑ if myoglobinuria causes renal impairment

LFTs
AST ↑
Albumin ↓
Otherwise normal

CK ↑
LDH usually elevated
ESR ↑
Immunoglobulins may be ↑, especially IgG
ANA often positive
Jo-1 positive 30% and is a marker for pulmonary fibrosis
Rheumatoid factor often positive

In older patients a basic search for malignancy with chest X-ray, mammogram, tumour markers and maybe a pelvic ultrasound is recommended, although some advocate that this is not indicated unless there is clinical suspicion of malignancy

DIAGNOSIS
Four of:

Proximal muscle weakness
Muscle pain
Fever, raised CRP or raised ESR
Raised CK
Positive biopsy
Positive EMG
Positive anti Jo-1 antibody
Non-erosive arthropathy

The above plus typical skin changes makes the diagnosis of dermatomyositis

EMG

Shows myopathy and denervation. The typical triad includes:

Short polyphasic motor units
Spontaneous fibrillation
High-frequency repetitive discharges

Muscle biopsy

Muscle fibre necrosis and inflammation with regeneration, but may be normal as the inflammation can be patchy and may be missed by biopsy

DIFFERENTIAL DIAGNOSIS

Connective tissue disorders – SLE, scleroderma, MCTD, rheumatoid arthritis
Other vasculitides – polyarteritis nodosa, giant cell arteritis/polymyalgia rheumatica
Myasthenia gravis
Muscular dystrophy
Endocrine myopathy – thyrotoxicosis, hypothyroidism, osteomalacia, Cushing's
Drug-induced myopathy
Inclusion body myositis
Infective myositis
Malignant myopathy
Neurogenic atrophy
Motor neurone disease

TREATMENT

Bedrest and limb splinting to prevent contractures
High-dose steroids
CK falls before muscle strength returns. Monitor both while reducing steroid dose
Physiotherapy once muscle strength begins to return
Immunosuppression with azathioprine or methotrexate may be required if steroids fail. IV immunoglobulin is an alternative second-line therapy

PROGNOSIS

Overall 20% mortality at 5 years
Poorer prognosis in children who also suffer long-term morbidity if they survive
Poor prognosis with cardiac involvement, dysphagia or pulmonary fibrosis

QUESTION SPOTTING

The difficulty will be in differentiating polymyositis with multisystem involvement from SLE or scleroderma. Polymyalgia can be differentiated by the muscle stiffness and the lack of wasting. Abnormal AST or CK in the absence of other abnormal LFTs points to a myositis. Questions may revolve around the choice of investigation or the interpretation of negative investigations (patchy involvement may cause EMG or biopsy to be negative).

CHURG–STRAUSS SYNDROME

Churg–Strauss syndrome is a combination of granulomatous necrotizing vasculitis of small to medium-sized vessels and eosinophilic pneumonia in association with asthma and peripheral eosinophilia. The disease tends to start with an allergic rhinitis with asthma. This usually develops into a blood, lung and gastrointestinal eosinophilia. The final stage is a systemic vasculitis when the asthma may recede. The syndrome is rare. There is slight male preponderance, and the mean age of onset is 40–50 years old. Commencement of leukotriene antagonists with consequent reduction in steroid dose may occasionally unmask the condition.

CLINICAL FEATURES
General
Seen once systemic vasculitis occurs:
Fever
Weight loss
Fatigue
Myalgia
Arthralgia

Respiratory (> 80%)
Allergic rhinitis and eosinophilic sinusitis – usually the first feature, and seen in young adulthood
Nasal polyposis
Asthma – typically severe and adult in onset
Haemoptysis

Nervous system (60%)
Mononeuritis multiplex
Polyneuropathy – distal and symmetrical or asymmetrical
Radiculopathies
Optic neuropathy
Cranial nerve lesions, including trigeminal neuropathy
Central nervous manifestations such as psychiatric disturbance, stroke and epilepsy have all been reported but are rare

Skin (60%)
Vasculitis rash – palpable purpura of the lower extremities
Subcutaneous granulomatous nodules
Livedo reticularis, bullous lesions, urticaria and maculopapular lesions all seen rarely

Renal (20–50%)
Focal segmental glomerulonephritis occurs but is less common and severe than polyarteritis nodosa

Gastrointestinal system (30–50%)
Abdominal pain – indicates eosinophilic mass lesions which may cause obstruction or ulceration and haemorrhagic diarrhoea
Fistulae, perforation also seen
Pancreatitis
Acute acalculous cholecystitis

Haematological
Peripheral eosinophilia
Autoimmune haemolytic anaemia (rare)

Cardiac
Myocardial infarction from coronary artery vasculitis
Heart failure from eosinophilic myocardial infiltration
Mitral regurgitation in the absence of heart failure, possibly due to myocardial fibrosis
Conduction defects

INVESTIGATIONS
FBC
Hb $\downarrow$ (normal MCV)
WCC $\uparrow$ or normal but eosinophils $\uparrow$ (> 1.5 $\times$ 10^9/L or > 10% of differential)
Platelets normal

U + Es
Na and K normal
Urea and creatinine $\uparrow$ if renal involvement

LFTs
Albumin $\downarrow$
Otherwise normal

ESR $\uparrow$
CRP $\uparrow$
Immunoglobulins often $\uparrow$ with $\uparrow\uparrow$ IgE
ANCA-positive in 60% (usually pANCA, but may be cANCA: compare with Wegener's granulomatosis, which tends to be cANCA-positive, and polyarteritis nodosa, which is usually ANCA-negative)

Rheumatoid factor may be positive or negative
ANA usually negative

Chest X-ray

Transient patchy infiltrates which disappear
rapidly with steroid treatment are typical but
the X-ray may remain normal. Occasional
nodules appear, but these rarely cavitate, unlike
Wegener's granulomatosis

DIAGNOSIS

Diagnostic criteria

At least four of the following:

Asthma
Eosinophilia > 10% on differential WCC
Mononeuropathy (including multiplex) or
  polyneuropathy
Non-fixed pulmonary infiltrates on CXR
Paranasal sinus abnormality
Positive biopsy

Biopsy

This can be from almost any involved tissue
including nerve, muscle or skin, but respiratory
tract gives the most characteristic appearance.
Extravascular eosinophils are characteristic.

DIFFERENTIAL DIAGNOSIS

As already alluded to, there is much overlap with
other vasculitides, especially:

Polyarteritis nodosa
Wegener's granulomatosis
Microscopic polyangiitis

Henoch–Schönlein syndrome
Shadowing on a chest X-ray with eosinophilia
Eosinophilic pneumonia
Loeffler's syndrome
Aspergillosis
Strongyloides infestation
Drugs: thiazides, hydralazine, tolbutamide,
  sulphonamides, penicillin, gold

TREATMENT

Steroids in high dose
Adjuvant immunosuppression with
  cyclophosphamide or azathioprine may be
  required for life-threatening disease
High-dose immunoglobulin and interferon-alpha
  have also been used

PROGNOSIS

25% 5-year survival without treatment
65% 5-year survival with treatment.
  Cardiovascular disease (especially myocardial
  infarction) remains the commonest cause of
  death

QUESTION SPOTTING

The typical question will involve a middle-aged
patient with late-onset asthma who develops
signs of systemic disease. If given part of the
white cell differential, always work out the
eosinophil count if possible, as this will give
diagnostic weight. The same can be done with
IgE if immunoglobulins are given.

GIANT CELL ARTERITIS (TEMPORAL ARTERITIS) AND POLYMYALGIA RHEUMATICA

Once thought to be two different diseases, giant cell arteritis (GCA) and polymyalgia rheumatica (PMR) are now widely believed to be different presentations of the same disease process. Patients may present with one or other of the two syndromes, or a combination of both, and the two conditions can appear in the same patient but at different times.

The aetiology of the condition is not known. Both humoral and cellular immunological mechanisms have been implicated. GCA affects only large arteries with an internal elastic component and may cause arterial occlusion. Blindness, which is the most worrying feature of the disease, is rarely due to central retinal artery occlusion, but more commonly due to arteritis of the posterior ciliary arteries.

Peak incidence is at 60–75 years of age and the male:female ratio is 1:3. The syndrome of GCA is 10 times less common than PMR. The disease is almost exclusive to Caucasians and those over 50 years old.

CLINICAL FEATURES
Polymyalgia rheumatica

SYMPTOMS
Pain and stiffness in the neck and shoulder and
  pelvic girdles – early-morning stiffness,
  bilateral and symmetrical
Low-grade fever
Anorexia
Malaise
Weight loss
The feet are never affected

SIGNS
Physical examination is often normal by afternoon
May show joint tenderness but muscles not
  always tender
No weakness

Giant cell arteritis

SYMPTOMS
Headaches and scalp tenderness

Visual disturbance – amaurosis fugax, transient
  blindness, scotomata, partial or complete
  visual loss in one eye. Diplopia and ptosis are
  also seen
Transient ischaemic attacks
Jaw claudication
Fever
Weight loss
Anorexia
Fatigue

SIGNS
Thickened tender, nodular and pulseless arteries

INVESTIGATIONS
FBC
Hb ↓ (MCV normal)
WCC normal or ↑
Platelets normal
ESR ↑ (usually > 50 mm/hour. May exceed
  100 mm/hour. Rarely may be normal or only
  slightly ↑)

U + Es
Normal

LFTs
ALP is often ↑

CRP ↑
ANA usually negative
ANCA usually negative
Rheumatoid factor negative (but watch out for
  the false-positive results seen more commonly
  with age)
EMG and nerve conduction studies: normal

DIAGNOSIS
Giant cell arteritis diagnosis requires three of:

Age > 50
New headache
Temporal artery tenderness or loss of pulse
ESR > 50 mm/hour
Vasculitis on temporal artery biopsy

Temporal artery biopsy shows inflammatory
  infiltrate of lymphocytes, plasma cells, giant

cells and eosinophils, with necrosis of the arterial media. The vessel may occlude altogether. Biopsy is negative in 30% of patients with symptoms of giant cell arteritis, due to the typical patchy nature of the inflammation. The biopsy is less reliable after steroids have been commenced, but remains positive for up to 48 hours. Only 10% are positive by 7 days

Polymyalgia rheumatica diagnosis requires three of:

Age > 65
ESR > 40 mm/hour
Bilateral upper-arm tenderness
Morning stiffness > 1 hour
Depression and/or weight loss
Duration of illness > 2 weeks

A rapid response to steroids is confirmatory of the diagnosis in both illnesses.

DIFFERENTIAL DIAGNOSIS

Multiple myeloma
Rheumatoid arthritis
Connective tissue diseases
Polymyositis
Neoplasia with paraneoplastic syndrome
Atherosclerotic disease
Depression

TREATMENT

Polymyalgia rheumatica

Steroids: prednisolone 10–20 mg/day for 1 month, then a reducing dose to maintenance of 5–7.5 mg/day. Steroids may be required for 3–4 years, but it is worth attempting withdrawal by 2 years.

Giant cell arteritis

Steroids: prednisolone 60–80 mg/day (80 mg if any ocular symptoms) for 2 months, then reduce dose. If dose reduction is difficult due to ongoing symptoms or persistently raised ESR, then azathioprine or methotrexate may be used as steroid-sparing agents.

PROGNOSIS

Relapses are common and may occur in up to 30%. Giant cell arteritis may be fatal if basilar artery occlusion occurs.

QUESTION SPOTTING

The diagnosis is almost exclusive to the over-50-year-old population. The typical patient will be a white 60–70-year-old woman with non-specific aches and pains, particularly in the morning. A history of headaches should give the diagnosis away. If the symptoms and ESR do not resolve rapidly with steroids, consideration of alternative diagnoses such as malignancy is imperative.

An inflammatory arthropathy of unknown aetiology, but with an autoimmune basis. There is a strong link to HLA B27. Onset usually occurs in young adults, and the disease is commoner in males (3:1).

CLINICAL FEATURES

Fatigue
Sacroiliitis – back pain and stiffness, worse in morning
Reduced chest expansion
Costochondritis
Tendinitis
Large-joint arthropathy (especially in the lower limb)
Aortitis
Cardiac conduction defects
Pulmonary fibrosis (upper zone)
Anterior uveitis

INVESTIGATIONS

FBC

May show normocytic anaemia

U + Es

Usually normal

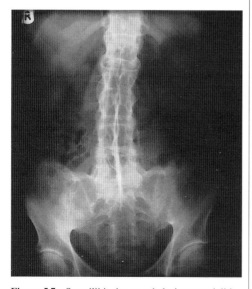

Figure 5.7 Sacroiliitis due to ankylosing spondylitis. Note the sclerosis along the sacroiliac joint lines. (Reproduced with permission from Kumar, Clarke (2001) *Clinical Medicine*, 5th edn. Saunders.)

LFTs

ALP may be slightly elevated

Ca usually normal
CK may be slightly elevated
ESR often elevated in active disease, but may be normal
CRP may be modestly elevated
HLA-B27 positive in 95% of sufferers

X-rays (Fig. 5.7)

Pelvic X-rays may show sacroiliitis – narrowed sacroiliac joint space, periarticular sclerosis
Spinal X-rays may show loss of the concave surface of the vertebrae and eventual fusion – 'bamboo spine'
Peripheral large joints may show sclerosis, erosion and loss of joint space

DIAGNOSIS

Is predominantly clinical. A combination of reduced lumbar spine movement, lower back pain and radiological evidence of sacroiliitis or enthesopathy is required.

DIFFERENTIAL DIAGNOSIS

Osteoarthritis
Diffuse idiopathic skeletal hyperostosis (DISH)
Fibromyalgia

Other seronegative arthropathies

Reactive arthritis
Reiter's disease
Psoriatic arthropathy (note lack of erosive changes in AS)
Arthropathy of inflammatory bowel disease
Seronegative rheumatoid arthritis

COMPLICATIONS

Aortic regurgitation
Thoracic aortic aneurysm
Respiratory failure due to thoracic deformity
Vertebral fracture
Cauda equina syndrome
Amyloidosis

TREATMENT

Physiotherapy – to maintain chest expansion and back suppleness
NSAIDs

Sulfasalazine – useful for peripheral joint involvement. Methotrexate can also be used for peripheral joint involvement

IV steroids for severe disease. Long-term oral steroids have little to offer

TNF inhibitors are effective, at least in the short term. They can be used in patients with active spinal disease that has not responded to at least two types of NSAID

Topical steroids may be used for uveitis

Joint replacement may be necessary in some cases (predominantly hip)

PROGNOSIS

Is generally good – especially if physiotherapy is instituted before deformity occurs

QUESTION SPOTTING

Consider the diagnosis in young patients with back pain. Occasionally the diagnosis may underlie upper-zone lung fibrosis or aortic regurgitation. Uveitis and large-joint arthropathy are other clues to the diagnosis.

ENDOCRINOLOGY

CUSHING'S SYNDROME

Chronic inappropriate hypersecretion of cortisol, as a result of several different disease processes:

1. High ACTH levels:
   Pituitary microadenoma (Cushing's disease)
   Ectopic ACTH (e.g. small cell lung cancer)
2. Primary hypercortisolaemia:
   Adrenal hyperplasia
   Adrenal tumour (carcinoma or adenoma)
   Exogenous steroids
3. Ectopic CRF production (very rare)

SYMPTOMS
Weakness, especially proximal (30–50%)
Easy bruising (60%)
Reduced libido
Dysmenorrhoea (80%)
Depression, psychosis (60%)
Weight gain (> 90%)

SIGNS
Moon face, buffalo hump (90%)
Centripetal obesity
Hirsutism (80%)
Red abdominal striae (50%)
Acne
Hyperpigmentation (if ACTH raised)
Ankle oedema (50%)
Hypertension (75%)
Proximal muscle weakness

OTHER FEATURES
Osteoporosis and fractures (20%)
Diabetes or impaired glucose tolerance (50%)
Renal calculi (15%)
Frequent infections
N.B.: Ectopic ACTH secretion by small cell lung cancer may produce a body habitus not dissimilar to Addison's disease, with weight loss and pigmentation

INVESTIGATIONS
FBC
Usually normal

U + Es
Na normal
K may be very ↓, especially if ectopic ACTH

Urea usually normal
Creatinine usually normal

LFTs
Normal

Calcium usually normal
Bicarbonate often elevated
Glucose often elevated
Chest X-ray can show evidence of small cell lung cancer
CT of adrenals may show adrenal adenoma or carcinoma (Fig. 6.1). If pituitary or ectopic ACTH production, bilateral adrenal enlargement will be seen. Note: 8% of population have 'incidentalomas'
MRI pituitary can show pituitary microadenomas

DIAGNOSIS
Is there hypercortisolism?
24-hour urinary free cortisol: elevated in 95% of Cushing's syndrome. False-positive rate is 1–5%
Low-dose dexamethasone suppression test:
0.5 mg dexamethasone given 6-hourly for 48 hours. Plasma cortisol then measured.
   Normal: < 50 nmol/L
Less discriminatory tests are:
Midnight cortisol: normal circadian rhythm is lost in Cushing's syndrome, thus 2400-hour cortisol is greater than 180 nmol/L. Infection

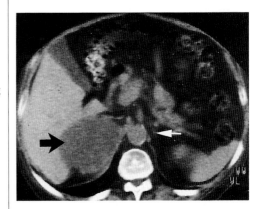

Figure 6.1 CT of abdomen showing large adrenal tumour as a cause of Cushing's syndrome. (Reproduced with permission from Forbes, Jackson (2003) *Colour Atlas and Text of Clinical Medicine*, 3rd edn. Mosby.)

and the stress of recent hospital admission will also give high readings

Short dexamethasone suppression test:
2 mg dexamethasone taken between 2200 and 2400 hours. Plasma cortisol taken at 0900–1100 hours. Normal ≤ 250 nmol/L

What is the cause?

Plasma ACTH measurement. High levels suggest pituitary or ectopic ACTH secretion. Suppressed levels indicate adrenal source or exogenous steroid. Levels above 300 ng/L are usually due to ectopic ACTH secretion

High-dose dexamethasone suppression test: measure 0900 hours cortisol at start, then give 2 mg dexamethasone 6-hourly for 48 hours. Suppression to less than 50% of basal level suggests pituitary origin for the high ACTH. Lack of suppression suggests an ectopic source

Venous sampling from inferior petrosal sinuses: if ACTH concentration is much higher ($\times 3$) in the sinuses than in the peripheral circulation, a pituitary source of ACTH is probable

DIFFERENTIAL DIAGNOSIS

Alcoholism – 'pseudo-Cushing's'

Severe intercurrent illness

Depression (can be very difficult to differentiate; depressed patients raise their cortisol in response to an insulin stress test; patients with Cushing's do not)

Obesity, with or without metabolic syndrome (hypertension and diabetes)

TREATMENT

Pituitary adenoma: surgery plus radiotherapy. Successful in 75–80%. Occasionally, bilateral adrenalectomy is needed for cases where the adenoma recurs or cannot be removed. Nelson's syndrome occurs as a result

Adrenal adenoma: surgery

Ectopic source: surgery, radiotherapy or chemotherapy

Metyrapone is useful prior to surgery, as it blocks cortisol production and thus allows control of BP, improves wound healing, stops weight gain and reduces the risk of infection. Ketoconazole is an alternative

QUESTION SPOTTING

Good discriminating features for Cushing's include:

Thin skin, easy bruising

Proximal myopathy

Facial plethora

Consider Cushing's if a hypokalaemic metabolic alkalosis is present

Another classic presentation is the patient who is a smoker with weight loss, pigmentation, hypertension and a metabolic alkalosis – small cell lung cancer being the diagnosis

ACROMEGALY

Excessive growth hormone secretion, usually from a pituitary adenoma (> 95%). Symptoms are caused by mass effect from the adenoma as well as by the effects of growth hormone. 3% of patients with acromegaly have GHRH secretion from tumours in the hypothalamus, adrenal, pancreas or from carcinoid tumours. Less than 2% of cases are due to GH-secreting islet cell tumours.

Overall, 6% of acromegalics have the MEN 1 syndrome

SYMPTOMS
Mass effect
Headache
Visual impairment
Diplopia

Hormonal
Deepening of voice
Enlarging hands, feet, jaw
Sweating
Joint pains (60–70%)
Snoring
Impotence (25–45%)
Dysmenorrhoea (30–85%)
Weakness
Numbness, paraesthesia

SIGNS
Mass effect
Cranial nerve palsies (III, IV, VI)
Bitemporal hemianopia

Hormonal
Frontal bossing
Prognathism, malocclusion
'Spade-like' hands
Thick, oily skin
Acanthosis nigricans
Carpal tunnel syndrome
Hypertension
Palpable thyroid
Palpable kidneys
Cardiac enlargement
Large tongue

INVESTIGATIONS
FBC
Usually normal

U + Es
Usually normal

LFTs
Usually normal

Calcium normal
Glucose often ↑ (10–20% are diabetic, 30–45% have impaired glucose tolerance)
Cholesterol normal
Triglycerides ↑
CK – may be elevated
IGF-1 ↑
Prolactin ↑ in 40%
LH, FSH may be ↓
Urinary calcium ↑

X-RAY
SXR may show enlarged pituitary fossa (Figure 6.2)
Thickened skull
Enlarged frontal sinuses
Malocclusion
Foot X-ray may show thickened heel pad
Hand X-ray shows large phalanges, phalangeal tufts
MRI brain often shows pituitary adenoma; most are macroadenomas (Figure 6.3)

DIAGNOSIS
IGF-1 levels almost always raised; low levels effectively rule out acromegaly
Glucose tolerance test (GTT): 75 g glucose load is taken after fasting. In normal individuals,

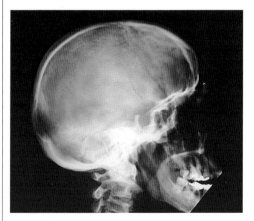

Figure 6.2 Acromegaly. A lateral skull X-ray showing enlarged pituitary fossa and enlarged jaw typical of acromegaly.

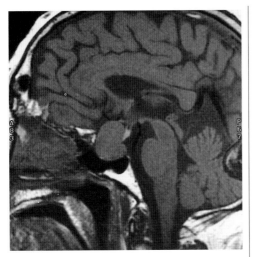

Figure 6.3 Acromegaly. An enlarged pituitary gland on a T1-weight sagittal MRI brain. The pituitary is clearly enlarged and extends both superiorly and posteriorly from the pituitary fossa.

GH levels are suppressed to < 2 mU/L. The GTT may also show evidence of diabetes or impaired glucose tolerance

MRI of the pituitary to detect the adenoma (Figure 6.3)

DIFFERENTIAL DIAGNOSIS

Acromegaly plus panhypopituitarism
Acromegaly as part of MEN 1
Haemochromatosis (diabetes + joint pains)
Other pituitary adenomas (mass effects), especially prolactinoma

COMPLICATIONS

Glucose intolerance or diabetes
Obstructive sleep apnoea
Panhypopituitarism
Cardiomyopathy (20–40%)

TREATMENT

Transsphenoidal hypophysectomy: 60% success rate; 1–9% diabetes insipidus
Radiotherapy postsurgery if control is inadequate (GH > 5 mU/L)
Bromocriptine, cabergoline, octreotide or lanreotide to control symptoms (successful in 70–90%) and as a holding measure. The dopamine antagonists bromocriptine and cabergoline are less effective than the somatostatin analogues
Pegvisomant is a new GH antagonist that can be used in patients resistant to the effects of somatostatin analogues; it is effective at reducing IGF levels to normal but should not be used in macroadenomas. There is a concern that the lack of blockade of negative feedback may accelerate growth of the adenoma in some cases

PROGNOSIS

Life expectancy is reduced in acromegaly, but suppression of GH levels to < 5 mU/L probably restores life expectancy to normal.

QUESTION SPOTTING

Although the clinical features are distinctive, beware coexistent hypopituitarism or other endocrine disease (e.g. part of MEN 1). Questions may revolve around choice of treatment or imaging modality.

ACUTE INTERMITTENT PORPHYRIA

An autosomal-dominant condition caused by inheriting an inactive allele of porphobilinogen (PBG) deaminase. This leads to reduced PBG deaminase activity and build-up of porphyrin precursors, particularly delta-aminolaevulinic acid. The features of the disease result from the neurotoxic effects of D-ALA on motor, sensory, central and autonomic nerves.

Attacks occur intermittently, being precipitated by intercurrent infection, fasting, pregnancy, parturition and a variety of drugs, including alcohol.

SYMPTOMS
Abdominal pain (95%)
Vomiting
Constipation
Depression and anxiety, hallucinations and psychosis (50%)
Weakness, often starting peripherally. May progress to respiratory paralysis and difficulty swallowing
Paraesthesia
Convulsions

SIGNS
Tachycardia, hypertension, postural drop (70%)
Pyrexia
Sweating
Mild abdominal tenderness
Bowel sounds usually normal
Lower motor neurone weakness

INVESTIGATIONS
FBC
Hb normal
WCC ↑ (neutrophilia)
Platelets normal

U + Es
Na ↓ (due to SIADH)
K ↓
Urea ↑

LFTs
Often abnormal

Abdominal X-ray normal or shows colonic dilatation
Urine shows proteinuria. Urine darkens on standing

DIAGNOSIS
Ehrlich's test: add one volume Ehrlich's reagent to one volume of urine. Sample turns red. Add two volumes of chloroform. Red colour stays in upper (aqueous) layer in AIP
Urinary D-ALA and porphobilinogen both raised
Erythrocyte PBG deaminase levels are decreased

DIFFERENTIAL DIAGNOSIS
SLE
Acute lead poisoning
Drug intoxication
Toxaemia of pregnancy
Atypical pneumonia
Alcoholic hepatitis (although the bilirubin will be very high in this condition)

COMPLICATIONS
Death can occur from respiratory paralysis or aspiration, and the autonomic instability is thought to be the underlying reason for sudden death in some cases.

Chronic abdominal pain, weakness and paraesthesia can occur as long-term neurological sequelae, and 40% of patients remain hypertensive between attacks.

TREATMENT
High carbohydrate intake – e.g. IV dextrose
Morphine for analgesia
Fluid replacement
Beta-blockade for tachycardia/hypertension
Chlorpromazine and a dark, quiet environment for psychosis and agitation
Monitor for respiratory embarrassment (FVC)
There is some evidence that using IV haem arginate reduces the duration and severity of attacks

QUESTION SPOTTING
AIP may present as abdominal pain and constipation but no tenderness. Look for a combination of low sodium (due to SIADH), raised WCC and deranged LFTs. Other clues are a past history of psychosis or fits, and patients who become very unwell after starting seemingly innocuous drugs, e.g. benzodiazepines.

ADDISON'S DISEASE

Addison's disease refers to primary failure of the adrenal cortex, with consequent loss of production of glucocorticoids and mineralocorticoids.

CAUSES
Autoimmune adrenalitis (70–80%) – antibodies can be found against the 21-hydroxylase enzyme in 90% of autoimmune cases
Tuberculosis
Metastatic malignancy, especially small cell lung cancer and lymphoma
Amyloidosis
Haemorrhage/infarction
Bilateral adrenalectomy
AIDS – caused by infections, e.g. CMV, PCP, fungi
Adrenoleukodystrophy

SYMPTOMS
Tiredness
Depression
Anorexia
Weight loss
Nausea and vomiting
Abdominal pain
Diarrhoea
Dizziness
Myalgia
Amenorrhoea (uncommon)

SIGNS
Pigmentation (90%) on sun-exposed areas, mucosal surfaces, axillae, palmar creases and in recent scars
Loss of body hair
Cachexia
Postural hypotension (lying BP may be normal)
Low-grade fever

Rare features
Benign intracranial hypertension
Proximal myopathy
Peripheral neuropathy

Addisonian crises
Characterized by dehydration and hypotension. Coma and fits may occur. Crises may be precipitated by surgery, trauma, infection or other major illness, particularly where gastrointestinal fluid loss is prominent

INVESTIGATIONS
FBC
Hb may $\downarrow$ after rehydration
WCC normal or $\uparrow$ (may show eosinophilia or lymphocytosis)
Platelets normal

U + Es
Na $\downarrow$ in 90%
K $\uparrow$ in 65%
Urea often $\uparrow$
Creatinine may be $\uparrow$

LFTs
Usually normal

Calcium may rise after rehydration
HCO_3 may be $\downarrow$ in crisis
Glucose $\downarrow$ in 50%
TFTs may show $\uparrow$ TSH and $\downarrow$ T_4. May be due to coexistent hypothyroidism or may revert to normal with corticosteroids
Adrenal antibodies: present in 90% of cases due to autoimmune adrenalitis. Rare in other causes of Addison's
Chest X-ray may show evidence of lung cancer or TB
Abdominal X-ray may show adrenal calcification from TB

DIAGNOSIS
Short Synacthen test. 250 µg tetracosactrin given IM. Cortisol and ACTH taken at 0, 30 and 60 min. Plasma cortisol should rise by at least 250 ng/L compared with baseline, reaching > 550 ng/L by 30 min
Failure to achieve these levels suggests adrenal insufficiency. A high ACTH level is good evidence of primary adrenal failure
Note also that renin levels are $\uparrow$, with normal or $\downarrow$ aldosterone
Basal cortisol and urinary free cortisol are usually low normal and are thus much less useful in making the diagnosis

ASSOCIATIONS

Autoimmune Addison's is associated with other
autoimmune diseases sharing the HLA B8,
DR3 haplotype, e.g.
IDDM
Pernicious anaemia
Thyroiditis/hypothyroidism
Vitiligo
Hypoparathyroidism
Primary ovarian failure

DIFFERENTIAL DIAGNOSIS

Beware syndromes which include Addison's
disease, e.g. Schmidt's syndrome,
polyglandular syndromes
Panhypopituitarism
Diuretic use (especially potassium-sparing
diuretics)
Psychological
Chronic fatigue syndrome

TREATMENT
Addisonian crisis

IV normal saline 2–4 L over 24 hours plus IV
hydrocortisone 200–400 mg in 24 hours. Correct
hypoglycaemia with IV dextrose. Treat
underlying infection or other precipitant of crisis.
Do not wait for results of a short Synacthen test
before treating; this could be fatal.

Maintenance

Oral hydrocortisone, e.g. 20 mg morning,
10 mg evening, or 10 mg/5 mg/5 mg. If postural
hypotension or electrolyte abnormalities
persist, fludrocortisone should be added in a dose
of 50–200 µg/day. A medic-alert bracelet, plus
patient education to double the dose of steroid
when unwell, are both essential.

QUESTION SPOTTING

Key features are a non-specific history of
tiredness, anorexia and GI symptoms
Dizziness with postural hypotension
Low sodium, with or without a high potassium
Also consider the diagnosis in any ill person with
low blood pressure, especially if the blood
pressure is resistant to treatment. There may be
a history of recent steroid use

HYPOPARATHYROIDISM

Underactivity of the parathyroid glands, or insensitivity to the effects of PTH (pseudohypoparathyroidism). Causes of hypoparathyroidism include:

Thyroid/parathyroid/neck surgery (> 90%)
Familial
Sporadic (autoimmune)
DiGeorge syndrome
Hypomagnesaemia
Wilson's disease – rare
Haemochromatosis – rare
Metastatic malignancy – rare

SYMPTOMS
Paraesthesia
Abdominal pain
Muscle spasm and tetany
Emotional lability
Memory impairment
Seizures
Diarrhoea

SIGNS
Chvostek's sign (occurs in 5% of normal
    population)
Trousseau's sign
Dry skin
Grooved nails

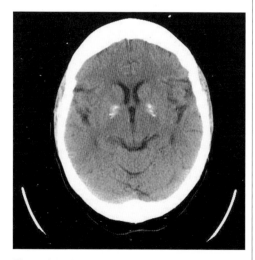

Figure 6.4 CT of the brain showing calcified basal ganglia in hypoparathyroidism.

Papilloedema
Cataracts
Somatic features associated with
    pseudohypoparathyroidism:
Round face, short neck
Short stature
Short metacarpals and metatarsals, especially
    4th and 5th
Osteitis fibrosa

INVESTIGATIONS
FBC
Normal

U + Es
Normal

LFTs
Normal (unless underlying liver disease)

Calcium ↓
PO_4 ↑
PTH ↓ or absent in hypoparathyroidism but ↑ in
    pseudohypoparathyroidism
CK may be ↑
Calcitriol ↓
Urine shows ↓ phosphate
ECG may show long QT interval
Hand X-ray shows short metacarpals
    (pseudohypoparathyroidism)
CT brain shows calcification of basal ganglia;
    other areas may also be affected

DIAGNOSIS
Low calcium plus raised phosphate in the
absence of other causes, e.g. renal failure,
malabsorption, osteomalacia
    Chase–Auerbach test: infusion of PTH,
causing:

↑ Urinary cAMP and PO_4 in hypoparathyroidism
No rise in urinary cAMP or PO_4 in complete
    pseudohypoparathyroidism
↑ in urinary cAMP only in partial
    pseudohypoparathyroidism

ASSOCIATIONS
Hypothyroidism
Diabetes mellitus

Gonadal dysgenesis
Dysmenorrhoea
Blue sclerae (uncommon)

Autoimmune hypoparathyroidism is associated with:

Pernicious anaemia
Addison's disease
Polyglandular endocrine syndromes
N.B.: Somatic features of
   pseudohypoparathyroidism without
   hypocalcaemia constitute a partially expressed
   disease phenotype:
   pseudopseudohypoparathyroidism

TREATMENT
Calcium plus calcitriol or 1-alpha calcidol

PROGNOSIS
Good, but cataracts may not be prevented by normalizing calcium

QUESTION SPOTTING
A typical case may present with tetany – particularly after thyroid or parathyroid surgery. Low calcium and high phosphate with normal renal function and no evidence of malabsorption point to the diagnosis. Calcified basal ganglia or cataracts should also alert you to the possibility of hypocalcaemia.

Look out for the typical body habitus of pseudohypoparathyroidism. Remember to look for other features of APS 1 if hypoparathyroidism is the diagnosis.

MULTIPLE ENDOCRINE NEOPLASIA

MEN syndromes come in at least two types: MEN 1 is caused by a mutation on chromosome 11, MEN 2 by a mutation on chromosome 10 (the *RET* oncogene). Both types display autosomal-dominant inheritance. MEN 2 is further divided into types a and b, based on the absence or presence of marfanoid features.

MEN 1 CLINICAL FEATURES

Parathyroid hyperplasia (almost 100%):

Symptoms due to hypercalcaemia
Pancreatic endocrine tumours (40–70%)
Gastrinoma (60%): peptic ulcers, indigestion, diarrhoea
Insulinoma (30%)
Glucagonoma
VIPoma
Non-functioning adenomas
Pituitary adenomas (30–50%)
Prolactinoma (65%)
GH-secreting (30%)
Others are rare:
Carcinoid (5–10%)
Adrenal tumours (5–40%): usually non-functioning
Adrenal cortical hyperplasia
Lipomas (1%)

MEN 2 CLINICAL FEATURES

Medullary C cell thyroid carcinoma (MTC) (100%)
Phaeochromocytoma (50%): bilateral in 70%
2a: Parathyroid hyperplasia in 80%; often asymptomatic
2b: Mucosal neuromas, marfanoid habitus, bowel neuromas – dysphagia, vomiting, megacolon, change in bowel habit. Parathyroid hyperplasia is rare

INVESTIGATIONS
MEN 1
FBC
Normal

U + Es
Normal

LFTs
Usually normal

Other Investigations
Calcium often raised
PO_4 often low
PTH often raised
Glucose normal, low or high (depending on pancreatic tumour)
Fasting gastrin raised in gastrinoma
Prolactin raised in prolactinoma
Insulin + C-peptide raised in insulinoma
Growth hormone, IGF-1 raised in acromegaly

MEN 2
FBC
Usually normal

U + Es
Usually normal

LFTs
Usually normal

Other Investigations
Calcitonin raised in MTC
Urinary catecholamines raised in phaeochromocytoma

DIAGNOSIS

Essentially clinical diagnosis based on two lesions occurring in a patient, or one characteristic lesion in a first-degree relative of someone known to have the condition
Pentagastrin stimulation test is used to look for the presence of MTC; raised calcitonin levels following the test suggest the presence of MTC

DIFFERENTIAL DIAGNOSIS

Other multiple neoplasia syndromes, e.g. Von Hippel–Lindau syndrome
Neurofibromatosis
Mixed MEN (phaeochromocytoma + prolactinoma)
Hereditary MTC or phaeochromocytoma

TREATMENT
MEN 1
Treatment is that of the individual tumours. First- and second-degree relatives should be screened

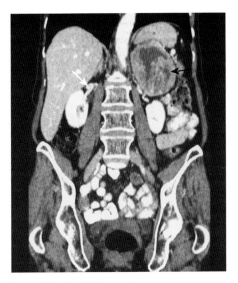

Figure 6.5 CT of abdomen showing a phaeochromocytoma. (Reproduced with permission from Boon, Colledge, Walker et al. (2006) *Davidson's Principles and Practice of Medicine*, 20th edn. Churchill Livingstone.)

every 6–12 months with a history, examination, calcium and prolactin levels, along with any tests for pancreatic or pituitary tumours suggested by the history and examination

Genetic analysis can also now be used to identify those with the defective gene

MEN 2

Again, the treatment is of the individual tumours, except for thyroid disease (see below)

Relatives of an index case should be genetically tested, and, if positive, should undergo screening, as should anyone with a tumour associated with MEN 2 or any of the somatic features of the disease

Screening should occur every 3–6 months in known cases and 6–12-monthly for carriers

History, examination, pentagastrin stimulation test, urinary catecholamines, PTH and calcium should be tested

To reduce the risk of MTC, thyroidectomy can be done when the pentagastrin test is first abnormal, or at age 5 (MEN 2a) or age 2–3 (MEN 2b) – these are the earliest recorded ages of tumour occurrence

QUESTION SPOTTING

Consider MEN in anyone with:

Hyperparathyroidism – especially if due to hyperplasia rather than adenoma
Unusual pancreatic tumour
Phaeochromocytomas
Multiple lipomas
Carcinoid

Also consider if a patient with a pituitary tumour presents with a second tumour

AUTOIMMUNE POLYGLANDULAR SYNDROMES

Three types are recognized:

APS 1

Caused by a mutation in the *APECED* gene (chromosome 21). Defined as two of:

Addison's disease
Hypoparathyroidism
Chronic mucocutaneous candidiasis
Ectodermal dystrophy is a characteristic feature, and the onset is usually in childhood

APS 2

Polygenic inheritance, with linkage to HLA DR3 and DR4. Adult onset. Defined as:

Addison's disease

plus either

Autoimmune thyroid disease or type 1 diabetes mellitus

Schmidt's syndrome (Addison's + hypothyroidism) therefore falls within the definition of APS 2

APS 3

Similar HLA linkage to APS 2. Defined as autoimmune thyroid disease plus at least one other autoimmune disorder in the absence of Addison's disease

FEATURES OF SYNDROMES
APS 1

Autoimmune features

Hypoparathyroidism 80%
Ovarian failure 60%
Alopecia 30%
Malabsorption 20%
Testicular failure 15%
Pernicious anaemia 15%
Vitiligo 15%
Addison's disease 10%
IDDM 10%
Autoimmune hepatitis 10%
Hypothyroidism 5%

Ectodermal features

Candidiasis > 95%
Enamel hypoplasia 80%

Nail dystrophy 50%
Keratopathy 35%
Tympanic membrane calcification 35%
Other associated manifestations reported include Sjögren's syndrome, asplenia, Turner's syndrome, vasculitis, hypophysitis and cholelithiasis

APS 2

Addison's disease 100%
Thyroid disease 70%
IDDM 50%
Vitiligo 5%
Gonadal failure 5%
Hypopituitarism < 1%
Alopecia < 1%
Pernicious anaemia < 1%
Candidiasis and hypoparathyroidism do not occur

INVESTIGATIONS

Results depend on which disease manifestations are present
Addison's: ↑ K, ↓ Na, may have ↓ glucose and ↑ calcium. Urea ↑ if dehydrated
Hypoparathyroidism: ↓ calcium, ↑ PO_4, ↓ PTH
IDDM: ↑ glucose
Pernicious anaemia: ↓ Hb, ↑ MCV, ↓ B_{12}. WCC and platelets may be ↓
Thyroid disease: hyperthyroid or hypothyroid pattern of TFTs
Hepatitis: abnormal LFTs, especially ↑ ALT
Autoantibodies to the affected organs are usually present

TREATMENT

Ketoconazole for candidiasis
Autoimmune syndromes are treated in the same way as isolated disease would be treated
Monitoring for the onset of associated disease manifestations is necessary

PROGNOSIS

Good with treatment; probably 90% survival at 20 years from diagnosis for APS 1

QUESTION SPOTTING

Any patient with candidal infection or hypoparathyroidism should raise the suspicion of APS 1.

For APS 2, cases of hypothyroidism that have extra features (e.g. a postural BP drop) should prompt consideration of APS 2. Similarly, look for evidence of hypothyroidism or other organ-specific autoimmune disease in any patient with Addison's – may be subtle, such as vitiligo.

HYPOPITUITARISM

Hypopituitarism is the partial or complete loss of anterior pituitary hormone secretion as a result of either pituitary or hypothalamic disease.

CAUSES
Congenital
Familial hypopituitarism – very rare inherited disorder
Isolated hormone deficiencies, e.g. Kallman's syndrome (isolated GnRH deficiency)

Neoplastic
Pituitary adenomas
Parapituitary tumours – meningiomas, gliomas, metastases, craniopharyngiomas

Vascular
Pituitary apoplexy
Sheehan's syndrome
Carotid artery aneurysm

Infective
Tuberculosis
Syphilis
Fungal
Abscesses

Trauma
Basal skull fracture
Pituitary surgery

Infiltrative
Haemochromatosis
Sarcoidosis
Wegener's granulomatosis

Other
Pituitary irradiation
Empty sella syndrome
Chemotherapy

The most common causes are pituitary tumours. Microadenomas rarely cause hypopituitarism, but with progressive enlargement of a pituitary adenoma, there is a sequential loss of pituitary function often in the context of excess secretion from the adenoma itself. In general, growth hormone (GH) is lost first, followed by luteinizing hormone (LH) and follicle-stimulating hormone (FSH). Adrenocorticotrophic hormone (ACTH) is lost later and finally thyroid-stimulating hormone (TSH)

CLINICAL FEATURES
This largely depends on the underlying cause and the hormonal axis lost. Below are the features expected for each deficiency.

Growth hormone deficiency
Children
Growth retardation
Adults
Reduced strength
Reduced muscle mass
Central obesity
Fatigue
Premature atherosclerosis

Gonadotropin deficiency
Men
Reduced libido
Erectile dysfunction
Impaired fertility
Loss of facial and body hair
Fine facial wrinkles
Gynaecomastia
Loss of bone mass
Loss of muscle mass and strength

Women
Altered menstrual function, ranging from anovulatory regular cycles through to amenorrhoea
Hot flushes
Reduced libido
Vaginal dryness with dyspareunia
Pubic and axillary hair is preserved unless there is also loss of ACTH
Postmenopausal women tend to present with either symptoms of the cause, e.g. headaches with visual field loss, or symptoms of other hormone deficiencies

Corticotrophin deficiency
Fatigue
Weakness
Headache
Dizziness
Anorexia
Nausea, vomiting
Abdominal pain
Altered mental activity
Loss of axillary and pubic hair
Pallor

Hypoglycaemia

Anaemia (MCV normal) with eosinophilia may be seen

Note that there is no hyperpigmentation as seen in primary adrenal failure, and that the typical findings of profound ↓ Na and ↑ K which are due to loss of aldosterone production in primary adrenal failure do not tend to be seen in hypopituitarism. Mild ↓ Na can occur due to ↑ vasopressin production

Thyrotrophin deficiency
Symptoms
Fatigue

Weakness

Weight gain

Puffiness

Constipation

Cold intolerance

Children may be growth-retarded, and with severe hypothyroidism, impairment of memory and mental activity can be noted

Signs
Bradycardia

Periorbital oedema

Slow relaxing reflexes

Prolactin deficiency or excess
Prolactin production is inhibited under normal circumstances, and loss does not usually cause any problems. However, hyperprolactinaemia is more common. This may either be due to a prolactin-secreting macroadenoma or due to loss of inhibition by dopamine, leading to increased prolactin production. A raised prolactin concentration is a good marker of pituitary dysfunction and may not necessarily indicate a prolactin-secreting adenoma unless the levels are very high.

Hyperprolactinaemia
Galactorrhoea

Menstrual dysfunction, especially secondary amenorrhoea

INVESTIGATIONS
FBC
Hb ↓ or normal (MCV normal or ↑ if hypothyroid)

WCC normal

Platelets normal

U + Es
Na normal or ↓ if ACTH or TSH-deficient

K usually normal

Urea and creatinine normal

LFTs
AST may be ↑ if thyroxine-deficient

Otherwise normal

Creatinine kinase may be ↑ with thyroxine deficiency

DIAGNOSIS
Hormone testing (clearly depends on which hormones affected)

ACTH ↓

TSH – often in the normal range despite low T_4

Prolactin – may be ↑ or ↓ as noted above.

T_4 ↓

Cortisol ↓

Oestradiol ↓

Testosterone ↓

LH ↓

FSH ↓

Dynamic testing (usually only required if partial loss of hormone makes diagnosis difficult)

Insulin stress test or glucagon stimulation test for growth hormone deficiency

Clomiphene test for gonadal function

Synacthen test for adrenal function

Imaging of pituitary fossa with MRI

DIFFERENTIAL DIAGNOSIS
Schmidt's syndrome/autoimmune polyglandular syndromes

Addison's disease

Hypothyroidism

TREATMENT
Replacement of hormone deficiencies

Treatment of underlying condition if possible

Points to note:
- Do not replace thyroxine until hypoadrenalism is excluded or treated as thyroxine may exacerbate cortisol deficiency
- Cortisol treatment may unmask a cranial diabetes insipidus, and this should be actively looked for after treatment commenced

- Cortisol replacement should be increased in times of stress such as surgery or infection
- Growth hormone has complicated interactions. Deficiency may make requirements of gonadotrophins higher for successful fertility in women and possibly men. Growth hormone replacement causes more conversion of T_4 to T_3 but this has no clinical significance. Growth hormone replacement may also reduce the availability of hydrocortisone, and may optimize glucose metabolism even if adequately replaced with cortisol, thyroxine and sex steroids

QUESTION SPOTTING

Some of the features are very non-specific, which can make diagnosis more difficult. The question may include a clue to the cause, such as previous trauma, headache or neurological disturbance. Consider this diagnosis if the patient is pale in the absence of anaemia or if there is a history of reduced libido, amenorrhoea or lethargy. Also watch out for thyroid function tests with a low T_4 and low-normal TSH.

Pituitary crisis may be the presenting syndrome – often in someone with a history of head trauma or pre-existing hypopituitarism stopping medications.

OSTEOMALACIA

Lack of effect of vitamin D, either because of vitamin D deficiency, failure to convert precursors into the active vitamin, or resistance to the effects of vitamin D. Osteomalacia is the result in adults; rickets the result in children. The end pathology is defective mineralization of osteoid.

CAUSES

Common
Dietary lack
Lack of exposure to sunlight
Chronic renal failure
Liver failure
Anticonvulsants (especially phenytoin, primidone, carbamazepine)
Malabsorption
Partial gastrectomy
Small-bowel pathology
Biliary pathology

Inherited
Vitamin D-resistant rickets
Fanconi's syndrome
Distal renal tubular acidosis
Vitamin D-dependent rickets

Other
Phosphate binders
Laxatives
Bisphosphonates
Hyperparathyroidism
Hypoparathyroidism
Paraneoplastic

N.B.: Vitamin D-resistant rickets is an X-linked condition where the renal tubule is insensitive to vitamin D. High urinary PO_4, low serum PO_4 but normal calcium and ALP result. Bone pain and weakness are uncommon, but the typical deformities of rickets occur, including short stature
   Vitamin D-dependent rickets is a rare inherited disease of two types:

1. Low levels of 1,25-hydroxyvitamin D, but normal levels of 25-hydroxyvitamin D. This block in conversion can be overcome by giving more 25-hydroxyvitamin D

2. High levels of 1,25-hydroxyvitamin D, but end-organ resistance. More 1,25-hydroxyvitamin D is given

SYMPTOMS
Bone pain, tenderness
Bone deformity
Weakness

SIGNS
Bony tenderness, pathological fractures
Proximal muscle weakness
Skeletal deformity (children), e.g. tibial bowing, rickety rosary, craniotabes, 'windswept' legs
Tetany (uncommon)
Enthesopathy; may lead to kyphosis and occasionally cord compression if gross deformity results

INVESTIGATIONS

FBC
Hb may be ↓ in GI tract disease
WCC usually normal
Platelets usually normal

U + Es
↑ Urea and creatinine in chronic renal failure

LFTs
ALP ↑

Calcium ↓ or low normal
PO_4 ↓
HCO_3 ↓
PTH ↑
Vitamin D ↓ in most cases

X-rays
Splayed metaphyses in children
Ragged appearance to growth plates
Looser's zones: commonest along femur, pubic bones, ribs, scapulae
Codfish (biconcave) vertebrae
Subperiosteal erosions on radial border of middle phalanges, resorption of clavicle ends and phalangeal tufts (due to secondary hyperparathyroidism)

DIAGNOSIS

Diagnosis can be confirmed by finding a low serum vitamin D level. Bone biopsy shows increased unmineralized osteoid

Bone scan may show multiple undiagnosed pathological fractures

DIFFERENTIAL DIAGNOSIS

For weakness and pains:

Polymyalgia rheumatica
Thyrotoxicosis
Cushing's syndrome
Polymyositis
Myeloma
Psychiatric pathology

TREATMENT

Replacement of vitamin D; usually precursor vitamin, but alfacalcidol or calcitriol in renal disease

Phosphate supplements may be needed in vitamin D-resistant rickets

QUESTION SPOTTING

Clues to the diagnosis are:

Elderly, housebound patients or Asian women
Anyone on anticonvulsants
Anyone with GI tract disease
Vague aching symptoms
Diffuse weakness
Low calcium with elevated ALP

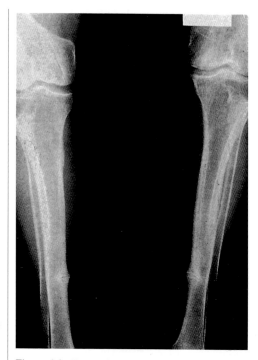

Figure 6.6　X-ray of lower legs showing Looser's zones in osteomalacia. (Reproduced with permission from Forbes, Jackson (2003) *Colour Atlas and Text of Clinical Medicine*, 3rd edn. Mosby.)

The important point with osteomalacia is not to stop once you have diagnosed the condition, but to go on and look for an underlying cause

HYPERPARATHYROIDISM

Inappropriately high levels of circulating parathyroid hormone (PTH). There are several causes.

PRIMARY
Single adenoma (85%)
Parathyroid hyperplasia (10%)
Multiple adenomas (5%)
Parathyroid carcinoma (< 1%)

SECONDARY
Due to low calcium levels, e.g. renal failure, low vitamin D levels

TERTIARY
Hyperfunction in the setting of secondary hyperparathyroidism

ECTOPIC
Due to release of PTH-related peptide (PTHrP) from tumours, e.g. cancer of the lung. These peptides do not cross-react with the normal PTH assay

The following comments apply mainly to primary hyperparathyroidism
Almost all features are due to hypercalcaemia

SYMPTOMS
Usually asymptomatic (> 70%)
Loin pain
Bone pain
Nausea
Vomiting
Polyuria, thirst
Arthritis
Mood swings, depression
Dementia, psychosis (uncommon)

SIGNS
Muscle hypotonicity
Band keratopathy
Hypertension (uncommon)
Proximal myopathy (uncommon)

OTHER FEATURES
Osteoporosis, fractures
Pseudogout
Nephrocalcinosis leading to renal failure
Peptic ulceration
Acute and chronic pancreatitis

INVESTIGATIONS
FBC
Normal

U + Es
Normal (unless chronic renal failure from nephrocalcinosis or dehydration)

LFTs
Bilirubin normal
ALT normal
ALP ↑ in 50%

Calcium ↑ (but may rarely be within normal range)
Phosphate ↓
ESR often ↑
PTH ↑ or inappropriately ↑ within normal range
Vitamin D usually normal
Chloride ↑
HCO_3 ↓

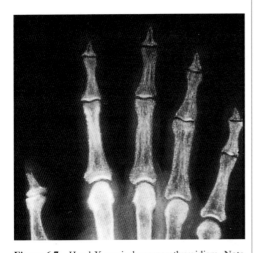

Figure 6.7 Hand X-ray in hyperparathyroidism. Note resorption of the distal phalanges and subperiosteal erosions more proximally. (Reproduced with permission from Forbes, Jackson (2003) *Colour Atlas and Text of Clinical Medicine*, 3rd edn. Mosby.)

Mg often ↓
Immunoglobulins may show monoclonal band
(even when no myeloma is present)

Urine
Calcium ↓
PO_4 ↑
ECG may show shortened QT interval

X-rays
Osteoporosis (especially at wrist)
Brown tumours (cysts)
Subperiosteal erosions, especially on radial
border of middle phalanges
'Salt-and-pepper' skull and loss of lamina dura
Resorption of phalangeal tufts
Nephrocalcinosis on abdominal X-rays

DIAGNOSIS
1. Elevated calcium
2. Inappropriately raised PTH in presence of
   elevated calcium

Note that the PTH sample should be
contemporaneous with the elevated calcium
level. If measures to lower calcium are
undertaken, the falling calcium level will trigger
PTH release, even in situations (e.g. malignancy)
where the PTH was previously suppressed. Thus
hyperparathyroidism will be wrongly diagnosed.

DIFFERENTIAL DIAGNOSIS OF HYPERCALCAEMIA
High PTH
Primary or tertiary hyperparathyroidism

Low PTH
Malignancy (lung, breast, kidney, ovary,
nasopharynx, myeloma, lymphoma,
oesophagus)
Granulomas (sarcoid, TB, leprosy,
histoplasmosis)
Drugs (lithium, vitamin A, vitamin D, milk
alkali, oestrogens, thiazides)
Endocrine (thyrotoxicosis, phaeochromocytoma,
VIPoma, addisonian crisis)
Also beware a low albumin level (calcium needs
correction), and prolonged cuffing prior to
blood collection

Familial hypocalciuric hypercalcaemia may also
mimic hyperparathyroidism, with an
inappropriately raised PTH. There are no
symptoms, however, and urinary calcium is
low (urinary calcium:creatinine clearance
ratio < 0.01)

TREATMENT
Surgery if any of the following:

Ca > 2.9 mmol/L
Osteopenia > 2.5 SD below normal on DEXA scan
Age < 50 years
Reduced creatinine clearance (30% or more)
Symptomatic disease
Urinary calcium > 10 mmol/24 hours

Surgery can be performed via a minimlly
invasive approach in some patients (if ultrasound
and technetium scanning both localize a single
adenoma
    Otherwise, the disease may be observed.
6-monthly calcium, yearly creatinine and DEXA
scanning every 2–3 years are advised. 25%
require surgery over a 10-year period

Bisphosphonates have been used in those not fit
for surgery

QUESTION SPOTTING
The old saying 'bones, stones, abdominal groans
and psychic moans' is still relevant, but most
cases are now picked up on routine blood
testing, and are often asymptomatic elderly
women
Look for evidence of MEN if you suspect
hyperparathyroidism

Pitfalls in interpreting raised calcium:

Check that specimen is uncuffed and that calcium
value is corrected for albumin level
Check that PTH was taken at same time as
calcium, and that calcium level was not falling
at the time
Check that urinary calcium is also raised before
diagnosing primary hyperparathyroidism

CARCINOID SYNDROME

Episodic release of 5-HT and other neuroendocrine mediators from tumours. The tumours are derived from neural crest cells, and often follow an indolent clinical course. They are usually found in the GI tract (90%) or in the lung (10%). Gut tumours cannot usually cause the carcinoid syndrome unless they have metastasized to the liver, as the liver is able to metabolize vasoactive mediators released into the portal vein by gut tumours. As a result, only 5–10% of carcinoid tumours produce the carcinoid syndrome.

Diversion of tryptophan away from niacin production into producing 5-HT can lead to pellagra in chronic cases.

SYMPTOMS OF AN ATTACK
Flushing precipitated by alcohol
Wheezing
Dizziness

Other symptoms
Diarrhoea
Nausea, vomiting
Abdominal pain, especially RUQ pain
Dermatitis

SIGNS OF AN ATTACK
Tachycardia
Hypotension
Facial oedema

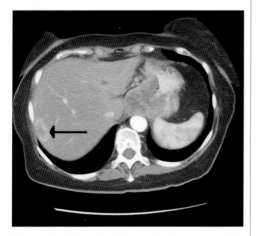

Figure 6.8 CT of the abdomen showing a carcinoid liver metastasis. This would give rise to the carcinoid syndrome.

Other signs
Telangiectasia
Red/blue discoloration of face
RUQ tenderness, hepatomegaly (from metastases)
Dermatitis (from pellagra)
Depression, psychosis, tremor (from pellagra)
Abdominal mass (unusual)
Tricuspid regurgitation and/or pulmonary stenosis (up to 50% of those with syndrome)
RV failure

N.B.: Bronchial carcinoids give rise to left-sided valve lesions

Other features
Arthritis
Sclerotic bone metastases (unusual)

INVESTIGATIONS
FBC
Usually normal unless GI bleeding

U + Es
Usually normal

LFTs
May all be raised (metastases)

Echocardiography may demonstrate valvular lesions
US or CT abdomen may demonstrate liver metastases
CT thorax useful if symptomatic but no liver involvement; may show bronchial carcinoid
^{123}I-MIBG tracer scan: can show presence of metastases anywhere in the body

DIAGNOSIS
24-hour urine collection showing raised levels of 5-HIAA. Need to avoid certain fruits prior to collection

ASSOCIATIONS
Cushing's syndrome (some tumours also secrete ACTH)
MEN type 1

DIFFERENTIAL DIAGNOSIS
Anxiety attacks
Perimenopausal symptoms

Paroxysmal tachycardia
Phaeochromocytoma
VIPoma
Other causes of right-sided heart lesion (e.g. endocarditis, rheumatic fever, amphetamine use, pulmonary hypertension)

TREATMENT

Surgery or embolization to bronchial tumours or solitary liver metastases. Rarely, liver transplant may be used successfully
Octreotide improves symptoms in 70%. Interferon alpha is an alternative – with significant side-effects
Nicotinamide to prevent pellagra
Radiotherapy may help pain from bone metastases. ^{131}I-MIBG is available in a few centres and may reduce tumour bulk
Chemotherapy is ineffective

PROGNOSIS

5-year median survival; some patients may survive for up to 20 years

QUESTION SPOTTING

Suspect carcinoid with:

Any right-sided heart lesion
Flushing episodes with low BP (compare with phaeochromocytoma, which elevates blood pressure)
Unexplained episodes of diarrhoea

DIABETES INSIPIDUS

A condition caused by either failure of the posterior pituitary to produce sufficient antidiuretic hormone (ADH) – cranial diabetes insipidus, or resistance of the kidney to the effects of ADH – nephrogenic diabetes insipidus. ADH acts on the collecting ducts to increase reabsorption of free water – failure of this system therefore leads to passing of large volumes of dilute urine, with resultant haemoconcentration.

CAUSES OF CRANIAL DI

Head injury
Post pituitary surgery
Tumour (e.g. pituitary macroadenoma, craniopharyngioma)
Cerebral infarction/haemorrhage
Sarcoidosis
Meningitis
Histiocytosis X
Can also occur as part of DIDMOAD syndrome (diabetes insipidus, diabetes mellitus, optic atropy and deafness)
Pregnancy (caused by placental vasopressinase)

Causes of nephrogenic DI:

High calcium
Low potassium
Drugs – especially lithium, demeclocycline
Chronic renal impairment
Renal tubulointerstitial disease
Inherited mutation in the aquaporin channel

SYMPTOMS

Thirst
Polyuria
Polydipsia
Nocturia
Dizziness, confusion, weakness may occur due to dehydration

SIGNS

Poor skin turgor and dry mucous membranes (if dehydration occurs)
Postural hypotension
Full bladder

INVESTIGATIONS
FBC
Hb may be high if dehydrated
WCC and Plts normal

U + Es
Na often elevated
K usually normal
Urea elevated if dehydrated
Creatinine usually normal unless underlying renal disease

LFTs
Usually normal

Calcium
Usually normal – may be elevated if severe dehydration
Glucose
Usually normal
Plasma osmolality is elevated
Urine osmolality is low; urinary sodium is also low

Skull X-ray
Normal unless previous macroadenoma has caused enlargement of the sella

MRI brain
May show reduced signal of posterior pituitary on T1-weighted images. May also show evidence of pituitary mass or bleed as a cause for posterior pituitary dysfunction

DIAGNOSIS
Is by water deprivation test. The patient is deprived of water for up to 8 hours; weight, urine output, plasma osmolality and urine osmolality are monitored. The test is stopped if more than 3% of body weight is lost
Normal response: urine output tails off; urine osmolality rises (usually to above 600 mOsm/kg) as plasma osmolality rises above normal (295 mOsm/kg)
Diabetes insipidus: urine output fails to tail off; urine osmolality stays low despite high plasma osmolality
If DI is diagnosed, a dose of DDAVP is then given and the test is continued for a further 4–6 hours. If urine osmolality rises and

urine volumes decrease, this suggests
cranial DI

Results are often not clearcut and may be
difficult to interpret. An alternative test is to
infuse hypertonic saline and chart the change
in plasma vasopressin levels

DIFFERENTIAL DIAGNOSIS

Psychogenic polydipsia
Hypercalcaemia
Hypokalaemia
Hyperglycaemia
Diuretic use
Alcohol ingestion

Note that drugs (especially lithium,
demeclocycline) can cause nephrogenic DI

COMPLICATIONS

Dehydration and electrolyte disturbance – may
be life-threatening in severe cases
Bladder distension and hydronephrosis

TREATMENT

Cranial DI can usually be treated by using
DDAVP – a synthetic analogue of vasopressin.

This can be administered nasally or orally.
Nephrogenic DI does not respond to this
therapy and can be very difficult to treat; treat
the underlying cause if possible

If patients are unwell, rehydrate using dextrose to
replace the lost free water and administer
DDAVP if cranial DI

PROGNOSIS

Quality of life is often reduced by DI. Prognosis
is good as long as fluid intake is not
compromised by intercurrent illness or frailty

QUESTION SPOTTING

Patients will often have had pituitary surgery or
trauma – you may be given the results of a water
deprivation test as part of the question. Take care
not to confuse diabetes insipidus with SIADH –
they are opposite conditions! Thirst and polydipsia
accompanied by elevated sodium suggest DI and
its differential diagnosis.

GRAVES DISEASE

An autoimmune condition in which stimulating autoantibodies bind to TSH receptors on the thyroid gland, causing enhanced release of thyroxine. Antibodies also cross-react with antigens in the retro-orbital area, causing restriction of extraocular muscle movement and proptosis. The condition is linked to the HLA DR3/B8 genotype, as are many other organ-specific autoimmune diseases. There is a 7:1 female-to-male preponderance, with most diagnoses being made between the ages of 30 and 50.

SYMPTOMS
Heat intolerance
Weight loss
Increased appetite
Tremor
Throat pain
Palpitations
Sweats
Anxiety
Tiredness/weakness
Diarrhoea
Diplopia
Sore eyes
Itching
Amenorrhoea

SIGNS
Thyroid enlargement/tenderness
Lid lag
Proptosis*
Oedema around the eyes*
Ophthalmoplegia*
Tachycardia/atrial fibrillation
Tremor
Hyperreflexia
Sweating
Warm peripheries
Proximal myopathy
Pretibial myxoedema* (uncommon)
Thyroid acropachy* (rare)
*Suggest Graves disease as opposed to other causes of hyperthyroidism

INVESTIGATIONS
FBC
Usually normal. Hb may be low

U + Es
Usually normal

LFTs
Usually normal

ECG shows sinus tachycardia; may show atrial fibrillation

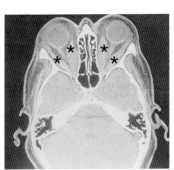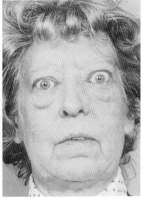

Figure 6.9 CT scan through orbits in case of exophthalmos. Note oedematous and enlarged extraocular muscle. (Reproduced with permission from Souhami, Moxham (2002) *Textbook of Medicine*, 4th edn. Churchill Livingstone.)

DIAGNOSIS

Is made on thyroid function tests – suppressed TSH level and raised T_4 level – along with a technetium thyroid scan showing diffuse enhanced uptake of tracer. Confirmation may be sought by screening for thyroid peroxidase antibodies and antithyroglobulin antibodies.

A few patients will have suppressed TSH but normal T_4 levels; T_3 is usually elevated in such cases (T_3 toxicosis).

DIFFERENTIAL DIAGNOSIS

Other causes of hyperthyroidism: toxic
  multinodular goitre, thyroid adenoma, early
  stages of thyroiditis
Anxiety
Phaeochromocytoma (tachycardia, sweats)
Malignancy (weight loss)
Drug abuse (e.g. cocaine)

COMPLICATIONS

Thyroid storm – severe tachycardia,
  hyperpyrexia, multiorgan failure, delirium/
  coma and seizures may occur
Atrial fibrillation
Thyrotoxic periodic paralysis (rare – affects those
  of South-east Asian descent)
Late hypothyroidism after treatment

ASSOCIATIONS

Other HLA DR3/B8 group autoimmune
  diseases, e.g.:
IDDM
Pernicious anaemia
Vitiligo

TREATMENT

Initial treatment is to block the effects of thyroxine using beta-blockers – usually propranolol (also slows conversion of T_4 to T_3), followed by chemical block of T_4 synthesis using carbimazole or propylthiouracil. Note that carbimazole and propylthiouracil cause agranulocytosis in 0.1% of patients

Definitive treatment may comprise:

Medical: partial blockade with dose of
  carbimazole or propylthiouracil titrated to T_4
  level, or block and replace (high-dose
  carbimazole/propylthiouracil with exogenous
  thyroxine added back in). After 18 months,
  treatment may be withdrawn, but relapse occurs
  in 50% of patients. Medical therapy is safe to
  use in pregnancy – propylthiouracil is usually
  used, and this is present at lower concentrations
  than carbimazole in breast milk
Radioiodine: ^{131}I can be given to ablate the
  thyroid partially. Although this is effective,
  hypothyroidism is a late complication,
  occurring in 10% at 1 year but often taking
  years to occur. Exacerbation of eye disease
  appears to be more common after radioiodine.
  Radioiodine cannot be used in pregnancy
Surgery: judging the amount of tissue to excise
  is difficult, and hypothyroidism often occurs
  after surgery, although this may not occur
  for several years. Other side-effects include
  recurrent laryngeal nerve damage and
  hypoparathyroidism. Medical therapy
  is needed to control hyperthyroidism prior to
  surgery in order to avoid a thyroid storm
Eye disease: if eye disease is severe,
  prednisolone can be used to reduce
  inflammation. An alternative for refractory
  disease is radiotherapy, with surgery being
  reserved for patients with threatened optic
  nerve compression. Lid surgery can be a useful
  adjunct if the cornea cannot be covered due to
  proptosis. If diplopia persists despite resolution
  of active inflammation, surgery to realign the
  ocular muscles may be required
Thyroid storm: manage in a high-dependency
  setting. Give propranolol, steroids, IV fluids
  (may need a CVP line as high-output cardiac
  failure is often a problem). Block the thyroid
  with propylthiouracil, then give Lugol's iodine
  to reduce release of thyroxine – failure to
  block thyroid first will lead to increased
  synthesis of thyroxine due to the abundance
  of iodine

PROGNOSIS

Excellent when treated. Thyroid storm is rare, but has up to a 50% mortality.

QUESTION SPOTTING

The diagnosis is likely to be obvious from the history; the questions are more likely to revolve around interpreting thyroid function tests, managing severe thyroid dysfunction or choosing a therapeutic modality. Watch for thyroid storm if presented with a very unwell person – look for a very rapid pulse, history of weight loss, fever > 40°C without an obvious source of infection, and a precipitant, such as surgery or radiotherapy without adequate thyroid blockade.

TURNER'S SYNDROME

Turner's syndrome is a genetic disease caused by failure to inherit the correct complement of sex chromosomes – the karyotype is 45 XO (i.e. only one X chromosome is inherited). A few cases have an incomplete or non-functional Y chromosome. Approximately 1 per 2500 women are affected.

CLINICAL FEATURES

Female phenotype
Short stature (short arms and legs)
Short fourth metacarpals
Webbed neck
Shield chest with immature breasts
Increased carrying angle at elbow (cubitus valgus)
Lymphoedema
May have a high arched palate
Cataracts, squint, ptosis

Cardiovascular problems

Coarctation of the aorta (leading to hypertension, radiofemoral delay)
Bicuspid aortic valve (may have associated murmur or signs of aortic stenosis later in life)
Aortic root dilatation and dissection
Partial anomalous venous drainage

Endocrine problems

Primary amenorrhoea
Hypothyroidism
Diabetes mellitus (increased risk of type 1 and type 2)

Other

Horseshoe kidney
Renal collecting system abnormalities
Osteoporosis

INVESTIGATIONS

FBC

Normal

U + Es

Normal unless chronic renal impairment due to diabetes, hypertension or chronic infection

LFTs

Normal

Other

Glucose may be elevated
Thyroid function tests may show high TSH and low T_4
FH/LSH usually very high in adulthood

ECG

May show left ventricular hypertrophy

CXR

May show abnormalities of aortic root

DIAGNOSIS

Is by karyotyping – this will show the XO pattern that is diagnostic of the disease. A blood sample or a cheek scrape can be used; prenatal diagnosis via amniocentesis is also possible.

DIFFERENTIAL DIAGNOSIS

Noonan's syndrome has similar manifestations but can affect males as well. Intellectual impairment and bleeding diatheses are sometimes seen; the karyotype in Noonan's syndrome is normal but the disease is transmitted in an autosomal-dominant manner
Other causes of primary amenorrhoea

COMPLICATIONS

Sequelae of hypertension
Aortic dissection
Renal infections and chronic renal impairment
Infertility
Diabetes mellitus
Hypothyroidism

TREATMENT

Oestrogen replacement – low doses help to develop secondary sexual characteristics. Menstruation often occurs after oestrogen replacement but this does not usually result in fertility

Growth hormone – relatively large doses are used to increase growth and final height

IVF can be used to allow pregnancy to occur

Control of hypertension

PROGNOSIS

Rates of cardiovascular death are three times higher than in the general population

QUESTION SPOTTING

Consider the diagnosis if someone presents with primary amenorrhoea. Another possible circumstance is associated with hypertension due to coarctation of the aorta. Also consider the diagnosis in early-presenting aortic stenosis.

KLINEFELTER'S SYNDROME

Klinefelter's syndrome is a genetic disease caused by failure to inherit the correct complement of sex chromosomes – the karyotype is 47 XXY (i.e. male, with an extra X chromosome inherited). Approximately 1 per 1000 men are affected.

CLINICAL FEATURES
Male phenotype
Low libido
Impotence
Sparse body hair
Fatigue
Long arms and legs
High-pitched voice
Mitral valve prolapse
Venous insufficiency and venous ulceration
Small testes
Gynaecomastia
Infertility
Osteoporosis
Intellectual impairment (not uncommon but often mild)

INVESTIGATIONS
FBC
Normal

U + Es
Normal

LFTs
Normal

Glucose normal
Thyroid function tests normal
FH/LSH usually very high in adulthood
Low testosterone levels with poor response to HCG administration

ECG
Usually normal

CXR
Usually normal

Echocardiography
May show mitral valve prolapse and mitral regurgitation

DIAGNOSIS
Is by karyotyping – this will show the XXY pattern that is diagnostic of the disease.
A blood sample or a cheek scrape can be used; prenatal diagnosis via amniocentesis is also possible.

DIFFERENTIAL DIAGNOSIS
Other causes of hypogonadism
Castration
Prolactinoma
Hypopituitarism
Kallman's syndrome
5 alpha-reductase deficiency
Anorchia
Other karyotypes can occur, e.g. 46 XX with Klinefelter phenotype; 48 XXXY
Consider drug therapy, liver disease, renal impairment, hyperthyroidism, prolactinoma and germ cell tumours as a differential for gynaecomastia

COMPLICATIONS
Increased incidence of germ cell tumours
Infective endocarditis on prolapsing mitral valve
Increased risk of breast cancer

TREATMENT
Is with testosterone replacement, starting at puberty. This does not lead to recovery of fertility

PROGNOSIS
Thought to have a normal lifespan. Testosterone therapy can help normalize the phenotype and thus aid the psychosocial distress that the syndrome can produce

QUESTION SPOTTING
Most likely to crop up as a differential for hypogonadism – look for tall individuals, small testes, lack of body hair and gynaecomastia.

Diabetes mellitus is caused by a relative or absolute lack of insulin. Type 1 diabetes is due to autoimmune destruction of the pancreatic islet beta cells; type 2 diabetes is due to a combination of peripheral insulin resistance and relative lack of insulin production by the beta cells. Over 2% of individuals in the western world have diabetes; 90% of these have type 2 DM.

SYMPTOMS
Thirst
Tiredness
Polyuria
Poor appetite (usually only with very high glucose)
Blurred vision
DKA may present with:
Drowsiness and confusion
Nausea and vomiting
Breathlessness
Abdominal pain
Hyperosmolar state may present with similar symptoms

SIGNS
Poor skin turgor
Cachexia (type 1 DM)
Ketones on breath (type 1 DM)
Diabetic emergencies:
Tachycardia
Hypotension
Pyrexia or hypothermia
Rapid respiratory rate (type 1 DM)
Confusion

INVESTIGATIONS
FBC
Hb elevated if dehydrated
WCC elevated in DKA
Plts usually normal

U + Es
Na may be low, normal or elevated in DKA. Invariably high in hyperosmolar states
K may be normal, low or elevated in DKA
Urea and creatinine raised if chronic renal impairment or dehydrated

Calcium: usually normal
Glucose: elevated
Amylase: may be mildly elevated in DKA
HbA1c: elevated

ECG
May show left ventricular hypertrophy; signs of old myocardial infarction

Urine
Glycosuria present if not well controlled.
Ketones may be present (especially in type 1 DM) if not well controlled

DIAGNOSIS
Diabetes is diagnosed by typical symptoms plus:

- Random glucose > 11.1 mmol/L or
- Fasting glucose > 7.0 mmol/L or
- Glucose level 2 hours after 75 g glucose tolerance test > 11.1 mmol/L

In asymptomatic patients, two readings taken on separate occasions are required to establish the diagnosis
Diabetic ketoacidosis is diagnosed by:

- Elevated glucose
- pH < 7.3
- Presence of ketones in blood

Hyperosmolar non-ketotic state is diagnosed by:

- Very high glucose
- High calculated plasma osmolality (> 320 mOsm/kg)
- Few ketones in blood

pH usually normal unless lactic acidosis or acute renal failure supervenes

DIFFERENTIAL DIAGNOSIS
Diabetes insipidus
Hypercalcaemia
Hypokalaemia
Renal tubular defect (as a cause of glycosuria)
Vasculitides (neuropathy and nephropathy)

Also consider possible underlying conditions:
Cushing's syndrome; exogenous steroids
Glucagonoma
Acromegaly

For diabetic emergencies:
Systemic sepsis
Acute abdomen
Respiratory infection, pulmonary embolism
Lactic acidosis; renal failure, drug intoxication
(as differential for metabolic acidosis)

COMPLICATIONS
Metabolic
Diabetic ketoacidosis (type 1 DM)
Hyperosmolar non-ketosis (type 2 DM)
Hypoglycaemia

Vascular
Ischaemic heart diseae
Peripheral vascular disease
Stroke
Diabetic cardiomyopathy
Impotence

Neurological
Sensory neuropathy (glove-and-stocking sensory
loss)
Diabetic amyotrophy
Acute painful neuropathy
Mononeuritis (e.g. cranial nerve palsies,
mononeuritis multiplex)
Autonomic neuropathy

Dermatological
Necrobiosis lipoidica (affecting shins)
Granuloma annulare
Xanthomata
Ulceration

Other
Diabetic nephropathy leading to renal failure
Diabetic retinopathy and visual loss
Recurrent infections, e.g. skin boils, *Candida*
infection
Charcot's joints (from neuropathy and
consequent damage)
Diabetic cheirarthropathy

TREATMENT
Type 1
Dietary modification plus insulin

Type 2
Dietary modification and weight loss. If this fails
to normalize blood sugar, add in metformin
(especially if overweight), sulphonylureas. If

these measures fail, consider adding in a
glitazone. If all of these fail, switch to insulin
(with metformin if overweight). Acarbose is
another possible therapy, but is often poorly
tolerated due to gastrointestinal side-effects.

With both types of diabetes, careful attention
should also be paid to:

Blood pressure: aim for 130/80 mmHg or better
Lipids: aggressive treatment with statins – aim
for LDL < 2.0 mmol/L and total cholesterol
< 4.0 mmol/L
Eyesight: yearly screening via retinal photography
Peripheral nerve function:
Renal function: check U + Es, check for
microalbuminuria
Foot care: regular podiatry input, especially if
peripheral neuropathy present

Diabetic ketoacidosis
Treat with rapid IV saline, potassium replacement,
and IV insulin, starting at 6 U/h. Aim to replace
5 L over 12–16 hours. Look for a precipitant (e.g.
infection) and treat. Patients may require NG tube
if drowsy (gastric stasis). If still acidotic and
ketotic despite normal glucose, give dextrose and
continue insulin to switch off ketogenesis. Cardiac
monitoring, and regular checks on potassium and
acid–base status are needed.

Hyperosmolar non-ketotic state
Treat with IV saline (despite very high initial
Na), IV insulin starting at 3 U/h. Aim to replace
fluids (5–10 L) over a longer period – 24–36
hours. Glucose may fall very quickly. A serious
underlying illness often precipitates the condition
– look for MI, stroke, infection and treat. Some
authorities suggest full-dose heparin as the risk of
thromboembolism is high.

PROGNOSIS
Life expectancy is considerably reduced in both
forms of the disease. Diabetes is the commonest
reason for requiring dialysis in the UK, and is a
leading reason for requiring lower-limb
amputation.

DKA has a good prognosis – mortality rates are
< 2%. Hyperosmolar state has a mortality of 20–
50%; most sufferers are old and frail, and often
have a serious underlying precipitant illness.

151

QUESTION SPOTTING

Diabetes is common and easy to diagnose. Questions will therefore often revolve around treatment decisions, e.g. how to optimize glycaemic control; how to treat diabetic emergencies. Also consider whether there is an underlying cause for the diabetes, e.g. Cushing's.

NEUROLOGY

7

SUBDURAL HAEMATOMA

Tearing of the veins in the arachnoid space, leading to accumulation of blood in the subdural space. Trauma is often mild, and is not recalled in 50% of patients with chronic subdural. The elderly, alcoholics, epileptics and those with cognitive impairment are especially at risk. Those taking anticoagulants are also at increased risk. Severe head trauma can produce acute, massive subdural bleeding.

SYMPTOMS

Headache (25%)
Vomiting (10%)
Drowsiness – may be intermittent
Limb weakness
Mood or personality change
Incontinence

SIGNS

Limb weakness/posturing (50%)
Dysphasia (20%)
Unequal pupils (15%)
Cranial nerve palsies (10–15%)

Fits (5–10%)
Extensor plantars (uncommon)

INVESTIGATIONS
FBC
Usually normal

U + Es
Usually normal

LFTs
Deranged in alcoholics
INR raised if on anticoagulants or alcoholic

SXR may show skull fracture – uncommon
CT brain shows bright crescent if haematoma; appears isodense with brain after 1–2 weeks (Fig. 7.1)

DIAGNOSIS
Is made on CT scan result. Beware missing the diagnosis when the blood is isodense with brain on CT at 1–2 weeks

DIFFERENTIAL DIAGNOSIS
Intracranial tumour
Thromboembolic CVA
Subarachnoid haemorrhage
Extradural haematoma
Metabolic derangement (renal failure, liver failure, infection)
Cerebral abscess
Fits

TREATMENT
Surgical evacuation of haematoma if focal signs, low GCS or significant midline shift – many older patients are not fit for surgery however
Small haematomas may resolve spontaneously

PROGNOSIS
Moderate to good outcome in 80% of patients with chronic subdural haematoma – many older patients do not recover fully, however
Worse outcome with lower GCS
Acute massive subdural bleeding has a 20–50% mortality rate

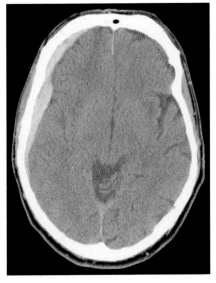

Figure 7.1 CT of the brain showing acute subdural haematoma.

QUESTION SPOTTING

Consider in any patient with neurological signs or reduced GCS, especially if:

They are on warfarin

They are elderly

There is a history of falls

They are alcoholic

A fluctuating level of consciousness or confusion is another pointer to the diagnosis

NEUROFIBROMATOSIS

Loss of function by mutations in one of the two NF tumour suppressor genes. The disease is inherited in an autosomal-dominant manner, but is expressed in different ways in different individuals – a wide variety of gene mutations has been described. NF 1 affects 1 in 3000 births; NF 2 affect 1 in 30 000 births.

FEATURES (TYPE 1)
Diagnostic
1. Café-au-lait spots (> 5, > 15 mm in adults)
2. Two or more Lisch nodules in iris
3. Axillary freckling
4. Cutaneous neurofibromas, plexiform neurofibromas
5. Bone deformity and fractures, pseudoarthrosis
6. Optic glioma

Body habitus
Relative macrocephaly
Relative short stature
Kyphoscoliosis
Limb gigantism

Other neoplasms
Phaeochromocytoma
Carcinoid
CNS tumours
Neurofibromas of the spine, nerve roots and cranial nerves
Juvenile CML
Rhabdomyosarcoma
Wilm's tumour

Other neurological manifestations
May have reduced higher cerebral function (up to 40%)
Glaucoma
Migrainous headaches
Epilepsy

Other systems
Arterial aneurysms
Renal artery stenosis: hypertension
GI bleeding, GI obstruction (neurofibromas)
Pulmonary fibrosis

FEATURES (TYPE 2)
Bilateral acoustic neuromas
Meningiomas
Schwannomas: cranial nerve, spinal, paraspinal

Gliomas, e.g. brainstem, cerebellum
Posterior lens opacification; cataract
Skin lesions (schwannomas or neurofibromas)
Retinal hamartomas
Peripheral neuropathy
Café-au-lait spots (usually < 5)

INVESTIGATIONS
FBC
Usually normal

U + Es
Usually normal

LFTs
Usually normal

CXR may show rib notching, normal or large lung fields. Neurofibromas may be visible.
MRI may reveal intracranial tumours, spinal tumours, and multiple high-signal areas (NF 1) of unknown aetiology
PFTs show normal FEV_1 and FVC with reduced TLco

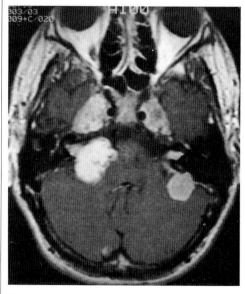

Figure 7.2 MRI of the brain showing multiple intracranial tumours in type 2 neurofibromatosis. (Reproduced with permission from Forbes, Jackson (2003) *Colour Atlas and Text of Clinical Medicine*, 3rd edn. Mosby.)

DIAGNOSIS

For NF 1

Two of features (1) to (6), listed above, or one plus an affected first-degree relative

For NF 2

Bilateral acoustic neuroma

or

Affected first-degree relative plus unilateral acoustic neuroma

or

Affected first-degree relative or unilateral acoustic neuroma or multiple meningiomas plus two of:

Meningioma
Glioma
Schwannoma
Neurofibroma
Posterior lens opacity in childhood

DIFFERENTIAL DIAGNOSIS

This depends on the context of the question. Possibilities are:

MEN 2 (for phaeochromocytoma)
Noonan's syndrome

For normal lung volumes with reduced TLco, consider:

Tuberous sclerosis
Lymphangioleiomyomatosis
Histiocytosis X

COMPLICATIONS

Plexiform neurofibromas may transform into sarcomatous lesions
Cutaneous neurofibromas almost never do
Renal artery stenosis and phaeochromocytoma may lead to hypertension
Most complications are due to mass effects from tumours (e.g. cord compression, intracranial mass effects) and skeletal malformation/fracture

TREATMENT

No treatment is curative; treatment is directed against specific lesions as they arise. Regular follow-up from birth or diagnosis is essential – this should include regular ophthalmological screening.

PROGNOSIS

Reduced life expectancy due to occurrence of tumours

QUESTION SPOTTING

Any previous neurological tumour should raise suspicion of neurofibromatosis, especially the presence of an acoustic neuroma
Also consider the diagnosis in a patient with what sounds like a phaeochromocytoma
Neurofibromatosis is also a cause of large lungs with a reduced transfer factor

BENIGN INTRACRANIAL HYPERTENSION (PSEUDOTUMOUR CEREBRI)

Raised intracranial pressure in the absence of an intracranial mass lesion, and no enlargement of the ventricles due to hydrocephalus. The CSF composition is normal. The cause is unknown in most cases, but it is important to exclude sagittal sinus thrombosis which may be associated with:

SLE
Pregnancy
Oral contraceptive pill
Essential thrombocythaemia
Protein S deficiency
Antithrombin III deficiency
Antiphospholipid syndrome
Paroxysmal nocturnal haemoglobinuria
Behçet's disease
Meningeal sarcoidosis
Mastoiditis

However, other drugs and conditions may predispose to benign intracranial hypertension per se, without obstruction to venous outflow.
   These include:

Hypovitaminosis A
Hypervitaminosis A
Empty sella syndrome
Drugs such as nalidixic acid, nitrofurantoin, corticosteroids and tetracyclines

A likely mechanism of disease is a reduction in the reabsorption of CSF by the arachnoid villi, although proof for this is lacking
   Benign intracranial hypertension is a rare disorder that is more common in women (over 90% being overweight) and particularly affects those between 18 and 40 years old

SYMPTOMS
Headache – throbbing, worse on waking, straining, coughing and sneezing
Visual disturbances
Transient and permanent visual loss
Photopsia – flashing lights
Blurring
Scotomata – enlarged blind spots are common
Diplopia due to sixth cranial nerve palsy (false localizing sign)

Colour vision is affected early in the disease
Pulsatile tinnitus
Retrobulbar pain

Note that cognitive function is preserved and seizures are rare, unlike mass lesions, hydrocephalus and viral and bacterial meningoencephalopathy

SIGNS
Papilloedema is almost always present – may be unilateral

INVESTIGATIONS
FBC
Normal

U + Es
Normal

Other blood tests normal
Visual field analysis with formal perimetry – to look for blind-spot enlargement, and scotomas. Most common are arcuate defects, nasal steps and global constriction of the visual fields
Skull radiography is usually normal

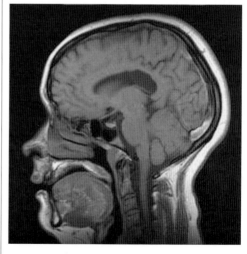

Figure 7.3 MRI of the brain showing dural sinus thrombus posteriorly.

DIAGNOSIS

CT head – should always be done before lumbar puncture

Shows normal or slit-like ventricles. Dural sinus thrombosis may be evident

LUMBAR PUNCTURE

Typically normal CSF composition, but with CSF pressure of > 20 cm H_2O. However, the opening pressure may be normal, but a continuous-pressure study may show pressure spikes

MR ANGIOGRAPHY (Fig. 7.3)

Sensitive for showing sinus thrombosis

DIFFERENTIAL DIAGNOSIS

Intracranial tumour
Sagittal sinus thrombosis
Subdural haematoma
Hydrocephalus
Sleep apnoea
Chronic meningitides (e.g. TB, cryptococcal)
SLE

TREATMENT

Aims to alleviate symptoms and preserve sight
Weight reduction – now of proven value
Carbonic anhydrase inhibitors, e.g. acetazolamide
Loop diuretics
Corticosteroids – beware of the complications in this group of already overweight patients

Repeat lumbar puncture – no proven benefit as the CSF pressure only remains low for about 1–2 hours after the puncture, but is still used on occasion

Surgical treatments

Lumboperitoneal shunt

Effective but complications of general anaesthesia, shunt obstruction and infection, amongst others, make this not without its risks

Optic nerve sheath fenestration

Fewer complications than lumboperitoneal shunt, but the procedure may cause blindness in the treated eye. Early improvement following this procedure may not be sustained. Patients must be followed up for several years with visual field perimetry in case of treatment failure

PROGNOSIS

BIH is not in fact benign. Permanent visual loss may be present in 50% and this may cause significant morbidity in as many as 10%. Although the symptoms of BIH tend to recede with time, the raised pressure may persist.

QUESTION SPOTTING

The typical question will include an obese women aged 20–40 years with visual symptoms or headaches. Dural sinus thrombosis and intracranial mass should be actively looked for. You are most likely to be asked questions regarding investigation, possibly in a patient with papilloedema.

Muscle weakness and fatiguability caused by autoimmune antiacetylcholine receptor antibodies that block the postsynaptic receptors at the neuromuscular junction as well as reducing their numbers. Although the mechanism is now well understood, the aetiology is not. There is a strong association with thymic abnormalities. Most are thymic hyperplasia, while the rest are thymomas. Thymectomy results in clinical improvement in many patients. A viral trigger has been suggested but has never been proven. The most promising theory is that the antibodies are induced by an infectious agent that in part resembles the acetylcholine receptor, causing cross-reactivity. There is an association with HLA B7 and DR2 haplotypes.

Onset is bimodal, with a peak in the second and third decades affecting mostly women, and a late smaller peak in the sixth and seventh decades mostly affecting men.

SYMPTOMS

Muscle weakness and fatiguability
Double vision (only presenting feature in 15%)
Nasal speech
Choking
Difficulty chewing
Difficulty swallowing
Difficulty breathing – may be life-threatening
  (myasthenic crisis)

SIGNS

Diplopia – ocular muscles may be the only
  muscles affected
Ptosis
Nasal speech
Flat facial features
Proximal limb weakness – may affect the neck
  extensors
Head drooping
Muscle fatigability
Reflexes are preserved

INVESTIGATIONS
FBC
Normal

U + Es
Normal

LFTs
Normal

ESR normal
CRP normal
ANA may be positive
Rheumatoid factor may be positive
Thyroid function tests – may demonstrate
  autoimmune thyroid disease
Fasting blood glucose – may indicate diabetes

Chest X-ray
Thymic enlargement (Fig. 7.4)
CT or MRI chest
Enlargement of thymus
Spirometry
Vital capacity ↓ is an indication for
  plasmapheresis

DIAGNOSIS

Antiacetylcholine receptor antibodies are highly
  specific, but only 85% sensitive (less in pure
  ocular disease)
Single-fibre EMG with repetitive stimulation
  shows fatiguability

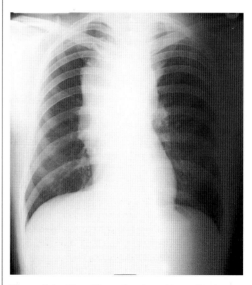

Figure 7.4 Chest X-ray showing wide mediastinum due to a thymoma. (Reproduced with permission from Forbes, Jackson (2003) *Colour Atlas and Text of Clinical Medicine*, 3rd edn. Mosby.)

Edrophonium (Tensilon) test should show clear improvement; the test is not always needed for diagnosis if clinical symptoms, EMG and antibodies suggest the diagnosis

DIFFERENTIAL DIAGNOSIS

Congenital myasthenic syndromes – rare
Drug-induced myasthenia, e.g. penicillamine (induces autoimmune myasthenia) or aminoglycosides, quinines, procainamide (exacerbation of myasthenia that recovers on drug withdrawal)
Hyperthyroidism – thyroid function should always be screened
Lambert–Eaton syndrome – may involve autonomic and sensory systems and rarely the extraorbital muscles
Guillain–Barré syndrome
Botulism
Progressive external ophthalmoplegia
Cranial masses causing ophthalmoplegia or cranial nerve palsies
Motor neurone disease

ASSOCIATIONS

There is an association with HLA B8 and HLA DR3 group autoimmune conditions, especially:

Graves disease
SLE
Rheumatoid arthritis
Pernicious anaemia

TREATMENT

Anticholinesterase drugs. Pyridostigmine. Cholinergic side-effects include diarrhoea and colic which may be reduced by simultaneous administration of propantheline

Thymectomy. Generally accepted that removal of thymus gives benefit to most patients with generalized myasthenia, and have evidence of thymic enlargement. Patients may show initial deterioration postoperatively, and so surgery should only be carried out electively in specialized centre. Plasmapheresis preoperatively should be carried out if the vital capacity is less than 2 L.

Steroids. Indicated in moderate to severe generalized disease and ocular myasthenia. Patients should be hospitalized due to common initial deterioration, which can be minimized by incrementing the dose. Bone protection is also needed

Azathioprine. Indicated if steroids fail or as a steroid-sparing agent. Action is very slow to begin, and may take up to a year to exert an effect

Ciclosporin. Same efficacy as azathioprine, but faster onset of action. This is balanced against frequent side-effects and high cost

Immunoglobulins and plasma exchange. Short-term treatment for myasthenic crisis or preoperatively. Exerts a rapid effect, but lasts only a few weeks. Immunoglobulin may have longer effects and does not require central venous access but is very expensive. Mechanism of action is not known

PROGNOSIS

Variable. If confined to the extraocular muscles, the prognosis is excellent
Young women tend to relapse early after thymectomy and elderly patients tend not to have remission at all

QUESTION SPOTTING

Usually the differential is with Guillain–Barré syndrome, or botulism. Look for clues such as worsening in the evenings. Initial muscle power is normal, and the reflexes are normal. There are never any sensory symptoms.

Other possibilities are myotonic dystrophy and bilateral third-nerve palsy. The disease may present as a myasthenic crisis triggered by a precipitant (e.g. gentamicin); the question may then revolve around management of the crisis.

MULTIPLE SCLEROSIS

Despite intensive research, much remains unknown about multiple sclerosis, but the main areas of investigation include lipid metabolism, autoimmunity and infection. The disease process centres around the destruction of myelin in the central nervous system (without involvement of the peripheral nervous system). This process may be either a direct immunological attack on the myelin sheath itself or on the oligodendrocyte cells which produce the myelin. These areas of demyelination known as plaques occur mainly in a perivenous and periventricular distribution and vary in size from 1 mm to 4 cm. There is weak linkage with HLA haplotype.

The pattern of disease is highly variable, making diagnosis and treatment difficult, but certain disease patterns seem to occur. The most common is the relapsing/remitting type – others include the acute, progressive and benign forms. Peak age for diagnosis is 20–40 years.

It is also likely that a subclinical form exists since demyelinated plaques can be seen at autopsy.

SYMPTOMS

Eye pain
Blurred vision
Double vision
Vertigo
Dizziness
Numbness
Weakness
Paraesthesia
Urinary retention or incontinence
Tremor – rare
Facial pain – trigeminal neuralgia – rare
Loss of memory – late

SIGNS

Reduced acuity
Blurred optic disc (usually unilateral)
Pale optic disc – starts in the temporal region of the discs
Nystagmus
Internuclear ophthalmoplegia
Increased muscular tone
Reduced muscular power
Increased reflexes and upgoing plantars

Positive Lhermitte's sign – tingling in the spine or limbs on neck flexion
Partial Brown-Séquard syndrome

INVESTIGATIONS
FBC
Normal

U + Es
Normal

LFTs
Normal

Vitamin B_{12} and folate normal

DIAGNOSIS
Is by clinical features (episodes separated in time and space), together with supporting evidence from:

CSF – IgG ↑ (oligoclonal bands on electrophoresis). Occasional ↑ IgM or IgA
Since low levels of immunoglobulin are seen in the CSF, contamination by blood is easy, and so it is useful to compare CSF with serum
MRI – multiple high signal plaques, particularly in the brainstem, and periventricular regions (Fig. 7.5). More sensitive than CT and now in

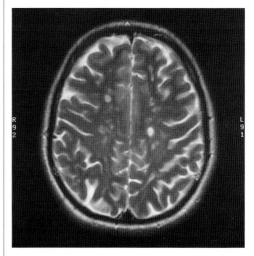

Figure 7.5 Multiple sclerosis. T2-weighted MRI of brain showing multiple areas of high attenuation typical of multiple sclerosis.

162

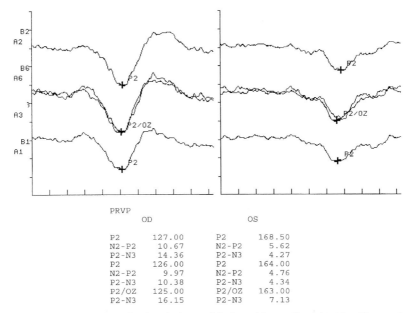

```
                              ms/div    uV/div
                              25.000     5.00

    A2 RO2 * VA :- N4.5 UC         B2 LO2 * VA :- N4.5 UC
    A6 ROZ * 2                     B6 LOZ * 2
    A3 ROZ * PATTERN REVERSAL      B3 LOZ * VISUAL EVOKED POTENTIAL
    A1 RO1 * HOWES N               B1 LO1 * 13 OCTOBER 95
```

PRVP

OD		OS	
P2	127.00	P2	168.50
N2-P2	10.67	N2-P2	5.62
P2-N3	14.36	P2-N3	4.27
P2	126.00	P2	164.00
N2-P2	9.97	N2-P2	4.76
P2-N3	10.38	P2-N3	4.34
P2/OZ	125.00	P2/OZ	163.00
P2-N3	16.15	P2-N3	7.13

Figure 7.6 Multiple sclerosis. The visual evoked potentials show delay on the right side with normal waveform and amplitude, and severe delay on the left.
Visual evoked potential (pattern) P100 latency
Right eye: 02 = 127.0 ms   Left eye: 02 = 168.5 ms
Right eye: 01 = 126.0 ms   Left eye: 01 = 164.0 ms
Right: delayed, good waveform and amplitude
Left: grossly delayed, good waveform and amplitude

routine use to assist in the diagnosis. Can be used to predict which patients with clinically isolated syndromes will progress to multiple sclerosis
Electrophysiological studies – visual, auditory and somatic sensory evoked potentials typically show delay without loss of amplitude

DIFFERENTIAL DIAGNOSIS

Brainstem and optic lesions may be seen in:

Sarcoid
Neurosyphilis
SLE
Behçet's disease

Spinal cord lesions may be confused with:
Cervical myelopathy with spondylosis (which may coexist)
Spinal cord compression
Subacute combined degeneration of the spinal cord
Other diseases which may cause diagnostic confusion:
Recurrent thromboembolic disease
Friedreich's ataxia
Acute disseminated encephalomyelitis
Neuromyelitis optica (Devic's syndrome)
Diffuse scleritis
Central pontine myelinolysis

TREATMENT

Supportive

Support groups

Physiotherapy

Baclofen, diazepam, or tizanidine for spasticity

Local injection of botulinum toxin can also be used

Corticosteroids have been shown to speed recovery from an acute relapse, but do not improve long-term outcome. High-dose oral steroids are probably as effective as intravenous

Interferon-beta may help in patients with relapsing–remitting disease

Glatiramer, intravenous immunoglobulins and azathioprine may all be of some benefit, but hyperbaric oxygen, linoleic acid supplements and a gluten-free diet have all been shown to be ineffective

Other treatments may be indicated such as sildenafil for erectile dysfunction, oxybutynin for bladder instability, isoniazid or clonazepam for ataxia and carbamazepine or amitriptyline for dysaesthesia

PROGNOSIS

Highly variable. Life expectancy is typically 20–30 years from onset of symptoms

20% of patients may have no second relapse after 15 years. 5% may show a rapidly progressive course with death within 5 years

QUESTION SPOTTING

Multiple sclerosis may be present in this form of question as part of the differential cause of complex neurological features. Remember it is the most common cause of neurological deficit that is separated in both place and time. It should always be considered as a diagnosis in patients presenting with painful blurring of one eye.

MYOTONIC DYSTROPHY

Autosomal-dominant disorder caused by increased trinucleotide repeats (AGC repeat) within the *DMPK* gene on chromosome 19. The number of repeats may increase from generation to generation, giving rise to increasingly severe disease (anticipation). The muscles involved are particularly those of the face, neck and distal extremities, but with increasing severity, more central muscles, including proximal limb muscles, muscles of the pharynx and larynx, and even the diaphragm may be involved. Myotonia is the inability of a contracted muscle group to relax quickly. Tends to present between 10 and 30 years of age, although features may be seen in the first decade.

CLINICAL FEATURES
Muscular features
Wasting of the involved muscles – gives a typical expressionless 'hatchet face' due to wasting of the temporalis, masseters and sternomastoids (prone to recurrent dislocation of jaw)
Bilateral ptosis
Myotonia
Weakness in the hands and wrists
Weakness of ankle dorsiflexion results in footdrop
Dysarthria
Dysphagia
Diaphragmatic weakness may lead to respiratory insufficiency
Diplopia if extraocular muscles involved (rare)

Endocrine
Impaired glucose tolerance or frank diabetes mellitus
Males: impotence, gonadal failure
Females: irregular menstruation and infertility

Cardiac
Conduction defects
AV block
RBBB
LBBB
Mitral valve prolapse
Cardiomyopathy
Sudden death

Gastrointestinal
Constipation
Diarrhoea
Abdominal cramps
Gallstones

Other
Frontal baldness
Cataracts – stellate
Somnolence
Progressive dementia
Hyperostosis of skull vault and small sella turcica
Abnormal immunoglobulin production may lead to increased infections

INVESTIGATIONS
FBC
Normal

U + Es
Normal

LFTs
May be elevated

Creatinine kinase – normal; (compare with myositis). May slightly ↑ late in the disease
IgG often ↓
Thyroid function normal

ECG
Conduction abnormalities including AV block, RBBB, LBBB

EEG
Often abnormal

DIAGNOSIS
EMG
Myotonic discharges – repetitive single motor unit potentials and low-amplitude short-duration, polyphasic motor unit potentials

Muscle biopsy
Typically type 1 muscle fibre atrophy. Occasional type 2 hypertrophy. Necrosis and degeneration are notably absent
Genetic testing for expanded repeats in the *DMPK* gene is now also available

DIFFERENTIAL DIAGNOSIS
Muscular dystrophies – Becker's muscular dystrophy, facioscapulohumeral muscular dystrophy

Polymyositis
Hypothyroidism

TREATMENT

Supportive – splints for footdrop
Myotonia may be treated with phenytoin; heated gloves may help
Methylphenidate or modafinil may be used for hypersomnolence
Cataract extraction if visual impairment.
Annual screening for diabetes and 12-lead ECG for conduction defects

PROGNOSIS

Highly variable. Younger onset of symptoms correlates with more severe disease. Sudden cardiac death occurs in 10–30% of patients. Respiratory failure occurs in 30% of patients due to muscle weakness and poor central drive.

QUESTION SPOTTING

Although more suited for PACES, myotonic dystrophy may appear in the written section. Typically, patients will be in their teens or 20s and will usually present with weakness or muscle stiffness (rather than myotonia). Look out for cardiac involvement and cataracts.

FRIEDREICH'S ATAXIA

Autosomal-recessive disease caused by expansion of trinucleotide repeats in the frataxin gene on chromosome 9q. The size of the repeat section correlates with the age of onset and the presence of cardiomyopathy and diabetes. The disease is characterized by neurodegeneration and cardiomyopathy. The neurodegeneration is thought to begin in the dorsal root ganglia, with loss of sensory neurones. Later, axonal sensory and motor neuropathy occur, with loss of the spinal tracts. There is cerebellar involvement with atrophy. Cognitive function is preserved throughout the disease. Mean age of onset is 14 years, with presentation usually before 25 years of age.

CLINICAL FEATURES
Neurological
Ataxia affecting gait and stance – often the first sign
Areflexia of legs (very rarely, increased reflexes)
Loss of vibration and position sense
Extensor plantars (65%)
Progressive muscular weakness and wasting with normal or decreased tone
Dysarthria (late) with hesitation and scanning speech
Optic atrophy (30%)
Retinitis pigmentosa
Sensorineural deafness
Bladder dysfunction
Flexor spasms (rare)
Loss of pain and light touch (10%)
Oculomotor disturbance – fixation instability, ↓ vestibulo-ocular reflex, jerky pursuit
Nystagmus (30%)

Non-neurological
Hypertrophic cardiomyopathy
Diabetes mellitus (10%)
Skeletal deformities (90%), e.g. pes cavus, equinovarus deformity, scoliosis

INVESTIGATIONS
FBC
Normal

U + Es
Normal
Glucose may be ↑

LFTs
Normal

Nerve conduction
Sensory potentials – reduced/absent (sensory axonal neuropathy)
Motor potentials – ↑ response or slowed conduction time
Visual, auditory and somatosensory evoked potentials show delay or absent potentials

CSF
Normal

ECG
T-wave inversion and non-specific changes

Echocardiography
Interventricular septal hypertrophy
Left ventricular hypertrophy
Reduced left ventricular dimensions
May see enlarged, hypokinetic ventricle in some cases

MRI
May confirm cerebellar atrophy

DIAGNOSIS
Is based on clinical features
PCR can show homozygosity for GAA repeat sequence

DIFFERENTIAL DIAGNOSIS
Hereditary motor-sensory neuropathies (no oculomotor disturbance, no cardiomyopathy and no dysarthria)
Refsum's disease
Vitamin E-deficiency ataxia
Ataxia-telangiectasia
Abetalipoproteinaemia
Multiple sclerosis
Myotonic dystrophy (as a cause of cardiomyopathy, diabetes and neurological dysfunction)

TREATMENT
Physiotherapy
Supportive treatments, including wheelchairs when required
Oral hypoglycaemics for diabetes

Corrective surgery for skeletal deformities

Propranolol has been used for hypertrophic cardiomyopathy; other therapies for HCM and dilated cardiomyopathy (e.g. antiarrhythmics) may be required

PROGNOSIS

Wheelchair-bound within 10–12 years, and death within 35 years is usual

QUESTION SPOTTING

The typical patient will be young and should show the cardinal features of progressive ataxia, lower-limb areflexia, reduced position or vibration sense in the lower limbs and dysarthria within 5 years of the onset of ataxia. These features are definitive for Friedreich's ataxia.

Note that Friedreich's ataxia is one of the causes of extensor plantars with absent tendon reflexes at the ankle.

GUILLAIN–BARRÉ SYNDROME

An acute polyneuropathy, usually demyelinating, which is thought to be caused by an autoimmune process triggered by a recent infection. It affects 2–3 per 100 000 per year, and usually takes the form of an ascending motor and sensory neuropathy which progresses over 1–3 weeks before beginning to resolve.

Agents that can trigger Guillain–Barré include:

Campylobacter jejuni
HIV
CMV
EBV
Enteroviruses
Mycoplasma species
Other upper respiratory tract pathogens
In 60% of cases, a prodromal illness (URTI or diarrhoea) precedes onset of symptoms by 1–2 weeks

SYMPTOMS
Limb weakness (usually starts in legs, and ascends)
Pain (usually in back)
Numbness, paraesthesia (usually distal)
Dizziness due to autonomic neuropathy
Constipation due to autonomic neuropathy
Nausea due to autonomic neuropathy
Sweating due to autonomic neuropathy

SIGNS
Tachycardia or bradycardia
Hypertension or hypotension (especially on standing)
Reduced muscle tone
Limb weakness
Reduced light touch/vibration/joint position sense
Reduced reflexes (may be preserved at first)
Papilloedema
Cranial nerve involvement (usually VII, less commonly bulbar, rarely ocular)
N.B.: Miller–Fisher variant (3%): ataxia, ophthalmoplegia plus reduced reflexes. Power is relatively spared in limbs
Diffuse cranial nerve involvement may also occur (polyneuritis cranialis)

INVESTIGATIONS
FBC
Usually normal

U + Es
Usually normal

LFTs
ALT ↓ (33%)
GGT ↓ (33%)

CK may be raised
ESR raised

Autoantibodies
GM1 positive in 25%. Associated with worse outcome
GQ1B associated with Miller–Fisher variant and ophthalmoplegia

CSF
Protein raised (may be normal in first 2 weeks)
WCC often normal. Almost always < 50 lymphocytes/cm

Nerve conduction studies usually show a demyelinating pattern. Some patients may display axonal loss with little or no evidence of demyelination

PFTs may show reduced FVC

DIAGNOSIS
Is primarily on clinical grounds. The presence of demyelination on nerve conduction studies, and a high protein with normal cell count in the CSF, are corroborating factors.

DIFFERENTIAL DIAGNOSIS
Drugs
e.g. neuromuscular junction blockers
Autoimmune
Myasthenia gravis
Eaton–Lambert syndrome
Vasculitis
Multiple sclerosis
Metabolic
Porphyria
Lead poisoning
Low K^+
High Mg^{2+}

Toxic
Snake/scorpion/fish toxins
Tick paralysis

Infection
Polio
Botulism

Other

Myopathy of critically ill (found in intensive-care patients)

COMPLICATIONS

Respiratory paralysis
Arrhythmias/cardiovascular instability
Pressure sores
Thromboembolic disease

TREATMENT

IV immunoglobulin for 5 days, unless illness mild or improving at diagnosis. Plasma exchange is an alternative
Subcutaneous heparin
Monitor FVC closely. If FVC < 20 ml/kg (approximately 1.5 L), consider elective intubation (needed in 25% of all patients)
Physiotherapy and later, occupational therapy
Analgesia for pain

PROGNOSIS

70–80% recover fully, although this may take months. Recovery usually starts within 2–4 weeks of onset
5–10% die, usually of cardiovascular problems, infection or thromboembolism
15% have some degree of significant residual disability

QUESTION SPOTTING

Usually occurs as a patient with rapid onset of weakness. Clues to the diagnosis are:

Relative sparing of the eye muscles
High CSF protein
Prominent autonomic symptoms
Prodromal illness

Consider the diagnosis in patients with a high CSF protein – especially if other constituents are normal or near normal. Protein may be up to 3–4 g/L; if it is above 4 g/L, consider Froin's syndrome (spinal block). The key management investigation is vital capacity – low vital capacity is an indication for ITU transfer

NORMAL-PRESSURE HYDROCEPHALUS

Normal-pressure hydrocephalus (NPH) is hydrocephalus in the absence of raised intracranial pressure (defined as 15 mmHg intracranial pressure). NPH may be caused by intracranial haemorrhage, head injury, intracranial surgery and meningitis, but 60% have no known cause. The mechanism of the disease is thought to be reduced reabsorption of CSF by the arachnoid villi. Despite the name, the intracranial pressure is not completely normal. There are transient increases in pressure, which may cause the ventricular enlargement.

The disease is rare in the under-60s. However it may occur as a consequence of one of the causes mentioned above. NPH is thought to account for as many as 5% of dementia in the older population; its true prevalence is unknown and other aetiologies for dementia often coexist.

CLINICAL FEATURES

Triad of (tend to occur in the given order):

Gait disturbance – slow, wide-based with short steps
Dementia – affects all function, including attention, memory, execution
Urinary incontinence

Other features include:

Apathy
Tremor (postural)
Increased tone in the legs
Hyperreflexia of the legs
Impairment of fine movement like handwriting
Dysphasia and apraxias are rare (compare with Alzheimer's disease)

INVESTIGATIONS
FBC
Normal

U + Es
Normal

LFTs
Normal

CSF
Normal composition

EEG
Normal

PET scanning using glucose markers shows hypometabolism (different pattern from Alzheimer's disease)

DIAGNOSIS

Intracranial pressure (ICP) monitoring shows peaks of pressure (B-waves) over a background of normal pressure. Drainage of 30–50 mL of CSF may cause clinical improvement
CT/MRI head shows hydrocephalus (Fig. 7.7) with no cause for obstruction to CSF flow. On T2 signal MRI periventricular oedema may be seen

DIFFERENTIAL DIAGNOSIS

Parkinson's disease – gait can appear similar
Alzheimer's disease – not associated with gait dysfunction in early stages
Multi-infarct dementia – neuroimaging should show evidence of infarction or ischaemia
Obstructive hydrocephalus

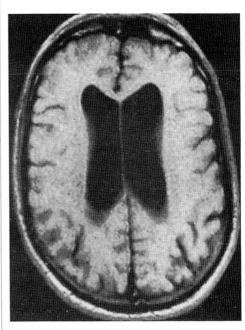

Figure 7.7 CT of the brain showing changes in normal-pressure hydrocephalus. Note gross ventricular enlargement and comparatively small sulci. (Reproduced with permission from Forbes, Jackson (2003) *Colour Atlas and Text of Clinical Medicine*, 3rd edn. Mosby.)

Subdural haematoma

Brain tumour (primary or metastasis)

TREATMENT

There is little evidence that medical therapy improves the condition

Lumbar puncture drainage of CSF. Improvement in symptoms (e.g. walking speed) after removal of CSF suggests that ventricular shunting may be of benefit

Ventricular shunting if recent-onset dementia, no evidence of multi-infarct dementia, large numbers of B-waves on ICP monitoring and no evidence of passive ventricular enlargement secondary to cerebral atrophy. Shunt complication rates are up to 30% and include subdural haematoma, epilepsy, shunt infection and occlusion

PROGNOSIS

Better prognosis if cause is known and recent onset and if shunting procedure performed. Long history, cerebral atrophy and vascular disease are all predictors of poor outcome

QUESTION SPOTTING

Unlikely to get the classic triad handed to you on a plate! Remember the order of occurrence. Exclude other causes of confusion in the elderly

VARIANT CREUTZFELDT–JAKOB DISEASE (vCJD)

Creutzfeldt–Jakob disease is a disease caused by prion protein (PrP) and is characterized by spongiform encephalopathy. Two forms are recognized: sporadic, which tends to affect patients aged 50–70, and variant, which tends to affect younger patients and may be related to bovine spongiform encephalopathy. PrP occurs in normal people as an alpha-helical structure but in vCJD, PrP undergoes posttranslational change to a beta-sheet form. This is resistant to proteases and accumulates in neural cells, disrupting function and leading to vacuolization and cell death.

CJD is rare; 850 deaths from the sporadic form were recorded in the UK from 1990 to 2005; vCJD is rarer still, with 153 deaths over the same period.

CLINICAL FEATURES

Psychiatric disturbance – depressed, apathetic, withdrawn, forgetfulness, depression. Often the first symptoms in vCJD
Sensory symptoms – dysaesthesia, paraesthesia. Commoner in vCJD
Ataxia
Dementia
Urinary incontinence
Involuntary movements
Myoclonus
Insomnia
Dysphasia
Dysarthria
Upgaze paresis also seen

Late

Immobility
Mutism
Cortical blindness
Note that sporadic CJD usually progresses very quickly; vCJD is slower

INVESTIGATIONS

FBC

Normal

U + Es

Normal

LFTs

Normal

EEG

Sporadic form shows periodic spike and slow-wave activity. vCJD shows normal or slow-wave activity, without typical spike activity

CSF

Protein normal or slightly ↑
Oligoclonal bands usually negative
Protein 14-3-3 may be positive (not specific for CJD; less sensitive for vCJD)
CT brain – normal

MRI brain – may be normal even late in the disease. Abnormal findings may include:
Mild generalized atrophy
Mildly enlarged ventricles
Sporadic: may see high signal in anterior basal ganglia
Variant: 90% have areas of high signal in the posterior thalamus (pulvinar) on T2-weighted imaging

DIAGNOSIS

Sporadic

Diagnosed clinically as rapidly progressive dementia plus typical EEG changes or positive protein 14-3-3 plus two of: myoclonus, akinetic mutism, pyramidal or extrapyramidal problems, cerebellar or visual signs

Variant

Progressive neuropsychiatric disorder, duration > 6 months, plus no diagnostic EEG changes plus bilateral high MRI signal in pulvinar area plus four of: early psychiatric symptoms, ataxia, dementia, myoclonus/chorea/dystonia, painful sensory symptoms

Brain biopsy before or after death
Tonsil biopsy may provide diagnosis in vCJD (not in sporadic), but low PrP yield

DIFFERENTIAL DIAGNOSIS

Wilson's disease
Schizophrenia
Syphilis
HIV
Progressive multifocal leukoencephalopathy
Alcoholism

Multi-infarct dementia and other causes of dementia

Gerstmann–Straussler syndrome – extremely rare familial form of spongiform encephalopathy

TREATMENT

Supportive. Trials of agents such as quinacrine and pentosan polysulphate are ongoing

PROGNOSIS

Death from sporadic CJD is usually rapid; most are dead by 6 months and death may occur within a few weeks. Mean time to death from diagnosis of vCJD is 7.5 months

QUESTION SPOTTING

Think of the diagnosis in any patient with a rapidly progressive neurological illness, especially if myoclonus or cognitive impairment is present. The typical onset for vCJD involves psychiatric disturbance. Sensory symptoms add weight to the diagnosis. Investigations are all normal and the EEG is not diagnostic; a normal EEG does not exclude sporadic CJD, and it is usually non-diagnostic in vCJD.

MOTOR NEURONE DISEASE

A chronic, progressive degenerative disease of unknown cause. Lower and upper motor neurones are progressively destroyed. Protein deposition and oxidative damage may play a part; genetic influences (e.g. the superoxide dismutase gene *SOD-1*) have also been implicated. The disease usually occurs in middle age; approximately 5 in 100 000 are affected.

DISEASE PATTERNS
Three main patterns of disease are commonly recognized:

Amyotrophic lateral sclerosis (mixed UMN and LMN signs affecting limbs and trunk)
Progressive muscular atrophy (mostly LMN signs; usually starts distally and spreads proximally)
Bulbar or pseudobulbar palsy (LMN and UMN signs respectively; affect cranial nerves VII, IX, X, XII)
A fourth subtype, primary lateral sclerosis, is rare. Ascending UMN weakness mostly affects the face

SYMPTOMS
Weakness
Dysphagia – especially to liquids
Dysarthria
Dysphonia
Sensory symptoms are invariably absent

SIGNS
Muscle weakness
Reduced or increased tone
Depressed reflexes (may be enhanced in ALS). Plantars may be extensor in ALS
Muscle fasciculations
Cognitive impairment (usually mild; occasionally precedes motor weakness)
Eye muscles are spared until very late in the disease, as are respiratory muscles and bladder/bowel function

INVESTIGATIONS
FBC
Usually normal

U + Es
Usually normal

LFTs
Normal

ECG
Normal

EEG
Normal

DIAGNOSIS
Is by a combination of clinical findings and EMG. This shows fibrillation and polyphasic motor responses, which suggest denervation. There are no EMG features that are diagnostic for MND. MRI of the brain and spine should be used to exclude structural causes for motor weakness.

DIFFERENTIAL DIAGNOSIS
Stroke disease (e.g. pseudobulbar palsy)
Multiple sclerosis
Muscular dystrophy
Cervical myelopathy
Mononeuropathy
Mononeuritis multiplex
Guillain–Barré syndrome (tends to be much more acute)
Myasthenia gravis (but note prominent eye muscle involvement)

TREATMENT
Riluzole prolongs survival by about 10% at 18 months
Baclofen can be used to treat spasticity
Physiotherapy, occupational therapy and speech therapy (with speaking aids) can help to maximize function and preserve independence for as long as possible
PEG feeding and NIPPV may be needed as the disease advances

PROGNOSIS
Usual time between symptom onset and death is 3–5 years.

QUESTION SPOTTING
May present as a progressive weakness, but may also occur in a question about respiratory failure. Look for the absence of sensory features and a normal or near-normal MRI brain and spine.

STROKE

Stroke is a sudden-onset focal neurological deficit, and is caused in most cases by either thrombus or embolism in the cerebral arteries, or by primary intracerebral haemorrhage in 10–15%. Stroke is the commonest neurological cause of death in developed countries – 10–15% of deaths are due to stroke, and 25% of those suffering a stroke are dead at 6 months. 150 000 people have a stroke each year in the UK. Hypertension is the most important risk factor; smoking, cholesterol and atrial fibrillation are other important risk factors.

SYMPTOMS

Symptoms and signs depend on the site of the stroke

Weakness
Numbness, paraesthesia
Dysphasia
Dysarthria
Dysphagia
Dyspraxia
Hemianopia
Falls
Change in personality
Reduction in cognitive function
Double vision
Dizziness

SIGNS

Reduced sensation
Reduced muscle power
Facial droop
Increased tone (may be reduced during first 48 hours)
Hyperreflexia (may have reduced reflexes in first 48 hours)
Impaired coordination
Dysphasia
Dysarthria
Dysphagia
Dyspraxia
Homonymous hemianopia/quadrantanopia
Chorea
Hemiballismus
Reduced level of consciousness (if massive stroke or bleed)
Diplopia/problems with conjugate gaze

Nystagmus
Ptosis/pupillary dilation

Other

Temperature may be elevated or reduced
BP usually elevated
Pulse may be elevated (occasionally bradycardic)
Respiration: may show Cheyne–Stokes pattern in large strokes

OCSP stroke classification

Total anterior circulation stroke (TACS): unilateral arm, face and leg weakness + homonymous hemianopia + higher-function disorder (e.g. apraxia, dysphasia)
Partial anterior circulation stroke (PACS): two of: unilateral weakness, hemianopia, higher function disorder
Lacunar anterior circulation stroke (LACS): pure motor or sensory deficit (two of arm, leg, face involved); mixed sensory and motor deficit without visual or higher-function loss; ataxic hemiparesis
Posterior circulation stroke (POCS): cerebellar signs without hemiparesis; cranial nerve signs (unless due to tentorial herniation); crossed motor signs (e.g. left-face and right-arm weakness); lone hemianopia or hemianopia with other posterior circulation signs

INVESTIGATIONS

FBC

Hb may be elevated as a cause (e.g. polycythaemia rubra vera)
WCC may be elevated after a large stroke
Plts may be elevated as a cause. Low in antiphospholipid syndrome
Clotting – APTT prolonged in antiphospholipid syndrome. Look for prolonged INR as a risk factor for intracerebral haemorrhage

U + Es

Usually normal; beware dehydration after stroke

Glucose

May be elevated as a stress response; check for hypoglycaemia mimicking stroke symptoms

LFTs
Usually normal

CK, troponins: may be mildly elevated after large stroke

ECG
May show underlying structural heart disease (e.g. previous MI, LVH). Acute massive stroke can cause ST elevation

DIAGNOSIS
Is on clinical grounds. A stroke is a focal neurological deficit of sudden onset; if the deficit resolves within 24 hours, it is termed a transient ischaemic attack. Beyond 24 hours, it is termed a stroke

CT brain should be done within 24 hours (or within 3 hours if thrombolysis is considered); lack of changes on CT does not exclude the diagnosis of stroke

MRI is an alternative, particularly for suspected posterior strokes

DIFFERENTIAL DIAGNOSIS
Causes of focal neurological deficit other than intracerebral haemorrhage and infarction include:

Subdural haematoma
Extradural haematoma
Subarachnoid haemorrhage
Cerebral tumour
Cerebral abscess
Dural sinus thrombosis
Hypoglycaemia
Multiple sclerosis
Hemiplegic migraine
Todd's paresis (post epileptic seizure)
Peripheral nerve lesions (especially if only a limited muscle group is affected)
   Consider underlying causes, e.g.
Arteriovenous malformation
Bleed into tumour
Cerebral vasculitis, giant cell arteritis

Also consider:

Antiphospholipid syndrome
Polycythaemia; thrombocythaemia

Thrombotic thrombocytopenic purpura
Other thrombophilic states (e.g. hyperhomocysteinaemia)
Infective endocarditis
Vertebral or carotid artery dissection
Aortic dissection
Severe hypotension giving rise to watershed infarction (e.g. post cardiac arrest)
Paradoxical embolism (via PFO)

TREATMENT
Acute
Manage all patients on an acute stroke unit

Give oxygen to maintain oxygen saturations > 95%, and ensure the airway remains patent

Do not reduce high blood pressure in the first few days after stroke; give fluids to maintain hydration

Assess swallow and place nil by mouth if swallow is at all compromised. If swallow does not recover in 48–72 hours, consider nasogastric feeding

Correct electrolyte imbalance and hypoglycaemia

Consider patients with ischaemic stroke on CT within 3 hours of symptom onset for thrombolysis

Neurosurgical consultation may be needed for patients with rapidly declining GCS or cerebellar haematoma

Postacute and secondary prevention
Stroke rehabilitation with a multidisciplinary team to maximize recovery and residual function

Start aspirin (and dipyridamole) within 24 hours for ischaemic stroke. Warfarin should be used instead for those patients in AF (unless contraindicated); start after 1–2 weeks poststroke

ACE inhibitors and diuretics reduce the risk of recurrent stroke regardless of initial blood pressure. Aim to keep blood pressure below guidelines (140/80 mmHg at time of writing)

Consider statin therapy to reduce overall vascular risk

If stroke is minor or recovery is good, consider carotid artery ultrasound with a view to carotid endarterectomy if severely stenosed

COMPLICATIONS
Epileptic fits
Cerebral oedema
Hydrocephalus (from bleeding)
Dehydration
Malnutrition
Aspiration
Pneumonia
Deep-vein thrombosis
Pressure sores
Cognitive impairment
Depression

PROGNOSIS
Dependent on OCSP category:

TACS: 60% dead at 1 year; 10–20% living independently

PACS: 15% dead at 1 year; 50% living independently

LACS: 5–10% dead at 1 year; 50–70% living independently

POCS: 20% dead at 1 year; 40–60% living independently

Impaired conscious level, incontinence and neglect are all poor prognostic signs for survival to discharge into the community

QUESTION SPOTTING
Questions are most likely to be asked regarding management of stroke syndromes, or will contain a stroke with an underlying cause. Think of uncommon causes, especially in young (< 60 years) patients with stroke, who will often not have traditional risk factors for the disease.

PARKINSON'S DISEASE

A progressive neurological disease caused by destruction of dopaminergic neurones in the substantia nigra. Lewy bodies are characteristically seen in the dopaminergic neurones. The disease becomes more common with age, affecting 2% of those aged over 80. A number of genetic mutations have been associated with the disease (e.g. synuclein, parkin), but the aetiology in the majority of cases remains obscure.

SYMPTOMS
Tremor
Difficulty starting to walk
Difficulty turning
Falls
Small writing
Stiffness, slow movements
Low mood

SIGNS
'Pill-rolling' tremor, present at rest
Bradykinesia
Mask-like face
Increased tone
Festinant gait; difficulty starting to walk
Dribbling
Impaired righting reflexes

Autonomic signs may also be present
Postural hypotension
Sweating
Constipation
Bladder dysfunction

Later features
Weight loss
Cognitive impairment
Hallucinations (may also be due to medication)

INVESTIGATIONS
FBC
Usually normal

U + Es
Usually normal

LFTs
Normal

CXR
Normal

ECG
Normal

CT, MRI brain
Usually normal

DIAGNOSIS
Is clinical. Bradykinesia plus at least one of tremor, rigidity and impaired righting reflexes are required. In idiopathic Parkinson's disease, arms are usually affected more than legs, and one side is usually affected more. The symptoms should respond well to a trial of L-dopa and the response should be sustained for at least 5 years.

DIFFERENTIAL DIAGNOSIS
Vascular parkinsonism (usually affects lower limbs; responds poorly to L-dopa)

Parkinson's plus syndromes (initial response to L-dopa not sustained):
Multisystem atrophy – cerebellar signs and marked autonomic features
Progressive supranuclear palsy – impaired vertical gaze

Lewy body dementia – prominent dementia early in course of illness, with hallucinations and fluctuating level of cognition. This may form part of a spectrum of disease with idiopathic PD
Drug-induced parkinsonism (e.g. antipsychotics)
Polymyositis
Alzheimer's disease
Benign essential tremor
Wilson's disease

TREATMENT
Treatment does not alter the course of the disease – it should only be started when symptoms are troublesome
Initial treatment comprises either:
L-dopa plus carbidopa
or
Dopamine agonists (e.g. cabergoline, ropinorole)

Side-effects include dizziness, nausea, vomiting, diarrhoea, extrapyramidal effects, hallucinations

Adjunctive treatments

COMT inhibitors (e.g. entacapone) and monoamine oxidase inhibitors (e.g. selegiline) – these prolong the effect of L-dopa

Amantadine – may help L-dopa-driven involuntary movements

Apomorphine – given by injection as rescue for patients with advanced disease who have 'frozen'. Can also be given as continuous infusion

Surgery

A few patients can benefit from either neurosurgical lesioning of areas of the basal ganglia to improve tremor or rigidity. A newer alternative is deep-brain stimulation of basal ganglial areas.

PROGNOSIS

The disease tends to progress slowly over a period of many years. After 10 years of therapy, many patients require increasing doses of L-dopa, and problems such as chorea occur. Keeping a balance between being able to move, involuntary movements and freezing becomes more and more difficult.

QUESTION SPOTTING

The diagnosis is usually obvious, although questions may revolve around the differential of parkinsonism. Questions are more likely to revolve around therapy or changes to therapy in an affected individual.

POLYNEUROPATHIES

Polyneuropathy refers to a loss of alteration of nerve function in multiple nerves, as opposed to one or a few discrete peripheral nerves. It has myriad causes, and can affect sensory nerves, motor nerves or both. The underlying lesion is either axonal loss or demyelination. Distribution varies with cause – e.g. alcohol and diabetes cause a glove-and-stocking sensory neuropathy; Lyme disease and sarcoidosis preferentially affect cranial nerves. Causes include:

INFLAMMATORY
Vasculitis
Guillain–Barré syndrome
Chronic inflammatory demyelinating polyneuropathy
Critical illness polyneuropathy

INFECTIVE
Diphtheria
HIV
Lyme disease
Botulism
Leprosy

DRUGS/TOXINS
Alcohol
Heavy metals (e.g. lead, gold, mercury, arsenic)
Many drugs (e.g. nitrofurantoin, vincristine, metronidazole, amphotericin)

NUTRITIONAL
B_1, B_6, B_{12}, niacin deficiency

METABOLIC
Diabetes mellitus
Porphyria
Renal failure
Liver failure

GENETIC
Refsum's disease
Hereditary sensorimotor neuropathy (including Charcot–Marie–Tooth disease)

OTHER
Malignancy
Amyloidosis
Motor neurone disease
Sarcoidosis

SYMPTOMS
Weakness
Numbness
Tingling
Loss of heat or cold sensation
Pain
Hyperaesthesia
Autonomic symptoms: disturbed sweating, dizziness, urinary retention, diarrhoea or constipation, impotence

SIGNS
Reduced tone
Reduced power
Reduced sensation
Reduced reflexes
Joint deformity
Ulceration
Orthostatic hypotension

INVESTIGATIONS
FBC
Anaemia in B_{12} deficiency
High MCV in alcohol excess and B_{12} deficiency
Basophilic stippling in lead poisoning

U + Es
Urea and creatinine elevated in renal impairment

LFTs
Elevated in liver disease and may be elevated in porphyrias

Glucose
Elevated in diabetes

ESR
Elevated in vasculitis

DIAGNOSIS
Is based on history, examination and nerve conduction studies. Further investigation is

invariably needed to elucidate the underlying cause, but nerve conduction studies, motor versus sensory symptoms, and the distribution of the neuropathy can help to subdivide the possible diagnoses (see below)

Axonal neuropathies cause a decrease in amplitude of the conducted impulse on nerve conduction studies; demyelination causes a delay in the conduction of the impulse

In some cases, biopsy of a nerve (e.g. sural nerve) may assist diagnosis (e.g. in amyloid, vasculitis)

CSF examination may reveal elevated protein (CIDP, Guillain–Barré syndrome)

DIFFERENTIAL DIAGNOSIS

Causes of predominantly motor polyneuropathy include:

Guillain–Barré syndrome
Lead poisoning
Dapsone
Tickbite paralysis
Porphyria
POEMS syndrome (polyneuropathy, organomegaly, endocrinopathy, M protein, skin changes)
Motor neurone disease

Causes of demyelinating polyneuropathy include:

Guillain–Barré syndrome
HSMN type 1
CIDP
Some drugs, e.g. chloroquine
POEMS syndrome
Diphtheria
Refsum's disease

Causes of prominent autonomic symptoms include:

Diabetes mellitus
Amyloid
Porphyria
Guillain–Barré syndrome

TREATMENT

Is usually that of the underlying condition. Even with correction of the underlying condition, nerve function may not recover

Neuropathic pain is difficult to treat, but may respond to atypical agents, e.g. carbamazepine, amitriptyline and gabapentin

Physiotherapy, occupational therapy and orthotic aids can help with motor weakness

A few neuropathies have specific treatments; CIDP is treated with steroids, plasma exchange or IV immunoglobulin; also see sections on porphyria, botulism and Guillain–Barré

COMPLICATIONS

Muscle weakness and loss of function
Ulceration
Joint damage
Chronic pain syndrome

PROGNOSIS

Dependent on the underlying condition

QUESTION SPOTTING

The polyneuropathy is likely to be part of an underlying disease process. You may be asked which investigations would yield the underlying diagnosis.

INFECTIOUS DISEASE

SYPHILIS

Syphilis is caused by the spirochaete *Treponema pallidum*. Transmission is mostly by sexual contact, and although congenital transmission may occur, it is now very rare. The organism enters the body via an abrasion during sexual contact, and there is an incubation period of about 3 weeks. The infection follows a typical pattern, but progression may halt at any stage. Tissue damage is caused by obliterative endarteritis.

The disease incidence fell throughout the 20th century until around 1985 when an increase was noted, thought to be associated with the spread of HIV. Late stages of syphilis are still very rare, probably due to the use of antibiotics in non-related conditions. Women show milder early symptoms (especially during pregnancy) and are less likely to develop neurosyphilis or cardiovascular syphilis.

CLINICAL FEATURES
Primary syphilis
Development of small painless papule, which ulcerates to form a painless, oval ulcer (the chancre). The site is usually the penis in heterosexual men, the anal canal in homosexual men and the vulva or labia in women. More rarely, the cervix may be involved or other sites such as the lip, mouth or hand. The ulcer is highly infectious.

Secondary syphilis
Secondary syphilis occurs 4–6 weeks after the chancre, lasts 2–6 weeks and resolves without any residual signs.

SYMPTOMS
Headaches and neck stiffness – due to low-grade meningitis
Slight fever
Malaise
Arthralgia
Myalgia
Rash – symmetrical, non-itchy, commonly on the trunk. It may also involve the palms, soles or face, where it should raise immediate suspicion of syphilis
Alopecia – rare
Laryngitis – rare

Bone pain due to periostitis – rare
Jaundice and abdominal pain secondary to hepatitis – rare

SIGNS
Generalized painless lymphadenopathy
Condylomata lata – papules occurring in moist areas, such as the perineum
Buccal snailtrack ulcers
Uveitis – seen in both secondary and tertiary syphilis
Nephrotic syndrome – very rare

Tertiary syphilis
Occurs after 2–20-year latent period. Patients are generally non-infectious, but may remain infectious (e.g. women may give birth to a child with congenital syphilis)

Cutaneous gumma
Inflammatory nodules which break down to become ulcers. These heal with scarring and are typically hypopigmented in the centre and hyperpigmented around the edges

Mucosal gumma
Destructive ulcers that involve the palate, pharynx and nasal septum causing perforation. Involvement of the tongue may lead to leukoplakia, and eventually malignancy

Osteoperiostitis
Thickening and irregularity of the long bones with severe pain

Liver
Irregular hepatomegaly secondary to multiple gummas

Eyes
Uveitis
Choroidoretinitis
Optic atrophy

Stomach
Gummatous infiltration

Lungs
Gummas may occur

Testis
Smooth painless enlargement secondary to gummas

Blood
Paroxysmal nocturnal haemoglobinuria
Cardiovascular syphilis
Aortitis (asymptomatic) – causes calcification of ascending aorta
Aortic aneurysm formation (saccular and often painful)
Aortic regurgitation
Coronary artery ostial stenosis
Neurosyphilis
Meningovascular syphilis – acute meningitis occurs early with cranial nerve palsies (may be bilateral) and papilloedema. Meningeal irritation may be minimal. Later, hydrocephalus, fits, strokes, radiculopathy and amyotrophic meningomyelitis occur
General paresis of the insane (GPI) – progressive dementia, with personality change which eventually leads to motor involvement and paralysis. Delusions occur but the classic grandiose delusions are actually rare
Tabes dorsalis – lightning pains, leg ataxia and bladder dysfunction is the classic triad. However, Argyll–Robertson pupils, loss of vibration and position sense and upper-limb pathology may all occur. Charcot joints occur
Extensor plantars with absent ankle reflex. (Also occurs in subacute combined degeneration of the spinal cord, motor neurone disease, Friedreich's ataxia, conus medullaris, multiple sclerosis and pellagra)

INVESTIGATIONS
FBC
Hb may be ↓ if paroxysmal nocturnal haemoglobinuria

U + Es
Normal

LFTs
AST may be ↑
ALT may be ↑
Bilirubin may be ↑
ALP may be ↑

CSF
Protein ↑ (> 0.4 g/L)
WCC ↑ (5–50/mm^3 CSF)

VDRL positive (in only 50%)
TPHA and FTA-ABS positive (but remain positive long after successful treatment)

DIAGNOSIS
Serology
Non-specific
RPR – rapid plasma reagin test
VDRL – Venereal Disease Research Laboratory test
Both of these tests have a high false-positive rate (e.g. SLE or pregnancy) but false-positive titres are usually lower than titres seen in syphilis infection. Both tests usually become negative following successful treatment as their titre follows disease activity

Specific
TPHA – *Treponema pallidum* haemagglutination test
FTA-ABS – indirect fluorescent test
Both of these tests are highly specific for the *Treponema* group but cannot differentiate one species from another (e.g. yaws). They do not mirror disease activity. TPHA is the most specific test in modern use, but is not as sensitive as FTA-ABS. Both tests remain positive long after successful treatment

DIFFERENTIAL DIAGNOSIS
Primary syphilis
Chancroid
Genital herpes
Drug reactions
Erosive balanitis

Tertiary syphilis
Gumma
Sarcoid
Tuberculosis
Leprosy
Lymphogranuloma venereum
Reticulosis
Donovanosis
Osteoperiostitis
Paget's disease
Osteomyelitis
Carcinoma
Leprosy

Causes of a false-positive VDRL

Autoimmune disease – especially SLE
Pregnancy
Drug addicts
Leprosy
Old age
Antiphospholipid syndrome

TREATMENT

Procaine penicillin for 10–14 days (tetracycline/erythromycin if true penicillin allergy). The Jarisch–Herxheimer reaction may occur 4–12 hours following first injection in 50% of primary syphilis, 90% of secondary and 25% of tertiary. It is a symptom that involves an inflammatory reaction in syphilitic tissue. However, this reaction may cause irreversible progression of clinical features in tertiary disease. The reaction does not relate to dose of penicillin. Steroids may be given to reduce the reaction. Trace sexual contacts (how far back depends on stage of disease)

QUESTION SPOTTING

Although syphilis is still rare in the UK, the incidence is rising and there is a strong rise in the HIV-positive population. Syphilis may come up in this section in conjunction with another disease such as HIV or as a cause of unusual cardiac/neurological symptoms and signs. Another cause of extensor plantars with absent ankle reflexes.

Watch out for the serology and think of other causes of a positive VDRL.

BRUCELLOSIS

Infection by *Brucella* spp., a genus of intracellular Gram-negative bacilli. Four species are known to cause human disease:

B. melitensis: sheep, goats
B. abortus: cattle
B. suis: pigs
B. canis: dogs

The infection has an incubation period of 1–8 weeks. Sources of infection include unpasteurized milk, soft cheese (e.g. goat's), animal faeces and urine. Routes of infection are inhalation, ingestion or via broken skin. At-risk groups include animal workers, e.g. farmers and vets.

SYMPTOMS

Fever (not always 'undulant') (90%)
Sweats (90%)
Myalgia (90%)
Joint and back pain (85%)
Headache (80%)
Weight loss (70%)
Anorexia
Constipation (45%)
Abdominal pain (45%)
Cough (25%)
Testicular pain (20% men)
Rash (15%)
Diarrhoea

SIGNS

Spine tenderness (50%)
Arthritis (40%)
Lymphadenopathy (30%)
Splenomegaly (25%)
Pallor
Hepatomegaly (20%)
Epididymo-orchitis (20%)
CNS signs (rare)
Meningoencephalitis
Cranial nerve palsies
Radiculopathy
Hemiplegia
Cardiac murmur – rare
Jaundice – rare
Signs of pneumonia – rare

Other manifestations

Cardiac
Endocarditis
Myocarditis
Pericarditis
Aortic root abscess
Gastrointestinal
Colitis
Peritonitis
Pancreatitis
Hepatitis (usually mild)
Skin
Subcutaneous nodules
Erythema nodosum
Maculopapular rash
Purpura
Ulceration
Eye
Endophthalmitis
Conjunctivitis
Keratitis
Neurological
Guillain–Barré syndrome
Transverse myelitis
Cerebral abscess
Musculoskeletal
Reactive arthritis, usually large-joint, polyarticular
Septic arthritis
Spondylitis
Osteomyelitis

INVESTIGATIONS
FBC

Hb may be ↓ (chronic infection)
WCC usually normal or neutropenic
Platelets usually normal

U + Es

Normal

LFTs

Albumin may be ↓
AST mildly ↑
ALP mildly ↑
Bilirubin mildly ↑
INR, APTT usually normal. DIC is rare

ESR ↑
CXR occasionally shows consolidation, hilar lymphadenopathy or effusions
Joint fluid shows elevated neutrophil count. High protein, low glucose. Organism cultured in 50%
Urine positive for culture in 50%
CSF in meningoencephalitis, shows elevated lymphocyte count, high protein, normal or low glucose, raised oligoclonal Ig. Organism can be cultured from CSF
Organ biopsy may show granulomas, which may caseate

DIAGNOSIS

Blood cultures positive in 50% (must incubate for 6 weeks)
Bone marrow cultures positive in 50–70%

Serology (agglutination tests)
Fourfold rise in titre over 4 weeks
or > 1:160 (non-endemic area)
or > 1:640 (endemic area)
Raised IgM titres denote recent infection. Raised IgG titres denote active infection. Assays can cross-react with cholera and tularaemia

DIFFERENTIAL DIAGNOSIS

Any cause of a PUO, especially granulomatous diseases, e.g. TB, sarcoid
Metastatic malignancy
Vasculitides
SBE
Pyogenic abscess
Typhoid

TREATMENT

Tetracycline (e.g. doxycycline) plus aminoglycoside (e.g. IM streptomycin). Therapy is continued for 1 month, then tetracyclines plus either rifampicin or co-trimoxazole is continued for 2 months. Relapse rate is 10%
Neurobrucellosis: add in rifampicin at start

N.B.: Jarisch–Herxheimer reaction may occur on starting antibiotics

PROGNOSIS

Good recovery when treated; untreated, illness may persist in a chronic form for many years. Neurological deficit may occur, and destruction of heart valves occurs with endocarditis, albeit rarely (2%)

QUESTION SPOTTING

Clues to the diagnosis are:

Pyrexia of unknown origin
Patient has been abroad (especially Malta, where it was first described!) and drunk unpasteurized milk
Back pain as a prominent symptom
Fever with a low neutrophil count
Granulomas on organ biopsy

TYPHOID FEVER

Typhoid fever is caused by the organism *Salmonella typhi*, a Gram-negative bacillus. The source is usually faecal contamination, but may be from sputum, vomitus or other body fluid. Following ingestion of an infectious dose, mucosal penetration in the distal ileum leads to a transient bacteraemia. The organisms multiply within mononuclear phagocytes in lymph nodes, the liver, spleen and bone marrow. Clinical manifestations begin within 1–3 weeks as a result of persistent bacteraemia. Haematogenous spread to Peyer patches in the ileum and to the gallbladder allows reintroduction of bacteria into the gut lumen to continue faecal–oral spread of the disease.

CLINICAL FEATURES
Early
SYMPTOMS
Fever (up to 39–40°C), gradual onset, rarely causes rigors and very little diurnal variation – 'ramping' continuous fever
Headache
Weight loss
Malaise
Anorexia
Myalgia
Arthralgia
Epistaxis is common early on
Constipation is a classical symptom, unlike infection with other *Salmonella*, but most patients also have loose stool at some point
Nausea and vomiting

SIGNS
Bradycardia relative to the fever is typical in about 50% of cases

Later – 1 week
SYMPTOMS
Cough
Bloody diarrhoea with ileal ulceration or fulminant colitis

SIGNS
Rash – rose spots on trunk
Abdominal distension
Mild splenomegaly may occur

Severe late – 2 weeks +
Delirium
Tremor
Ataxia
Ocular complications
Coma
Death

INVESTIGATIONS
FBC
Hb normal or ↓ (normal MCV)
WCC often normal or ↓
Platelets often ↓

U + Es
Na ↓
K ↓
Urea and creatinine ↑ if nephritis

LFTs
AST normal or ↑
ALT normal or ↑
Bilirubin normal or ↑
ALP normal or ↑
Albumin normal or ↓

ESR ↑
Clotting frequently prolonged
Serology (Widal reaction) usually rising antibody titre to O and H antigens. Not reliable
DNA probes and PCR test have been developed but are not widely available

DIAGNOSIS
Positive culture for *Salmonella typhi* from bone marrow (highly sensitive – days 7–10 best), blood (80% sensitive – days 7–10 best), rose spots (70% sensitive), and urine/stool (low sensitivity – positive in second to third weeks).

COMPLICATIONS
Gastrointestinal
Intestinal perforation and haemorrhage (< 5% and usually terminal ileum)
Hepatitis, cholecystitis, pancreatitis

Cardiovascular
Pancarditis
Asymptomatic ECG changes
Sudden cardiac death
DVT

Respiratory
Pneumonia
Bronchitis
Respiratory tract ulceration

Neurological
Delirium
Psychosis
Depression
Meningoencephalitis
Focal neurological signs
Guillain–Barré syndrome

Renal
Nephritis
Rarely renal failure

Haematological
Deranged clotting
Anaemia
Haemolysis
Haemolytic–uraemic syndrome

TREATMENT
Fluid management
Antipyretics
Observation for complications
Antibiotics – ciprofloxacin first-line or
  amoxicillin/choramphenicol/co-trimoxazole
  second-line, though resistance increasing
Dexamethasone has a place in severe typhoid
  (shock or coma) where mortality reaches as
  high as 50%
Surgery if intestinal perforation

Carrier status
Excretion of S. typhi in asymptomatic individuals
for 3 months after treatment is relatively
common. Up to 3% of patients continue to
excrete S. typhi in their stool for more than
1 year and are defined as chronic carriers (and
may excrete bacilli indefinitely). The gallbladder
is usually the site of persistent infection. Urinary
carriage is associated with Schistosoma
infection and nephrolithiasis. Acute typhoid
may recur, and there is an increased incidence of
cholangiocarcinoma. Treatment of carriers
is with 4 weeks of ciprofloxacin and
cholecystectomy is rarely required.

Prophylaxis
Prevention with one of the three available
  vaccines is recommended for travellers to
  endemic areas
Treatment of water by heat or chemicals and
  careful hygiene are essential

QUESTION SPOTTING
Typhoid fever is one of the diseases that must be
excluded in travellers returning home from
tropical or less well-developed countries (along
with malaria). The cardinal symptoms are fever
and headache. Rash, bradycardia, constipation
are clues. Blood results may resemble Legionella
but a ↑ WCC occurs in typhoid only in
complications such as perforation.

TUBERCULOSIS

Caused by the organism *Mycobacterium tuberculosis*, tuberculosis (TB) is still a major cause of morbidity and mortality worldwide. Although primarily an infection of the lungs, the disease can spread to involve virtually any other organ. Spread is usually by droplet and is particularly prevalent in overcrowding, poor social conditions and poor nutrition. More recently, an increase in TB has been seen in the HIV-positive population.

The classic pathology of TB is the caseating granuloma. The necrotic centre is surrounded by epithelioid cells and Langhans giant cells with multiple nuclei. The granuloma may heal completely, and may calcify. Even calcified lesions may reactivate later if immunity becomes impaired.

The pattern of TB infection may be described as follows:

PRIMARY INFECTION
Usually in childhood
Usually pulmonary, but occasionally, the primary infection may be at the ileocaecal region of the gastrointestinal tract or the tonsils
Usually some lymph node spread
In most people this primary infection heals, but may leave some active bacilli

POSTPRIMARY TB
Primary TB may reactivate during a period of lowered immune resistance, to cause postprimary TB, which may in itself cause progressive or miliary TB

PROGRESSIVE TB
Failure of primary or postprimary TB to heal initially leads to progressive TB. This may also occur following reinfection

MILIARY TB
Rarely, primary or postprimary TB may spread via the blood to become widespread. This is miliary TB which is universally fatal if untreated. Miliary TB tends to affect younger people, especially young adults

CLINICAL FEATURES
Primary tuberculosis

SYMPTOMS
Are rare
Fever
Lethargy
Wheeze
Cough
Conjunctivitis

SIGNS
Are rare
Erythema nodosum
Small pleural effusion
Lymphadenopathy

Postprimary

PULMONARY SYMPTOMS
Tiredness
Malaise
Fever
Weight loss
Night sweats
Cough
Haemoptysis
Chest pain

PULMONARY SIGNS
Finger clubbing if advanced
Erythema nodosum
Pulmonary crackles may be heard

Non-pulmonary features

CNS
Meningitis
Tuberculoma

Eye
Phlyctenular conjunctivitis – tuberculous allergic hypersensitivity
Iritis
Choroidoretinitis

Cardiac
Pericardial effusion
Cardiac tamponade
Constrictive pericarditis ± pericardial calcification

Lymph nodes

Lymph node swelling
Sinus formation

Musculoskeletal

Osteomyelitis
Vertebral collapse (Pott's vertebra)
Psoas abscess

Gastrointestinal

Ascites
Obstruction
Peritonitis

Genitourinary

Renal TB
Cystitis
Dysuria, frequency, sterile pyuria
Epididymitis
Endometrial TB
Salpingitis and tubal abscess

Adrenals

Addison's disease

Skin

Lupus vulgaris
Erythema nodosum

Bone marrow

Anaemia
Thrombocytopenia

Miliary tuberculosis

SYMPTOMS

High fever
Drenching night sweats
Weight loss
Cough (rare)
Shortness of breath (rare)

SIGNS

Tachycardia
Anaemia
Hepatomegaly
Splenomegaly
Pulmonary crackles rare until late

INVESTIGATIONS

FBC

Hb ↓
WCC normal or ↑ if miliary TB
Platelets ↓

U + Es

Abnormal if renal TB

LFTs

May show impairment if high tubercle load

ESR ↑
CRP ↑

Chest X-ray

No absolute diagnostic features, but suggestive features include:

Nodular shadows in upper lobes
Bilateral upper-lobe shadows
Cavitating lesions in upper lobes
Calcified lung lesions
Fibrotic changes
Pleural effusions
Mediastinal enlargement
Previous thoracoplasty – see example chest X-ray (Figure 8.1)

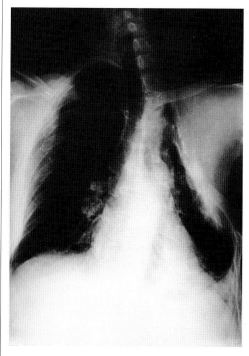

Figure 8.1 TB with previous thoracoplasty. This chest X-ray shows the typical appearances of previous thoracoplasty following TB infection. Although it is rarely done now, there are still many patients alive who have had this procedure.

Immunological

The tuberculin test looks for cell-mediated response to different concentrations of tuberculin injected intradermally. More than 10 mm response at 48–72 hours is positive. A positive result occurs if immunity is present, i.e. previous infection, current infection, previous BCG. A large response or response to 1 tuberculin unit is suggestive of current infection. False-negative tests occur in immune suppression, e.g. miliary TB, AIDS, lymphoma, sarcoid.

Sputum examination for acid-fast bacilli with Ziehl–Nielsen stain or immunofluorescence. Bronchoalveolar lavage fluid may be used.

An enzyme-linked immunosorbent assay with greater sensitivity and specificity has recently been developed. Its use in clinical practice looks promising and will probably replace the tuberculin skin test in the future.

DIAGNOSIS

Culture of *Mycobacterium tuberculosis*
   to confirm diagnosis and obtain sensitivities.
   Culture possible from sputum, bronchoalveolar lavage or biopsy of lymph node or pleura
Early-morning urine culture in difficult cases
Treatment should be commenced in those
   suspected to have active TB infection on clinical and radiological grounds and who have positive sputum smears

DIFFERENTIAL DIAGNOSIS

Atypical mycobacteria (non-tuberculous mycobacteria) are usually low-grade pathogens in humans. Clinical and radiological features are usually indistinguishable from mycobacterial TB. Disseminated infection can occur in the immunocompromised. Examples include *M. avium* complex and *M. kansasii*.

COMPLICATIONS

Pneumothorax
Empyema
Tuberculous enteritis
Respiratory failure
Right ventricular failure
Fungal colonization of lung cavities
Chronic osteomyelitis – see example of spinal
   TB (Pott's disease) (Figure 8.2)

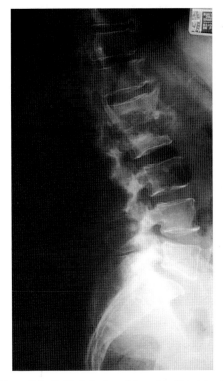

Figure 8.2 Pott's infection of the spine. This lateral spine X-ray shows chronic infection in the L2 disc space. This has expanded and eroded into the adjacent lumbar vertebrae with destruction of the endplates. There is also evidence of a poorly defined soft-tissue mass around the joint space.

TREATMENT
Prevention

BCG vaccination given to 12–13-year-olds in the UK if they show a negative tuberculin test. Gives immunity for approximately 7 years, thus preventing TB when most susceptible to miliary TB. BCG may also be given to infants of high-risk groups such as Asian immigrants

Treatment

Standard treatment comprises 2 months of:
   pyrazinamide, isoniazid, rifampicin (add ethambutol if risk of drug resistance). Then 4 months of: isoniazid and rifampicin
Full compliance is essential. Taken properly, this regimen is almost 100% effective. If compliance is not certain, patients should be

treated as inpatients for the initial 2 months with the standard triple or quadruple therapy, then twice-weekly streptomycin 1 g IM with 15 mg/kg isoniazid and pyridoxine 10 mg orally, supervised, for a further 10 months

Common side-effects of treatment
- Rifampicin: orange urine, orange staining to contact lens, oral contraceptive pill inactivation. Hepatitis – stop if bilirubin rises
- Isoniazid: neuropathy, hepatitis, pyridoxine deficiency, agranulocytosis
- Pyrazinamide: arthralgia, hepatitis
- Ethambutol: optic neuritis (colour vision first to be affected and is an indication to stop this treatment)

PROGNOSIS
Cure can be expected for almost any stage of TB infection if therapy is followed correctly, and the organism is not multidrug-resistant. Drug resistance is an increasing problem, and requires specialist care. Single-drug resistance is common (10%) but multidrug resistance is still rare (0.2%, but this may be an underestimate). Alternative drugs to the standard therapy include: p-aminosalicylic acid, capreomycin, cycloserine, clarithromycin, ciprofloxacin.

QUESTION SPOTTING
TB should be considered and actively looked for in patients with persistent cough, haemoptysis, pleural pain in the absence of acute illness or pneumothorax, especially if there is any evidence of immunosuppression. The typical patient will be in a high-risk group – poor nutrition, alcoholic, ethnic immigrant or immunosuppressed, e.g. AIDS, lymphoma. If the patient has no risk factors, then there must be a history of close contact with active infection.

Infection with the human immunodeficiency virus, types 1 and 2. HIV attaches to cells bearing the CD4 surface protein (mostly T-helper lymphocytes and antigen-presenting cells), and uses reverse transcriptase to copy the viral RNA into DNA, which then integrates with the host cell genome. Replication and new virus formation then take place. Over a period of years, the virus slowly erodes the cell-mediated immune response, eventually allowing secondary infections and malignancies to occur. The modes of transmission and epidemiology are well covered elsewhere.

FEATURES OF INFECTION
Seroconversion illness (after a 2–6-week incubation)
Fever
Sore throat
Arthralgia
Morbilliform rash
Lymphadenopathy
Candidiasis

Rare manifestations
Guillain–Barré syndrome
Encephalopathy

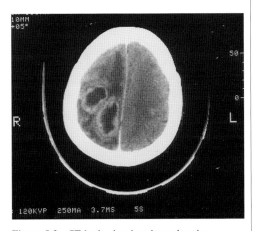

Figure 8.3 CT brain showing ring-enhancing lesions – due in this case to *Toxoplasma* infection. (Reproduced with permission from Forbes, Jackson (2003) *Colour Atlas and Text of Clinical Medicine*, 3rd edn. Mosby.)

Seventh cranial nerve palsy
Flare of psoriatic arthropathy

INVESTIGATIONS
FBC may show ↓ lymphocyte count
CD4$^+$ T-cell count may be ↓
Atypical lymphocytes on blood film
Antibodies to HIV usually take 3 months to form
HIV PCR and p24 antigen are positive during
  seroconversion illness

CD4 count 350–800 × 10^6/L
Reactivation of VZV, leading to shingles
Persistent lymphadenopathy

CD4 count 200–350 × 10^6/L
Tuberculosis
TB meningitis
Oral hairy leukoplakia
Candidiasis
Pneumonia (usually conventional organisms)
Non-specific symptoms: fever, myalgia, weight
  loss, fatigue, diarrhoea

CD4 count < 200 × 10^6/L
Pneumocystis carinii pneumonia
Cerebral toxoplasmosis
Kaposi's sarcoma
Oesophageal *Candida*
Diarrhoea, including *Cryptosporidium*

CD4 count < 50 × 10^6/L
Mycobacterium avium-intracellulare complex
  (MAC)
Cryptococcal meningitis
Histoplasmosis
CMV retinitis, colitis, oesophagitis,
  radiculopathy, encephalitis
Non-Hodgkin's lymphoma (high-grade, B-cell)
Dementia
Progressive multifocal leukoencephalopathy
  (JC virus)

SYMPTOM COMPLEXES AND PROBABLE CAUSES IN HIV
Neurological
Depression (30%)
Dementia (30%) – from HIV, or progressive
  multifocal leukoencephalopathy
Even in asymptomatic disease, CSF often shows
  raised WBC, protein and IgG

Meningitis
TB
Cryptococcus. Note need to perform India ink staining on CSF
Syphilis
Lymphoma
Other aseptic meningitis

Encephalitis
Cytomegalovirus
Herpes simplex virus
Varicella-zoster virus

Space-occupying lesions
Toxoplasmosis (Fig. 8.3)
Lymphoma

Transverse myelitis (HIV)
Often painless, slowly progressive
Spastic/ataxic paraparesis
Reduced joint position sense, vibration and light touch
Sensory level usually absent
Mononeuritis multiplex (HIV)
Peripheral neuropathy (HIV or medications)

CMV polyradiculopathy
Bowel and bladder dysfunction
Reduced power and reflexes in lower limbs
CSF shows ↑ WCC, ↑ protein and low/normal glucose, plus CMV particles

Respiratory
Pneumocystis carinii

Pneumonitis
CMV or non-specific
Diagnosis often via BAL at bronchoscopy
Kaposi's sarcoma

Pleural effusion
Cough, SOB, haemoptysis
Respiratory failure may occur
Diagnosis via bronchoscopy or thoracoscopy
Tuberculosis
Cough, sputum, fever
CXR is often atypical in HIV infection
ZN stain is often negative
Tuberculin test is often negative
MAC infection often gives systemic symptoms

Gastroenterological

Mouth
Aphthous ulcers
Oral hairy leukoplakia

Oesophagus
Cytomegalovirus
Herpes simplex virus
Candida

Diarrhoea
Salmonella; leads to septicaemia in 20–40%
Campylobacter
MAC; requires stool culture and jejunal biopsy for diagnosis. May lead to a systemic illness including fever, weight loss, lymphadenopathy and hepatomegaly
Cryptosporidium parvum; may need bowel biopsy to diagnose
Microsporidium; found on stool culture
CMV; causes bloody diarrhoea, abdominal pain and tenderness, and may lead to perforation or toxic dilatation. Can be diagnosed on rectal biopsy
Sclerosing cholangitis
Pancreatitis (especially as a drug side-effect)
Appendicitis (especially from CMV infection)

Dermatology
Multiple warts (human papilloma virus)
Varicella-zoster infection, often of multiple dermatomes. May disseminate
Molluscum contagiosum. Often very large lesions that do not regress spontaneously
Fungal nail and skin infections
Seborrhoeic dermatitis is increased
Psoriasis. Tends to be more aggressive, and psoriatic arthropathy is much more common
Pruritic papular eruption
Eosinophilic folliculitis
Squamous cell carcinoma of the skin is more common

Kaposi's sarcoma
Starts as pink macules, then darkens to red/purple and becomes raised
Also occur in GI and respiratory tracts

May cause local oedema from lymphatic invasion

Common places include genitalia, inner thigh, trunk, feet, face, hard palate and conjunctivae

Diagnosed by biopsy. Radio-, chemo- and cryotherapy are all used to treat

Differential diagnosis includes TB, MAC, *Bartonella* infection

Other problems

Anogenital carcinoma

High-grade B-cell non-Hodgkin's lymphoma

CMV retinitis

Causes reduced visual acuity and field loss with floaters

Yellow/white areas are seen on the retina, with areas of haemorrhage ('eggs and bacon'). Retinal detachment sometimes occurs. Treatment is with ganciclovir. Differential diagnosis includes HIV, HSV, VZV and *Toxoplasma*

DIAGNOSIS

Diagnosis is based on detecting anti-HIV antibodies in serum. P24 antigen and PCR to detect HIV RNA should be used to detect suspected acute infection. HIV RNA, detected by PCR, gives an estimate of viral load.

TREATMENT

Highly active antiretroviral therapy (HAART) is the mainstay of treatment at present, typically involving two reverse transcriptase inhibitors plus a protease inhibitor. This can substantially delay the onset of the AIDS complex, delay death and reduce viral load to undetectable levels in many patients

Important side-effects include (vary between drugs):

Pancreatitis: (didanosine) ddI, lamivudine

Neuropathy: (zalcitabine) ddC, ddI, ritonavir

Anaemia and granulocytopenia: zidovudine

Myositis: zidovudine

Ulcers: ddC

Rash: nevirapine

Deranged LFTs: ritonavir and nearly all antiretroviral therapies

GI upset: protease inhibitors

There is also considerable current interest in the increased cardiovascular risk caused by HAART – this is at least partly due to side-effects of insulin resistance and dyslipidaemia

PROGNOSIS

Improving. The average time from an AIDS-defining illness to death is now well over 3 years. 25% of patients are predicted to live for more than 15 years from the time of infection

QUESTION SPOTTING

The presenting problem is likely to be an AIDS-defining illness, e.g. *Pneumocystis* infection. A less likely scenario would be a patient known to be HIV-positive developing a symptom complex, e.g. meningitis, or the presentation of a seroconversion illness

Look for risk factors:

Promiscuity

Haemophilia (may have a prolonged APTT)

Previous blood transfusions

Presence of hepatitis B or C (i.e. viruses transmitted in the same way)

Businessman, especially if a history of foreign travel

African or Asian travel

Also remember to look for other HIV-related conditions when you have identified the major problem

Isolated lymphopenia from the FBC should also raise suspicion in at-risk groups

GONORRHOEA

Infection with *Neisseria gonorrhoeae*, a Gram-negative diplococcus, is almost always spread by sexual contact, and can colonize and infect the genitourinary tract, anus, rectum, pharynx and conjunctivae. Systemic infection occurs in less than 1% of cases.

FEATURES
Males
5% are asymptomatic
Dysuria
Urethral discharge
Rectal discharge

Females
More often asymptomatic
Cervical discharge (40%)
Dysuria (12%)

Other features
Epididymo-orchitis (2%)
Prostatitis, seminal vesiculitis
Periurethral abscesses
Endometritis
Salpingitis
Meningitis – rare
Fitz-Hugh–Curtis syndrome (perihepatitis):
RUQ pain
Shouldertip pain
Fever
Tender hepatomegaly
Hepatic rub
Right-sided pleural effusion
Septicaemia (dermatitis/arthritis syndrome)
Large-joint polyarthritis. Effusions may be present. Septic monoarthritis may occur
Tenosynovitis
Fever
Rash: maculopapular at first, becoming pustular, then haemorrhagic, and finally necrotic

INVESTIGATIONS
FBC
Hb normal
WCC may be ↑
Platelets normal

U + Es
Normal

LFTs
Elevated in septicaemia or perihepatitis

ESR may be elevated
ECG normal

CXR shows small right-sided effusion (Fitz-Hugh–Curtis syndrome)
Joint X-ray usually normal
Joint fluid straw-coloured or purulent

DIAGNOSiS
Culture; urethral swab in men, endocervical swab in women
Disseminated infection
Blood culture (25–75% sensitivity)
Joint aspirate (25–75% sensitivity)
Skin lesions (5–10% sensitivity)

DIFFERENTIAL DIAGNOSIS
Disseminated infection
Meningococcal septicaemia
Lyme disease
Secondary syphilis
SBE
Vasculitis

Fitz-Hugh–Curtis syndrome:
Chlamydia infection
Viral hepatitis
Right basal pneumonia

Urethritis
Chlamydia infection
Non-specific urethritis
Foreign body in urethra

TREATMENT
Simple infection
If organism is penicillin-sensitive in population, use penicillin + probenecid (single dose).
Otherwise, use ciprofloxacin or ceftriaxone single dose. *Chlamydia* often coinfects, and should be eradicated (e.g. 1 week of doxycycline)

Disseminated infection

Parenteral cephalosporins for 48 hours, then
   oral cephalosporin for 1 week
Test for other STDs
Trace sexual contacts
Test for cure at 4 and 10 days postantibiotics;
   cure rate is very high

QUESTION SPOTTING

Will tend to present as either Fitz-Hugh–Curtis
syndrome or arthritis/dermatitis syndrome

Clues to the presence of an STD (in the
examination) are:

A businessman (who travels)
A history of a new relationship
Recent foreign travel or holiday

LYME DISEASE

Infection by *Borrelia burgdorferi*, a spirochaete transmitted by ticks of the *Ixodes* genus. Rodents are the main reservoir for infection; some birds are also infected. Disease appears to be more virulent in the USA than in Europe; in particular, arthritis is very uncommon in European infection. Infection tends to peak around June to October.

FEATURES

Symptomless in up to 90%

Immediate (stage I)

Erythema migrans (90%): rash slowly (over
  weeks) spreads outwards from tick bite;
  centre may then clear. Multifocal rashes may
  occur
Fever
Flu-like illness
Headache
Arthralgia
Regional lymphadenopathy

Delayed (stage II) (weeks)

Carditis (10%)

AV block
Myocarditis
Pericarditis

Neurological features (10–20%)

Meningitis
Cranial nerve palsies; especially VII nerve; may
  be bilateral
Radiculopathy
Encephalopathy
Peripheral neuropathy
Borrelia lymphocytoma: bluish nodule on nipple
  or ear

Chronic (stage III) (months to years)

Acrodermatitis chronica atrophicans (Europe
  only)
Migratory large-joint oligoarthritis, especially in
  knees; often swollen but not hot or painful
Chronic neurological problems –
  polyneuropathy, cerebral vasculitis

Other features

Conjunctivitis occurs uncommonly (< 5%)
Gastrointestinal and pulmonary involvement is
  extremely uncommon

INVESTIGATIONS

FBC

Usually normal

U + Es

Normal

LFTs

Mild ↑ of AST and ALT

ESR normal or ↑
Normal glucose
CSF shows pleocytosis
Synovial fluid shows moderately high WCC,
  mildly elevated protein

ECG

May show ST elevation (pericarditis)
T-wave changes (myocarditis)
Long PR interval or higher-grade AV block

DIAGNOSIS

Culture in patients presenting with rash: 100%
  specific and 55–85% sensitive
Culture in patients without rash: CSF, blood,
  urine and joint fluid all have a very
  poor yield
Serology: rising titres are unreliable, particularly
  in populations where Lyme disease is endemic,
  e.g. forestry workers. Antibodies persist for
  years. False positives occur in a number of
  other diseases, including ehrlichiosis and
  babesiosis. Seroconversion takes up to 6
  weeks. However, negative antibody tests are
  rare in chronic disease

N.B.: Some features of Lyme disease may be
due to coinfection with *Ehrlichia* or *Babesia*
species; this is an area of some controversy
at present

DIFFERENTIAL DIAGNOSIS

Viral infections: pericarditis, encephalitis,
  meningitis, arthritis
Sarcoidosis, especially bilateral VIIn palsy
Syphilis
Ehrlichiosis
Babesiosis
Lymphoma
Vasculitides
Reiter's disease and reactive arthritis

TREATMENT

For mild disease, oral penicillins or tetracyclines

For cardiac or neurological disease, IV
  ceftriaxone or IV penicillin

PROGNOSIS

Usually excellent once treated. Cardiac problems
usually resolve, but mild neurological deficit may
remain

QUESTION SPOTTING

Clues to the diagnosis are:

Bitten by a tick, or visited a known endemic area

Typical rash (too much of a giveaway in
  MRCP!)

AV block in a young or middle-aged patient

Bilateral VIIn palsy, or VIIn palsy with arthritic
  symptoms

Indolent meningitis/encephalitis

MALARIA

Caused by the parasite *Plasmodium*, of which there are four species: *vivax, ovale, falciparum* and *malariae*. Infection occurs following introduction of sporozoites via the female *Anopheles* mosquito. The parasite life cycle length depends on the species: 48 hours for *P. falciparum*, 48–72 hours for *P. vivax* and *P. ovale* and 72 hours for *P. malariae*.

The different species also tend to have different capacities to infect the red cell.

P. falciparum will infect any red cell, especially young ones, and therefore tends to have the most severe effects. *P. vivax* and *P. ovale* tend to infect reticulocytes and immature red cells. *P. malariae* infects senescent red cells.

Patients with sickle-cell disease, beta-thalassaemia, phosphate kinase deficiency, glucose-6-phosphate deficiency or Duffy-negative red cells show resistance to malaria infection.

Incubation period of 10–14 days except for *P. malariae* (18 days to 6 weeks), which may be modified if antimalarial chemoprophylaxis is used so that the clinical disease may not present for months after infection.

SYMPTOMS

Fever up to 41°C
Headache
Myalgia
Shortness of breath due to anaemia and/or
    metabolic acidosis
Confusion
Coma
Convulsions
Chest pain
Abdominal pain
Diarrhoea

SIGNS

Hepatomegaly
Splenomegaly
Meningism
Dysconjugate gaze
Extensor plantars
Hypotension

INVESTIGATIONS

FBC

Hb ↓
WCC ↑ (neutrophilia), normal or sometimes ↓
Platelets normal or ↓

U + Es

Na normal or often ↓
K normal
Urea and creatinine ↑ if renal failure

LFTs

ALP ↑
ALT ↑
Bilirubin ↑
Albumin ↓

Clotting
Prolonged clotting times if DIC
ESR ↑
CRP ↑
Haptoglobins ↓
Reticulocytes ↑

Urinalysis

Blood and protein if glomerulonephritis or acute tubular necrosis

DIAGNOSIS

Thick and thin blood films stained with Giemsa stain. *P. falciparum* only shows ring forms in the early stages, whereas the other species show all stages of the erythrocytic cycle. Multiple infection of a single erythrocyte suggests *falciparum*. 3–4 stains over a period of days may be required. Diagnosis may be difficult if the patient has been partially treated.

Serological blood tests are available that may be used in conjunction with blood films.

ASSOCIATIONS

Anaemia due to:
Haemolysis (both of infected and non-infected
    red cells)
Dyserythropoiesis
Sequestration secondary to splenomegaly
Folate deficiency
Herpes simplex

COMPLICATIONS

Glomerulonephritis and nephrotic syndrome seen in children, especially with *P. malariae* and this may be fatal

Acute tubular necrosis with oliguria, uraemia and haemoglobinuria (black-water fever)

Metabolic acidosis, septic shock

Splenic rupture

Cerebral oedema

TREATMENT

Antipyretics such as paracetamol and salicylates

Fluids if dehydrated or shocked

Exchange transfusion if heavy parasitaemia

Phenobarbital may be used to prevent fitting

Specific treatment for acute attacks

Consult *British National Formulary* or Tropical Diseases Centre for most up-to-date information. Currently:

P. vivax, *P. ovale* and *P. malariae*

Chloroquine 600 mg of the base, then 300 mg 6 hours later, and then 150 mg twice daily for 2 days

P. falciparum

Widespread resistance to chloroquine so treatment is quinine for 7 days followed by either tetracycline 250 mg/6 hours, doxycycline 100 mg/12 hours or clindamycin 300 mg/6 hours for 7 days

An alternative is artemetherlumefantrine (Riamet) 4 tabs twice daily. Or atovaquone + proguanil (Malarone) 4 tabs once daily (both for 3 days with food)

Eradication of liver forms

Essential for *P. vivax* and *P. ovale* which may represent at a later date unless eradicated with primaquine

Prevention

Passive prevention of mosquito bites is strongly recommended with repellents, mosquito nets and clothing to cover exposed skin

Chloroquine in area of low resistance. Chloroquine and proguanil or mefloquine if resistance high. Mefloquine is contraindicated in first trimester of pregnancy, lactation, epilepsy, cardiac conduction disorders and psychiatric disorders

DIFFERENTIAL DIAGNOSIS

Fevers

Pneumonia

Ascending cholangitis

Pyelonephritis

Hepatitis

Infective endocarditis

Infectious mononucleosis

Splenomegaly

Visceral leishmaniasis

Schistosomiasis

Tuberculosis

Brucellosis

Typhoid

Haematological and inflammatory causes

QUESTION SPOTTING

History of travel which is not necessarily recent and appropriate prophylaxis may well have been taken. Consider in non-specific flu-like prodromes with anaemia, jaundice and hepato-splenomegaly but absence of rash and lymphadenopathy. Should also be a differential in culture-negative fever which is resistant to antibiotic therapy.

TOXIC SHOCK SYNDROME (TSS)

Localized infection, usually by *Staphylococcus aureus*, producing an exotoxin which causes widespread cytotoxic effects on multiple organ systems. TSS toxin 1 (TSST 1) is the toxin responsible in 75% of cases. Similar syndromes have been reported with *Staphylococcus epidermidis* and streptococci as causative organisms.

First described in 1978 in children who suffered *Staphylococcus aureus* infections and then was commonly associated with tampon use following an epidemic in 1981. Recognized risk factors nowadays also include postoperative wound infection, postpartum toxic shock, nasal packing, common bacterial infections, viral infections with influenza A and varicella, diabetes mellitus, HIV and chronic cardiopulmonary disease.

SYMPTOMS
Fever
Myalgia
Vomiting and diarrhoea
Confusion and drowsiness
The local source of infection may be from tampons, conjunctivitis, abscesses or burns

SIGNS
Fever
Low BP, tachycardia
Macular rash, progressing to desquamation
May have tender muscles
May have a reduced conscious level
Vaginal discharge

INVESTIGATIONS
FBC
Hb usually normal
WCC often ↑
Platelets may be ↓

U + Es
Na usually normal
K may be ↑
Urea and creatinine ↑ in renal failure

LFTs
May be ↑

Calcium may be low
CK often raised and can point towards rhabdomyolysis
Clotting usually normal, but DIC can occur
Blood cultures almost always negative

ECG
Bundle branch block, first-degree block; VT and ST segment changes may all be seen
CSF virtually never shows growth

DIAGNOSIS
Firm diagnosis is based on all five of:

1. Temperature > 39°C
2. Macular rash
3. Systolic BP < 90 mmHg, or diastolic postural drop
4. Source of localized TSST producing infection
5. Evidence of toxic action on three systems:
   - Diarrhoea/vomiting
   - Myalgia/raised CK
   - Drowsiness/confusion
   - Raised urea/creatinine
   - Reduced platelets

DIFFERENTIAL DIAGNOSIS
Septicaemic shock
Weil's disease
Measles
Rickettsial infections
Malaria

TREATMENT
Remove source of infection (tampon, abscess)
IV flucloxacillin
Supportive therapy for shock and renal failure. Shock is often resistant to fluid replacement and necessitates use of inotropic/vasopressor support

PROGNOSIS
Mortality rate is less than 3% in staphylococcal TSS but significantly higher with streptococcal TSS at 30–70%

QUESTION SPOTTING

If you are lucky, there will be clues, e.g. tampon use, conjunctivitis or abscesses. If there are no clues, suspect the diagnosis in a young woman with a septic shock/multiorgan failure picture with no apparent cause. A triad of rash, hypotension and fever should make you consider TSS.

LEPTOSPIROSIS (WEIL'S DISEASE)

Infection with the spirochaete *Leptospira interrogans*. This is harboured by a wide variety of animals, but rats are the most common source of human infection. Severe disease involving hepatic and renal failure is known as Weil's disease. Anyone exposed to contaminated water or handling infected animals is at risk of infection; the organism can enter via broken skin or mucous membranes. The incubation period is 2–20 days. At-risk groups include farmworkers, sewer workers, vets and watersports participants.

N.B.: Only 10–15% of infections result in severe liver and renal disease.

PHASE 1: INFECTION (LASTS 4–7 DAYS)

SYMPTOMS

Fever and chills ($>$ 85%)
Headache ($>$ 85%)
Myalgia ($>$ 85%)
Abdominal pain
Vomiting, diarrhoea
Delirium, hallucinations, psychosis
Arthralgia
Cough, sore throat, haemoptysis

SIGNS

Fever
Tachycardia
Hypotension
Splenomegaly (15–25%)
Hepatomegaly
Lymphadenopathy (15%)
Lung crackles
Meningism
Skin rash: purpuric, urticarial or maculopapular
Conjunctival suffusion

PHASE 2: IMMUNE RESPONSE (LASTS 4–30 DAYS)

SYMPTOMS

Headache, photophobia, neck stiffness (50–90%)
Sore eyes

Fever
Skin rash
Jaundice

SIGNS

Jaundice
Meningism
Reduced conscious level
Cranial nerve palsies, radiculopathy, focal weakness, fits and nystagmus may all occur
Hepatomegaly
Uveitis

INVESTIGATIONS

FBC
Hb often $\downarrow$ (haemolysis, bleeding)
WCC usually $\uparrow$
Platelets may be $\downarrow$

U + Es
Urea and creatinine often $\uparrow$ (65%)

LFTs
Bilirubin may be very $\uparrow$
ALT slightly $\uparrow$
ALP $\uparrow$

Reticulocytes may be $\uparrow$
Haptoglobins may be $\downarrow$
ESR $\uparrow$
LDH $\uparrow$
CK may be $\uparrow$
PO_4 $\uparrow$ if renal impairment severe
Urate $\uparrow$ if renal impairment severe
Clotting abnormal (liver disease or DIC)
D-dimers $\uparrow$ (in DIC)
Blood film may show fragmented RBCs and polychromasia

Urine proteinuria (usually $<$ 1 g/24 hours). Microscopic haematuria and leukocytes
CSF pleocytosis. Glucose normal, protein slightly raised

DIAGNOSIS

Blood cultures and CSF may grow organisms on days 0–10 of illness
Urine culture may be positive from second to fourth week

Serology (agglutination testing): positive from week 2. Titres of > 1:100 are diagnostic

PCR testing for Weil's disease is also now available

DIFFERENTIAL DIAGNOSIS

Other haemorrhagic fevers (e.g. dengue)
Yellow fever
Viral hepatitis
EBV infection
Brucellosis
Atypical pneumonias
Malaria
Aseptic meningitis
Relapsing fever
Hepatorenal syndrome
Paracetamol overdose
Carbon tetrachloride toxicity
Amanita phalloides poisoning
Toxaemia of pregnancy
HUS/TTP
Incompatible blood transfusion

COMPLICATIONS

Liver failure
Acute renal failure
DIC, microangiopathic anaemia
ARDS
Cardiac arrhythmias
Jarisch–Herxheimer reaction on starting antibiotics

TREATMENT

Support for vital organs
IV penicillin or tetracyclines
Prophylactic antibiotics may avoid infection if given after exposure to water known to be infected

PROGNOSIS

Good recovery in most cases; renal function usually recovers fully. Between 5 and 20% mortality seen in patients with full-blown Weil's disease. Higher mortality rates are seen in pregnancy and the elderly.

QUESTION SPOTTING

Clues to the diagnosis are:
Exposure to rodents, sewers or watersports
A job as a vet or farmworker
Presence of meningism
Combined hepatic and renal dysfunction
Myalgia and conjunctival suffusion as a prominent symptom
A biphasic illness (may be asymptomatic for 1–3 days between infectious and immune phases)

BOTULISM

Ingestion of a 150 kD, heat-stable toxin produced by *Clostridium botulinum*. Ingestion of the bacterium itself is unnecessary. The most common source is canned foods which have not been adequately heat-treated (spores are heat-resistant and require temperatures of up to 120°C to ensure eradication).

Botulinum toxin is absorbed via mucous membranes, and spreads haematogenously to neuromuscular junctions, where it inhibits cholinergic transmission irreversibly. Recovery therefore requires new motor end-plate formation.

SYMPTOMS
Onset 2–48 hours after ingestion
Nausea, vomiting
Double vision
Blurred vision
Dry mouth
Constipation
Urinary retention
Muscle weakness
Difficulty breathing
Dysarthria

SIGNS
Conscious level preserved
Descending paralysis; cranial nerves affected first
Convergent strabismus
Fixed mid-range or dilated pupils
Ptosis
Reduced tone and power
Reflexes preserved at first
Labile BP; may be low
Note that fever is unusual

INVESTIGATIONS
FBC
Usually normal

U + Es
Usually normal

LFTs
Usually normal

ECG may show non-specific ST/T abnormalities
Nerve conduction studies normal
EMG shows reduced amplitude discharges, but may increase after tetanic stimulation

PFTs
FVC may drop quickly
FEV_1 drops in parallel
Anti-AChR antibodies negative
Anti-calcium channel antibodies negative
CSF protein may be slightly elevated. No increase in cell numbers
Tensilon test may be weakly positive

DIAGNOSIS
Demonstration of toxin in faeces, blood or food by mouse bioassay

DIFFERENTIAL DIAGNOSIS
Guillain–Barré syndrome (especially Miller–Fisher variant)
Myasthenia gravis
Poliomyelitis
Tick paralysis
Familial periodic paralysis
Drug-induced neuromuscular block
Shellfish poisoning

TREATMENT
Deaths usually occur from respiratory paralysis, thus close monitoring of the FVC and mechanical respiratory support is crucial. Antitoxin against A, B and E toxins (those usually responsible) probably reduces death rates. Some centres also give penicillin to clear any clostridia which may have colonized the gut.

Respiratory support may have to be given for between 30 and 100 days; ventilator failure, tracheostomy complications and infection may supervene.

PROGNOSIS
Mortality in the UK with appropriate support is currently 5–10% after, following improvement in recognition and early intensive support.

QUESTION SPOTTING

Clues are:

Descending paralysis

No sensory involvement

No impairment of consciousness

Afebrile

The tensilon test is usually normal (excluding myasthenia), and the CSF protein is not greatly raised (in contrast with Guillain–Barré syndrome).

HEPATITIS

This is inflammation of the liver. Often, episodes are subclinical and cases are detected by demonstrating deranged liver enzymes. Other times patients present with fulminant liver failure. This section will discuss hepatitis A, B, C, D and E viruses. However one must remember that bacterial infections, drugs, chemicals and toxins should always be part of the differential diagnosis. Hepatitis viruses A and B and alcohol are the commonest causes in the UK.

SYMPTOMS
Commonly asymptomatic. Antibodies to hepatitis A, B or E are commonly found in asymptomatic individuals
Prodrome (over 2–14 days) of:

Anorexia
Malaise
Nausea
Myalgia
Fever
Jaundice
Itching (unusual in viral hepatitis)
Dark urine and yellow stools
Arthralgia

SIGNS
May be none
Jaundice
Hepatomegaly
Splenomegaly
Lymphadenopathy
Chronic liver disease signs are uncommon
Extrahepatic manifestations more common in hepatitis B

DIFFERENTIATION
Incubation (weeks)
Hepatitis A: 2–6
Hepatitis B: 4–26
Hepatitis C: 6–12
Hepatitis D: 3–20
Hepatitis E: 2–9

Transmission
Hepatitis A: faecal–oral
Hepatitis B: blood products, IV drug use, sexual intercourse, direct contact and vertical transmission
Hepatitis C: blood products, IV drug use, sexual intercourse. Unknown in 40%
Hepatitis D: superinfection or coinfection with hepatitis B
Hepatitis E: faeces

Chronicity
Hepatitis A: no
Hepatitis B: 5–20%
Hepatitis C: 20–60%
Hepatitis D: 30–50%
Hepatitis E: no

Carrier
Hepatitis A: no
Hepatitis B: 10%
Hepatitis C: 50%
Hepatitis D: 5%
Hepatitis E: no

Risk factors
Hepatitis A: institutions, children, travel to Middle East and Far East
Hepatitis B: Middle/Far East, haemophilia, unprotected sex, dialysis, IV drug use and being born to hepatitis B-positive mother
Hepatitis C: IV drug use, transfusion, haemophilia
Hepatitis D: similar to hepatitis B
Hepatitis E: North India, Mexico and Middle East. Higher mortality in pregnancy

INVESTIGATIONS
FBC
Usually normal
Raised WCC consider bacterial infection
Low platelets consider alcoholic hepatitis

U + E
Normal
Coagulation
Raised INR and APTTR in cirrhosis

LFTs
Bilirubin ↑
ALT ↑
AST ↑
ALP ↑
Albumin ↓

DIAGNOSIS
Hepatitis A
Raised serum transaminases from
days 22 to 40
IgM from day 25
IgG detectable for life

Hepatitis B
HBsAg (surface antigen) 1–6 months.
More than 6 months indicates
carrier status
HBeAg (e antigen) 6 weeks to 3 months.
Indicates infectivity
Anti-HBsAg (antibodies to surface antigen)
indicates vaccination

Hepatitis C
AST:ALT enzyme ratio is usually less than 1
until cirrhosis sets in
Anti-HCV antibodies

HCV-PCR
Liver biopsy if PCR-positive to assess damage
and need for therapy

Hepatitis D
Anti-HDV antibody

Hepatitis E
Serology

DIFFERENTIAL DIAGNOSIS
Common
Alcohol

Uncommon
EBV
Drugs, e.g. paracetamol overdose
Autoimmune disease
Ischaemia (shock liver)

Rare
Herpes simplex
CMV
Coxsackie A and B
Echovirus
Leptospirosis
Measles
Mycoplasma
Lassa fever
Yellow fever
Mushroom toxins

COMPLICATIONS
Hepatitis A
Usually self-limiting
Fulminant hepatitis (rare)

Hepatitis B
Fulminant hepatitis (rare)
Chronic hepatitis
Cirrhosis
Hepatocellular carcinoma (HCC) ($10\times$ increased
risk) ($60\times$ risk if HBsAg- and HBeAg-
positive)
Glomerulonephritis
Vasculitis (e.g. polyarteritis nodosa)

Hepatitis C
HCC
Cirrhosis
Cryoglobulinaemia

TREATMENT
Supportive treatment and avoidance of alcohol
should be mainstay of treatment of all viral
hepatitis infections.

Hepatitis A
Interferon-alpha for fulminant hepatic failure

Hepatitis B
Interferon-alpha for chronic infection. Also
antivirals such as lamivudine and adefovir are
used

Hepatitis C
Interferon-alpha and ribavirin in chronic
infection
Interferon-alpha in acute infections may reduce
progression to chronic disease

Hepatitis D
Interferon-alpha has not been successful

Hepatitis E
No specific treatment available

IMMUNIZATION
Hepatitis A
Havrix Monodose gives 1-year immunity for
those at risk

Hepatitis B
Specific anti-HBV immunoglobulin

Hepatitis C
None

Hepatitis D
None

Hepatitis E
None

QUESTION SPOTTING

May be incidental findings of deranged liver enzymes, mild symptoms or fulminant hepatic failure in those with risk factors such as foreign travel to the Far and Middle East, IV drug use, haemophilia.

You may be asked to interpret serological markers of hepatitis B infection.

ANTHRAX

Bacillus anthracis, a Gram-positive rod usually spread by handling infected carcasses, but has achieved high media profile as some have attempted to use it in biological warfare. Anthrax means coal in Greek after the appearance of its cutaneous form. It can infect via skin, GI tract and inhalation. The toxin is composed of three entities (protective antigen, lethal factor and oedema factor) which are thought to trigger tumour necrosis factor and interleukin-1 in a cascade that leads to tissue oedema and microvascular haemorrhage.

CLINICAL FEATURES
Cutaneous
Spores inoculate through skin abrasions or lacerations and the incubation period is 2–5 days

The disease begins as a papule initially which then becomes a 1-cm vesicle within 2 days

Oedematous, necrotic lesions occasionally develop which are painless and non-pruritic

Rupture occurs after a week, leaving a characteristic black eschar lesion despite antibiotic therapy

Inhalational
Inhaled spores are carried via macrophages to hilar and mediastinal lymph nodes. Incubation is 1–6 days

Initial stage
Flu-like symptoms; myalgia, malaise and fatigue with a dry non-productive cough and fever. Occasionally symptoms improve before the second stage

Second stage
Usually lasting about 24 hours with hypoxia, cyanosis and respiratory distress

Crackles in the chest ± effusions

Mild fever

Diaphoresis

Hepatosplenomegaly

Stridor (due to enlarged mediastinal adenopathy)

Meningism (50%)

Coma

Death

Intestinal
Abdominal pain and fever followed by nausea, vomiting and diarrhoea after ingesting contaminated food

Extremely rare and mortality rate of 50% from volume loss (GI haemorrhage, interstitial and intraperitoneal)

INVESTIGATIONS
FBC
Normal or raised WCC

U + Es
Normal unless shock supervenes

LFTs
Normal

CXR
Mediastinal adenopathy is common in inhalational anthrax. Usually associated with pleural effusions. Pulmonary infiltrates are unusual and should prompt consideration of other diagnoses

CSF
Haemorrhagic macroscopically, few polymorphs and large number of Gram-positive bacilli are seen in meningitis. *B. anthracis* readily grows on blood agar and staining with methylene blue or Giemsa differentiates the organism from other *Bacillus* species

DIAGNOSIS
Based on typical clinical features along with *Bacillus anthracis* isolation from cutaneous lesions, blood or lymph nodes

Always warn the labs if suspecting anthrax in order for them to take the appropriate biohazard precautions

DIFFERENTIAL DIAGNOSIS
Cutaneous
Tularaemia

Diphtheria

Staphylococcal infection

Orf

Rickettsia infections

Plague
Primary syphilis

Inhalational
Pulmonary tularaemia
Mediastinitis

Intestinal
Shigella
Amoebic dysentery

TREATMENT
Penicillins, doxycycline and quinolones are effective in the treatment of anthrax

Intravenous therapy and intensive care are usually required in inhalational anthrax

Postexposure prophylaxis, usually with oral ciprofloxacin, is given to prevent inhalational anthrax. The eschar lesion becomes sterile in 2 days and takes 2–3 weeks to pass through its developmental/resolution cycle

PROGNOSIS
Most anthrax cases are cutaneous (95%) and have an excellent outlook. Approximately 5% are inhalational and carry a mortality rate around 95%. Less than 1% are gastrointestinal.

QUESTION SPOTTING
History of handling animals or animal products (e.g. contaminated wool, hair or animal hides) or of military personnel may be given in the scenario

Widened mediastinum, haemorrhagic pleural effusion and fever in the absence of thoracic surgery or oesophageal rupture

HAEMATOLOGY

HYPOGAMMAGLOBULINAEMIA

Is a deficiency in one or several classes of Ig. All types lead to a predisposition to repeated infections, which may become chronic. It can be subclassified into:

PRIMARY
X-linked agammaglobulinaemia
Common variable immunodeficiency (CVID)
Selective IgG subclass deficiency
IgA deficiency
Thymoma with hypogammaglobulinaemia
Transient infantile hypogammaglobulinaemia
Transcobalamin II deficiency

SECONDARY
Chronic lymphocytic leukaemia
Myeloma
Protein-losing enteropathy
Nephrotic syndrome
Myotonic dystrophy
Drugs: gold, phenytoin, penicillamine (the latter two usually IgA-selective)

X-LINKED (BRUTON'S) AGAMMAGLOBULINAEMIA
This disease is rare. Patients usually start to develop infections once the maternal IgG disappears from the blood stream at 3 months onwards. IgG levels are detectable but are < 50 mg/100 ml. T cells are present in normal numbers and function normally, but there are no mature B cells. Lack of the *BTK* gene prevents maturation of pro-B cells. X-linked immunodeficiency with hyper-IgM (XHM) is a related disorder where maturation progresses to production of IgM, but B cells are unable to switch class to produce other Igs.

COMMON VARIABLE IMMUNODEFICIENCY
Onset at any age, but peak incidence is in the third decade. There is no HLA matching. There is a slight increase in incidence of selective IgA deficiency in relatives
IgA is often virtually abs. IgG levels vary but are usually < 200 mg/100 mL. IgM may be low or even raised
30% have lymphopenia and associated splenomegaly

T cells are often functionally immature, as may be the macrophages. There may therefore be a reduced level of cellular immunity, but the infections associated with T-cell deficiencies are rare. T cells fail to stimulate differentiation of B cells into plasma cells

SELECTIVE IgG SUBCLASS DEFICIENCY
May be either inherited or acquired. The most important type is the IgG_2 subclass which is involved in immunity to polysaccharides and deficiency has been associated with poor response to polysaccharide vaccines and an increase in certain pulmonary infections. However most patients have normal lives and life expectancy. IgG_4 deficiency is seen in 15% of the population; its clinical effects are however unclear.

SELECTIVE IgA SUBCLASS DEFICIENCY
Very common, with an incidence of 1:700 in Caucasians. The disease is usually sporadic but may be inherited as a defect in chromosome 18. Associations include ataxia telangiectasia; coeliac disease (may be due to the common association with HLA DR3 but may be directly due to the deficiency itself), rheumatoid arthritis, Still's disease and epilepsy, due to the use of gold, penicillamine and phenytoin.

It is important to check for IgA deficiency prior to truncal vagotomy as this reduces gut motility and causes bacterial overgrowth in these patients, leading to chronic diarrhoea and malabsorption.

Patients with IgA deficiency should be tested for IgA autoantibodies (the presence of which is a contraindication to blood transfusion or gammaglobulin treatment, as this can cause anaphylaxis unless depleted of IgA).

MOST COMMON PATHOGENS
Streptococcus – pneumonia, meningitis, septic arthritis
Haemophilus influenzae – pneumonia, meningitis, septic arthritis
Staphylococcus – pyoderma and septic arthritis (especially in children)

Mycoplasma pneumoniae – pneumonia and arthritis
Campylobacter – gastrointestinal infection
Giardia – gastrointestinal infection
Ureaplasma urealyticum – chronic urinary tract infection
Herpes zoster – shingles
Enteroviruses – diarrhoea, chronic meningitis and myositis

SYMPTOMS

Vary according to infective organism
Watch for symptoms of meningism, septic arthritis, pneumonia, infective diarrhoea, urinary tract infections, shingles and myositis
No symptoms directly due to hypogammaglobulinaemia

SIGNS

Lymphadenopathy
Pulmonary crackles from chest infections, bronchiectasis and fibrosis
Splenomegaly associated with nodular lymphoid hyperplasia

INVESTIGATIONS
FBC

Hb normal
WCC variable. May be ↑ in infection or ↓ if X-linked agammaglobulinaemia
Platelets normal

U + Es

Normal

LFTs

Normal unless infection or sclerosing cholangitis occurs (associated with XHM)

Rheumatoid factor negative
Urinary protein normal
Faecal ^{51}Cr transferrin normal (compare with protein-losing enteropathy)

Synovial fluid:
Mononuclear infiltrate
Positive culture if septic arthritis

DIAGNOSIS

Immunoglobulins ↓
Protein electrophoresis is normal or has ↓ γ band

Note that XHM immunodeficiency may show elevated levels of IgM

DIFFERENTIAL DIAGNOSIS

Selective class hypogammaglobulinaemia
Lymphoma
Leukaemia
Rheumatoid arthritis, including Felty's syndrome
Other causes of bronchiectasis, including cystic fibrosis
Other causes of chronic diarrhoea

COMPLICATIONS

Bronchiectasis
Pulmonary fibrosis
Cor pulmonale
Malabsorption
Gastric carcinoma ($\times$ 50 risk)
Non-erosive arthritis – symmetrical polyarthritis which usually spares hands and feet
Tenosynovitis
Achlorhydria (30%). Some of these lack intrinsic factor and develop pernicious anaemia
Autoimmune disease (including coeliac disease in IgA deficiency – note that usual antibody tests will not work)
Lymphoreticular malignancy

TREATMENT

IV gammaglobulin – frequency and dose depend on the clinical experience of the patient. Is of little use in selective IgA deficiency (oral IgA has been used to reduce diarrhoea)
Antibiotics for acute infection
Physiotherapy for bronchiectasis
Antibiotic prophylaxis with low-dose penicillin is advised
Avoid live vaccines

QUESTION SPOTTING

Watch for recurrent infections and arthritis, especially if there is lymphadenopathy or splenomegaly. If the albumin and the total protein are given, always work out the globulins to exclude hypogammaglobulinaemia. Need to exclude Felty's syndrome (↑↑ rheumatoid factor, leukopenia, anaemia and thrombocytopenia. Immunoglobulins raised)

PAROXYSMAL NOCTURNAL HAEMOGLOBINURIA

An acquired clonal abnormality of bone marrow stem cells, thought to produce deficiency of glucosylphosphatidylinositol (GPI) in cell membranes. This lipid acts as an anchor for several membrane proteins, including those which protect cells against complement-mediated lysis (e.g. CD59 and CD55). Thus red cell, white cell and platelet lines become hypersensitive to complement lysis, causing intravascular haemolysis. Platelets can be activated inappropriately, leading to thrombotic complications, and the bone marrow reveals hypoplasia of all three cell lines. The disease usually affects younger adults.

SYMPTOMS
Tiredness
Shortness of breath
Dark urine due to haemoglobinuria. This is classically worse overnight, but may occur at any time
Headache
Abdominal pain

SIGNS
Jaundice (usually mild)
Splenomegaly
Hepatomegaly (if Budd–Chiari)
Purpura (if severe)

INVESTIGATIONS
FBC
Hb ↓
MCV slightly ↑
Reticulocytes ↑
WCC ↓
Neutrophil ALP score ↓
Platelets ↓

U + Es
Usually normal

LFTs
Bilirubin ↑ (unconjugated, so not found in urine)

Fe often ↓
TIBC often ↑
Haptoglobins absent

LDH elevated
Marrow biopsy shows hypoplastic marrow in many cases. Low iron stores
Urine shows haemoglobin in urine. Haemosiderin is also detectable in urine (derived from tubular cells taking up haem pigment from circulation)

DIAGNOSIS
Is by flow cytometry to detect the absence of CD59 and CD55 antigens on haematopoietic cells

ASSOCIATIONS
Aplastic anaemia (this precedes PNH in 25%)
Myelofibrosis
Acute myeloblastic leukaemia (rare)

COMPLICATIONS
Thrombotic disease, usually venous. There is a predilection to portal vein thrombosis and Budd–Chiari syndrome, as well as DVT and PE
Pigment gallstones (secondary to long-standing haemolysis)
Bacterial infections (due to granulocytopenia)

TREATMENT
Bone marrow transplant if disease is severe (especially if leukaemia or aplastic anaemia occurs)
Supportive treatment with blood transfusion, iron supplements (secondary iron deficiency is common due to loss of haemoglobin in the urine)
Venous thrombosis necessitates therapy with warfarin, but prophylaxis is not used
Steroids may reduce the rate of haemolysis in some patients

PROGNOSIS
10-year median survival, but 10–15% remit spontaneously

QUESTION SPOTTING
Think of PNH when:
Venous thromboemboli occur, especially in conjunction with pancytopenia
There is a past history of aplastic anaemia
The history of haemoglobinuria is often long, unlike many other causes of haemolysis

VITAMIN B$_{12}$ DEFICIENCY

Vitamin B$_{12}$ is absorbed in the terminal ileum, and body stores may last between 3 and 5 years in the absence of dietary B$_{12}$. Deficiency chiefly affects haematopoietic cell turnover and neural tissues. The mechanism of neuronal dysfunction is unclear; the effect on bone marrow is due to defective DNA synthesis. B$_{12}$ deficiency is common in older people; prevalence may be as high as 15% depending on the cutoff used. Neurological symptoms may occur even in the absence of anaemia or an absolute macrocytosis.

CAUSES
Dietary (e.g. vegans)
Lack of intrinsic factor
Pernicious anaemia
Gastrectomy
Gastric carcinoma
Small-bowel dysfunction
Bacterial overgrowth
Crohn's disease
Ileal resection
Fish tapeworm
HIV infection
Tropical sprue
Radiation enteritis
Transcobalamin II deficiency

SYMPTOMS
Sore tongue (glossitis)
Diarrhoea (if intestinal dysfunction is cause)
Indigestion

Weight loss
Tiredness, SOB
Easy bruising
Numbness and tingling in limbs
Unsteadiness, limb weakness
Memory loss
Visual loss

SIGNS
General
Pale
Bruising occasionally seen
Red, shiny tongue
Skin pigmentation (occasional)
Pyrexia (up to 38°C)
Splenomegaly (mild)

Neurological
Optic atrophy (Fig. 9.1)
Altered sensation in limbs
Limb weakness
Reduced ankle reflexes
Extensor plantars
Loss of vibration and joint position sense
Cognitive impairment

INVESTIGATIONS
FBC
Hb ↓
MCV markedly ↑
Reticulocytes ↓
WCC often ↓
Platelets often ↓

U + Es
Normal

LFTs
Bilirubin may be ↑ (haemolysis)
ALT mildly ↑
ALP ↓
Clotting normal

Ferritin ↑
Fe ↑
LDH elevated (haemolysis)
Haptoglobins low or absent
Cholesterol low

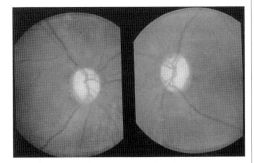

Figure 9.1 Optic atrophy due to vitamin B$_{12}$ deficiency. (Reproduced with permission from Souhami, Moxham (2002) *Textbook of Medicine*, 4th edn. Churchill Livingstone.)

Blood film
Macrocytic RBCs
Hypersegmented ($>$ 5) neutrophils

Bone marrow
Megaloblasts
Giant metamyelocytes

DIAGNOSIS
B$_{12}$ deficiency
Low serum B$_{12}$ with normal or low folate

Pernicious anaemia
Parietal cell antibodies are positive in 90% of
cases. Intrinsic factor (IF) antibodies are
present in 50% and are specific for pernicious
anaemia

To differentiate lack of intrinsic factor from
small-bowel disease:

Schilling test
1 µg radiolabelled B$_{12}$ is given orally
1 mg unlabelled B$_{12}$ is then given IM to saturate
the body stores and mobilize the oral dose
Urine is collected for 24 hours
Normal subjects should excrete $>$ 10% of the
radioactive dose
If the test is abnormal, IF is given orally with the
radiolabelled B$_{12}$. If the test corrects to normal,
lack of IF (i.e. a gastric problem) is to blame

DIFFERENTIAL DIAGNOSIS
Usually of other causes of megaloblastic
anaemia, most commonly folate deficiency,
which may coexist. Also consider alcohol
abuse, drugs (e.g. cytotoxics), myelodysplasia,
reticulocytosis
Causes of neurological disease – especially
syphilis, multiple sclerosis, multi-infarct
disease

TREATMENT
Intramuscular B$_{12}$ injections. Haematological
response is evident within a few days;
neurological symptoms may reverse entirely
over a few months provided B$_{12}$ deficiency is
not long-standing
Correct hypokalemia prior to giving vitamin B$_{12}$
Supplemental iron may be needed if iron stores
are low (due to enhanced red cell production)

ASSOCIATIONS
Associations with pernicious anaemia
IDDM
Addison's disease
Vitiligo
Hypothyroidism
Graves disease
Primary ovarian failure
Hypoparathyroidism
IgA deficiency
Hypogammaglobulinaemia
Gastric carcinoma
Lambert–Eaton syndrome
Myasthenia gravis

QUESTION SPOTTING
Pernicious anaemia is perhaps less likely than
one of the small intestinal causes. Note that B$_{12}$
deficiency is one of the causes of absent ankle
reflexes plus extensor plantars.
    Look out for anaemia or pancytopenia plus
neurological signs, perhaps complicating a case
of Crohn's disease or several years after
radiotherapy for cervical cancer.

MYELODYSPLASIA

Generally thought of as a group of preleukaemic disorders, with neoplastic change and ineffective haematopoiesis due to enhanced apoptosis. There are abnormalities of peripheral blood and bone marrow function, which may eventually evolve into an acute myeloid leukaemia.

Although there are many classifications, the simplest is primary (no known cause), and secondary, as a result of treatment with alkylating agents with or without radiotherapy for the treatment of myeloma, lymphoma and other cancers. The FAB classification is widely used and recognized, and can be seen in Table 9.1.

The patient is usually over 50 years of age (mean age of onset is 69 years) and men and women are equally affected.

SYMPTOMS

May be asymptomatic
Tiredness
Shortness of breath
Easy bruising, excessive bleeding
Recurrent infections
Fever

SIGNS

Anaemia
Bruising
Splenomegaly (10–20%)

INVESTIGATIONS

FBC

Hb ↓
MCV ↑ or normal
WCC ↑ or ↓. Monocytosis may be present
Platelets ↓ but may be normal or elevated
Reticulocytes ↓

Blood film – anisopoikylocytosis, polychromasia, punctate basophilia, abnormal neutrophils and blasts may be present. Giant platelets may be seen

U + Es
Normal

LFTs
Normal

Bone marrow aspiration
Erythroid lineage: abnormal nuclear shape with nuclear fragments, and ring sideroblasts
Myeloid lineage: ↓ granules in neutrophils and myelocytes. Hyposegmented (Pelger cells) or hypersegmented neutrophils. Blasts
Megakaryocytic lineage: micromegakaryocytes, megakaryocytes with abnormal nuclei

Bone marrow trephine
Shows hypercellularity with little or no fat space. Clusters of blasts can be seen. Fibrosis is not a feature of primary myelodysplasia, but may be seen in secondary. Occasional patient may have a hypocellular marrow

DIFFERENTIAL DIAGNOSIS

Anaemia secondary to folate/vitamin B_{12} deficiency
Anaemia secondary to chronic diseases such as liver/renal disease or chronic inflammation
Overt leukaemias such as AML
Myeloproliferative diseases

TREATMENT

Correct any deficiency of haematinics (iron, B_{12}, folate)
Supportive therapy with red cell and platelet transfusions

Table 9.1 FAB classification of myelodysplasia

Type	Peripheral blood	Bone marrow
Refractory anaemia (RA)	< 1% blasts	< 5% blasts
Refractory anaemia with ring sideroblasts (RARS)	< 1% blasts	< 5% blasts, > 15% sideroblasts
Refractory anaemia with excess blasts (RAEB)	< 5% blasts	5–20% blasts
Refractory anaemia with excess blasts in transformation (RAEBt)	> 5% blasts	21–30% blasts
Chronic myelomonocytic leukaemia (CMML)	> 1.0×10^9/L monocytes	< 30% blasts plus promonocytes

Erythropoietin, with or without G-CSF, can sometimes reduce or eliminate the need for transfusion

Antibiotic therapy for infection

CMML can be treated palliatively with hydroxycarbamide

Bone marrow transplantation is the only curative therapy, but only 40–60% are disease-free after 5 years, and only young, fit patients tolerate this therapy

Intensive chemotherapy without BMT is occasionally used for severe disease, but has little evidence and long-term outcomes are still poor

PROGNOSIS

Highly variable. Median survival is about 20 months, but ranges from 3 to 60 months depending on prognostic factors. The International Prognostic Scoring System (IPSS), based on number of cytopenias, karyotype and percentage of blasts, provides an alternative to the FAB system

One-third die of unrelated conditions

One-third die of leukaemic transformation

One-third die of marrow failure without transformation

QUESTION SPOTTING

Typically, patients will be in their 60–80s and will present with symptoms of anaemia, infection or bruising. Diagnosis comes from bone marrow examination in most cases.

SICKLE-CELL DISEASE

Hereditary disorder of haemoglobin structure where valine has been substituted for glutamic acid at position 6 of the haem β chain, caused by a point mutation. The abnormal HbS is insoluble in the deoxygenized form, polymerizes, and makes the red blood cell inflexible and take up the classic sickle shape. This is initially reversible, but after repeated sickling episodes, the cell becomes fixed in the sickled shape. The sickled red blood cells have a shortened lifespan due to increased fragility, and this leads to a chronic haemolytic anaemia. The cells can aggregate, increasing blood viscosity, and cause arterial occlusion and tissue infarction. Sickling is precipitated by hypoxia, acidosis, infection, dehydration and cold. Many crisis episodes have no obvious precipitant.

The disease is common in but not exclusive to peoples of equatorial African ancestry. Sickle disease is caused by inheriting abnormal haemoglobin genes from both parents. The most common cause of this is SS disease. However other abnormalities, such as HbC, and the β-thalassaemias can occur in conjunction with HbS to give HbSC disease, which has a similar course to HbSS disease, but with a slightly increased risk of thrombosis, and sickle-cell/thalassaemia disease. People with only one abnormal HbS gene have the sickle-cell trait which gives a usually harmless carrier state and which also gives some resistance to malaria.

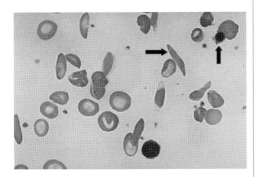

Figure 9.2 Blood film showing sickle cells, target cells and nucleated red cells. (Reproduced with permission from Boon, Colledge, Walker et al. (2006) *Davidson's Principles and Practice of Medicine*, 20th edn. Churchill Livingstone.)

The sickle-cell gene occurs with a frequency of up to 30% in Africa, southern Europe and some parts of India.

CLINICAL FEATURES

All clinical features arise from the two main features of the disease – haemolysis and vaso-occlusive disease

Haemolysis

Anaemia – though this is rarely symptomatic except during crisis, as HbS releases oxygen to the tissues more easily, and there is increased cardiac output

Bone marrow enlargement may lead to frontal bossing

Hyperdynamic circulation may lead to heart failure and cardiomegaly

Gallstones common (pigment) (up to 40% of 20-year-olds with sickle-cell disease)

Haemolysis increased by certain drugs, infection, or in association with G6PD deficiency.

Aplastic anaemia can occur as a result of certain viral infections, especially parvovirus B19

Vaso-occlusive disease

Bone pain (70%) with dactylitis and avascular necrosis and impaired growth in children. Painful, swollen joints

Acute chest syndrome (40%) – fever, cough, dyspnoea and pleuritic pain caused by combinations of infection, infarction, pulmonary sequestration and fat embolism

Leg ulcers (20%). Rare in HbSC disease

Genitourinary – priapism (10–40%), impotence

Renal (5–20%) – papillary infarcts causing pain and haematuria; renal tubular defects, chronic renal failure, enuresis

Cerebral – strokes (10%) (commonest in childhood, and rare after 14 years of age), fits and cognitive impairment

Late puberty (average menarche 2.5 years late) may give rise to above-average adult height

Spleen – upper abdominal pain, acute enlargement (acute splenic sequestration), chronic enlargement (hypersplenism) and eventually splenic fibrosis (asplenia) leading to increased risk from capsulated bacteria, especially pneumococcal septicaemia, and

223

Salmonella or *Staphylococcus aureus* osteomyelitis

Liver (2%) – abnormal liver function tests with upper abdominal pain

Watch out for secondary haemochromatosis from iron overload due to multiple transfusions

Bowel ischaemia causing abdominal pain

Retinopathy – retinal detachment and proliferative retinopathy (rare in HbSS but up to 50% in HbSC).

Complications during pregnancy such as acute chest syndrome, and crisis (maternal mortality 1%). Spontaneous abortion common

INVESTIGATIONS
FBC
Hb 6–9 g/dL steady state, but 3–4 g/dL during crisis

WCC normal

Platelets normal

Reticulocytes 5–15% steady state, 20–30% during crisis or low if aplastic crisis

U + Es
Na normal

K normal

Urea and creatinine ↑ if renal failure

LFTs
Bilirubin ↑

AST may be ↑

ALP may be ↑

Albumin may be ↓

LDH usually elevated

Haptoglobins usually absent

Folate deficiency may give rise to megaloblastic anaemia with low reticulocyte counts, ↑ MCV and ↓ Hb

ABGs
po_2 ↓

pco_2 ↓

pH ↓

Chest X-ray
Infection

Infarction

Avascular necrosis of ribs

Infiltrates

Fibrosis

Bone X-rays to demonstrate avascular necrosis (especially femoral heads)

Liver ultrasound may show gallstones

DIAGNOSIS
Blood film (Fig. 9.2) may show sickled cells and hyposplenism. Sickling can be induced by sodium metabisulphite

Hb electrophoresis confirms diagnosis

TREATMENT
Sickle crisis
Oxygen

Adequate pain relief, e.g. intravenous opiates

Vigorous rehydration

Broad-spectrum antibiotics

Consider exchange transfusion (especially if chest syndrome with hypoxia, stroke, or priapism) to reduce HbS below 20%

Other management
Prophylactic penicillin for prevention of pneumococcal infection. Vaccination against *Streptococcus pneumoniae* and *Haemophilus influenzae*

Aggressive management of blood pressure to prevent strokes

Folate supplements in pregnancy and severe haemolysis

Transfusion is only required on a regular basis if severe anaemia or frequent crises.

Transfusions are often given prior to elective surgery and exchange transfusion may be needed before emergency surgery

Splenectomy may be required for hypersplenism

Hydroxycarbamide reduces the frequency of crises and the need for blood transfusion. It enhances production of HbF, protecting against sickling, and is useful for patients with frequent crises or high transfusion requirements. It is still unclear whether hydroxycarbamide increases the risk of leukaemia in the long term in patients with sickle-cell disease

Bone marrow transplantation is used in a few cases. Hazards are high, and it is only indicated for patients under 16 years of age, with severe complications and an HLA-matched donor (only about 1% of patients)

PROGNOSIS

Approximately 120 000 babies per year are born in Africa with sickle-cell disease but < 2% survive to 5 years old. Highest mortality is in the first year of life, especially the second 6 months, when HbF levels have fallen. In industrialized nations, the prognosis is much better, and some patients survive to normal ages. However there is much variability from patient to patient.

QUESTION SPOTTING

With the diverse complications of this disease, sickle-cell disease is ideal for questions. Think about it as a cause of abdominal pain and gallstones. The nationality of the patient in the question may not be given.

Consider in any patient of Afro-Caribbean origin. Also consider in chest pain and shortness of breath in a young patient with anaemia – especially if any evidence of haemolysis.

MIXED ESSENTIAL CRYOGLOBULINAEMIA

Mixed cryoglobulinaemia is caused by immune complexes that precipitate at low temperatures (cryoglobulins). There are two components, a polyclonal IgG as antigen, and either a monoclonal IgM (type II) or a polyclonal IgM (type III), with anti-IgG Fc specificity, i.e. rheumatoid factor activity. IgA or IgG can occasionally take the place of IgM. Females tend to be affected more frequently.

CAUSES OF MIXED ESSENTIAL CRYOGLOBULINAEMIA

Type II
Hepatitis C (90%)
Hepatitis B
SBE
EBV
CMV

Type III
Lyme disease
Syphilis
Coccidiomycosis
Malaria
SLE
Rheumatoid arthritis
Systemic sclerosis
Sjögren's syndrome

FEATURES
Lower-limb purpura (95–100%)
Arthralgia (70–90%); N.B.: arthritis is
    uncommon
Hepatitis; usually chronic (60–70%)
Sensorimotor peripheral neuropathy (20–70%)
Membranoproliferative glomerulonephritis
    (30–50%) leading to hypertension, nephrotic
    syndrome and renal impairment
Leg ulcers (30%)
Raynaud's syndrome (20%)
Abdominal pain (20%)
Sjögren's syndrome (15–40%)
Other features include hyperviscosity
    syndrome, pulmonary vasculitis and
    pleuropericarditis

INVESTIGATIONS
FBC
Hb may be ↓
WCC variable
Platelets variable

U + Es
Urea and creatinine may be ↑

LFTs
ALT, ALP often ↑

ESR raised
Igs may be ↓
Complement: low C1q, C2, C4 and
    total complement activity.
    Normal C3, C9

Autoantibodies
ANA positive in 5%
Antimitochondrial positive in 5%
Anti-smooth-muscle positive in 13%
Extractable nuclear antigens positive in 3%
Rheumatoid factor invariably positive

CXR
Chest X-ray may show patchy shadowing or
    pleural effusions

DIAGNOSIS
Is on clinical grounds, together with the demonstration of cryoglobulins. Analysis of the cryoprecipitate then determines which category of cryoglobulinaemia is present.

DIFFERENTIAL DIAGNOSIS
Other vasculitides, e.g. Wegener's, PAN,
    Churg–Strauss, SLE
SBE
Other causes of liver disease
Amyloidosis
Sarcoidosis

COMPLICATIONS
Liver cirrhosis
B-cell non-Hodgkin's lymphoma (5–10%)
Renal failure
Hyperviscosity syndrome

TREATMENT

Treat the underlying cause

Interferon and ribavirin for hepatitis C

High-dose steroids, with or without
cytotoxics for underlying vasculitic
disease

Plasmapheresis for life-threatening
manifestations or hyperviscosity syndrome

Rituximab may also be of use in controlling the
underlying B-cell proliferation

PROGNOSIS

50% survival at 10 years

QUESTION SPOTTING

The triad of cutaneous vasculitis, renal
involvement and arthralgia should raise the
diagnosis. Other clues are:

Deranged LFTs

Risk factors for hepatitis C infection

Abnormalities of haemoglobin synthesis which result in reduced output of one or other of the globin chains in adult haemoglobin. Each adult haemoglobin has four chains, two α and two β. Abnormalities of α-chain production occur following mutations on the short arm of chromosome 16, whereas those of the β-chain occur with mutations of chromosome 11. However the α-chain genes are duplicated. Thalassaemias may arise from over 200 different mutations, resulting in loss of α- and β-chain production either as a direct mutation of the globin chain or affecting translation or transcription processes.

Thalassaemias are common and are distributed across the Mediterranean region (especially beta-thalassaemia), the Middle East, the Indian subcontinent and South-east Asia (especially alpha-thalassaemia). It is not uncommon to see combinations of abnormalities such as thalassaemias and sickle cell, to give sickle-cell thalassaemias.

BETA-THALASSAEMIA SYNDROMES

The disease has a wide range of presentations and severities depending on whether there is no β-chain production ($\beta0$) or reduced production ($\beta+$). It also depends on whether the individual is homozygous or heterozygous for a defect or has more than one defect. The imbalance of α- and β-chains leads to precipitation of α-chains, causing ineffective erythropoiesis and haemolysis.

The syndromes tend to be divided into:

Thalassaemia major (Cooley's anaemia)
Thalassaemia intermedia
Thalassaemia trait or minor

Thalassaemia major

Clinical Features
Severe anaemia
Splenomegaly
Hepatomegaly
Bony changes due to bone marrow expansion – so-called 'hair-on-end' appearance and frontal bossing (Fig. 9.3)
Growth retardation
Failure to thrive
Recurrent infections
Digital ulceration
Gallstones

Thalassaemia intermedia
Tends to present with milder symptoms, and is often caused by mild $\beta+$ syndromes where β-chain production is mildly impaired or in combination with alpha-thalassaemia

Patients present later with:
Moderate anaemia (Hb 7–10 g/dL)
Splenomegaly
Bony deformities
Recurrent leg ulcers
Recurrent infections
Gallstones

Thalassaemia trait or minor
An asymptomatic condition. Patients may have mild anaemia or normal haemoglobin levels. However, they do have abnormalities on investigation such as microcytic (MCV 50–70 fl) hypochromic (MCH 20–22 pg) red cells (iron stores are normal) and often a raised HbA_2 and sometimes HbF fractions.

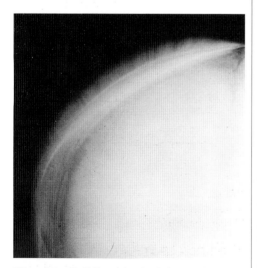

Figure 9.3 Skull X-ray showing hair-on-end appearance in beta-thalassaemia. (Reproduced with permission from Kumar, Clarke (2001) *Clinical Medicine*, 5th edn. Saunders.)

INVESTIGATIONS
FBC
Hb ↓ (variable amount)

MCV and MCH ↓↓ – out of proportion to anaemia

WCC and platelets normal unless coexistent hypersplenism

U + Es
Normal

LFTs
Bilirubin ↑ if severe

TIBC may be saturated and ferritin high because repeated transfusions cause iron overload

Blood film
Hypochromia

Microcytosis

Nucleated red cells

Basophilic stippling

Target cells

Raised reticulocyte count

Skull X ray: may show frontal bossing and marrow expansion

DIAGNOSIS
Is by Hb electrophoresis. This shows:

HbF ↑

HbA_2 ↑ or normal

HbA ↑ or absent

DIFFERENTIAL DIAGNOSIS
Other haemoglobinopathies, e.g. sickle-cell disease, G6PD disease, hereditary spherocytosis

Vasculitis, e.g. SLE

Iron deficiency

Lead poisoning

Sideroblastic anaemia

TREATMENT
Transfusions to maintain Hb at 9–10 g/dL

Iron chelation with desferrioxamine.

Desferrioxamine is associated with ocular and acoustic nerve complications with long-term treatment and may lead to growth retardation and bone disease if given in large doses. Oral chelators are now available (e.g. deferiprone); controversy over their safety remains

Folic acid therapy

Splenectomy if hypersplenism

Bone marrow transplantation should be considered in early life before iron overload or other complications occur

Iron therapy is contraindicated

PROGNOSIS
50% of patients die by the age of 35 years, often due to iron overload from repeated transfusions, and suboptimal iron chelation.

ALPHA-THALASSAEMIA SYNDROMES
Unlike the beta-thalassaemias, these all arise from gene deletions. As the alpha genes are duplicated, four scenarios may arise:

Single gene deletion (–a/aa)
Asymptomatic carrier. Minority show ↓ MCV and MCH

Two gene deletions (–a/–a or —/aa)
Alpha-thalassaemia trait – microcytosis with or without mild anaemia. Low MCV and MCH but asymptomatic

Three gene deletions (—/–a)
HbH disease (Hb β4) – moderate haemolytic anaemia (Hb 7–10 g/dL) and splenomegaly, hepatomegaly, jaundice, leg ulcers, gallstones and folate deficiency. HbH is seen in older red cells on blood film

Four gene deletions (—/—)
Hb Barts (Hb γ_4) – no α-chain production. Hb γ_4 is not able to carry oxygen, and infants are either stillborn at 28–40 weeks, or die soon after birth. They are pale and oedematous with huge spleens and livers – hydrops fetalis.

TREATMENT
Nil specific

Folic acid if necessary

Avoid iron therapy

QUESTION SPOTTING
Could appear with sickle cell or alone. The key for thalassaemia is that the MCV and MCH are disproportionately low for the degree of anaemia. Also suspect this disease in Mediterranean or patients of arab origin.

ANTIPHOSPHOLIPID SYNDROME (HUGHES' SYNDROME)

Presence of an antibody which may either target phospholipids in cell membranes, or may react with β_2 glycoproteins bound to phospholipids in cell membranes. Antiphospholipid antibodies may be found in isolation (primary disease) or may accompany other autoimmune diseases, e.g. SLE.

CLINICAL FEATURES
Recurrent miscarriages

VENOUS THROMBOSIS
Deep-vein thrombosis
Pulmonary embolus
Pulmonary hypertension
Budd–Chiari syndrome
Dural sinus thrombosis

ARTERIAL THROMBOSIS
CVA/TIA
Mesenteric/peripheral thrombosis
MI
Endocarditis
Livedo reticularis

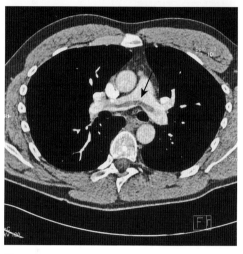

Figure 9.5 Massive central pulmonary embolus caused by antiphospholipid syndrome. (Reproduced with permission from Boon, Colledge, Walker et al. (2006) *Davidson's Principles and Practice of Medicine*, 20th edn. Churchill Livingstone.)

LESS COMMON FEATURES
Pyoderma gangrenosum
Acrocyanosis
Haemolytic anaemia
Transverse myelopathy

INVESTIGATIONS
FBC
Hb occasionally ↓
WCC normal
Platelets usually ↓

U + Es
Normal

LFTs
Normal unless syndrome is part of another disease

INR normal
VDRL often positive
Anticardiolipin antibody often positive

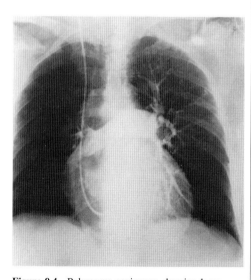

Figure 9.4 Pulmonary angiogram showing large central embolus. (Reproduced with permission from Souhami, Moxham (2002) *Textbook of Medicine*, 4th edn. Churchill Livingstone.)

DIAGNOSIS
Diagnostic criteria are one of:
Recurrent miscarriage
Arterial or venous thrombosis

Immune thrombocytopenia

plus

Anticardiolipin antibodies
or
Prolonged APTT or dilute Russell's viper venom test not correctable with normal plasma

Antiphospholipid antibodies may occur transiently with some infections and drug therapies (see below); the persistent presence of antiphospholipid antibodies is required to make the diagnosis

ASSOCIATIONS
Autoimmune disease
Rheumatoid arthritis
SLE
Giant cell arteritis
Systemic sclerosis
Sjögren's syndrome
Psoriatic arthropathy

Infections, especially
Syphilis
Malaria
Hepatitis C
HIV

Drugs
Phenytoin
Hydralazine
Quinidine

Other
Early, severe pre-eclampsia
IV drug abuse
Behçet's disease
Sickle-cell anaemia
Guillain–Barré syndrome

DIFFERENTIAL DIAGNOSIS
Other causes of thrombophilia, including:

Factor V Leiden mutation
Protein C deficiency
Protein S deficiency

Antithrombin III deficiency
Hyperhomocysteinaemia
Polycythaemia
Essential thrombocythaemia
Paroxysmal nocturnal haemoglobinuria

TREATMENT
Treatment with warfarin (target INR 2.5) for 6 months after first arterial or venous thrombotic episode. Patients suffering a further event whilst maintained at INR 2.0–3.0 should receive warfarin to target INR of 3.5 (range 3.0–4.0) and remain on warfarin for life
Low-dose aspirin is efficacious in reducing the risk of recurrent miscarriage

PROGNOSIS
Patients with a single episode of thrombus are at high risk of recurrent episodes without treatment, with a median time to second episode of 18 months.

QUESTION SPOTTING
Any combination of:

Abortion
Venous/arterial thrombosis
Low platelets
Livedo reticularis

should prompt consideration of the antiphospholipid syndrome, as should thrombosis in the presence of a positive VDRL. The syndrome may accompany SLE or another autoimmune disease as part of a dual diagnosis. Other clues are low platelets or long APTTR

A heterogeneous group of disorders caused by a proliferation of various cells in the lymphoid system, classified as Hodgkin's disease (HD) or non-Hodgkin's lymphoma (NHL). Further classification of HD can be seen in Table 9.2 and the staging of this disease, which is important for treatment, is seen in Table 9.3. NHL has a complicated classification which depends on the rate of cell division, the cell type involved and the behaviour of the disease. It can be divided into T- or B-cell, low- or high-grade. The details of these classifications are not important for the MRCP examination.

Hodgkin's disease has been linked to Epstein–Barr virus infection, as well as some carcinogens and the HLA DB1 haplotype. Several factors have been linked to NHL, including:

EBV (Burkitt's lymphoma)
HTLV-1
Helicobacter pylori (GI lymphoma)
Autoimmune disease
Genetic defects (e.g. Fanconi syndrome, xeroderma pigmentosum)

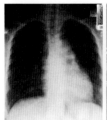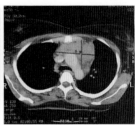

Figure 9.6 Chest X-ray and CT chest showing large mediastinal lymphadenopathy in Hodgkin's disease. (Reproduced with permission from Kumar, Clarke (2001) *Clinical Medicine*, 5th edn. Saunders.)

Immunosuppression (e.g. HIV, immunosuppressive drugs)
Radiation

CLINICAL FEATURES
Hodgkin's disease
Lymphadenopathy (especially cervical, axillary; also mediastinal and para-aortic)
Fever, sweats
Weight loss
Pruritus
Alcohol-induced lymph node pain
Recurrent infections
Anaemia
Bruising/bleeding
Splenomegaly/hepatomegaly
Extranodal involvement is rare; paraneoplastic phenomena may occur rarely (e.g. cerebellar signs, Guillain–Barré syndrome)

Non-Hodgkin's lymphoma
As above, plus extranodal organ-specific involvement:
Rash (e.g. mycosis fungoides)
Thyroid, testicular, salivary masses; jaw mass (Burkitt's lymphoma)
Abdominal pain/obstruction/malabsorption (GI lymphoma)
Meningism/cranial nerve palsies (CNS lymphoma)

INVESTIGATIONS
FBC
Hb usually normal but may be ↓
WCC ↓ or ↑ (↓ is poor prognostic sign).
Eosinophilia may occur

Table 9.2 Rye classification of Hodgkin's disease

Type	Frequency	Prognosis
Nodular sclerosing	70%	Good
Lymphocyte depleted	2%	Poor
Mixed cellularity	20%	Good
Lymphocyte predominance	5%	Good
Other	3%	

Table 9.3 Ann Arbor staging system

Stage	
I	Single LN region (I) or extralymphatic organ (Ie)
II	2 or more LN regions on same side of diaphragm (II) or 1 or more LN regions with an extralymphatic organ (IIe)
III	LN regions on both sides of the diaphragm (III)
IV	2 or more extralymphatic organs (IV)
Subtype	
A	Asymptomatic
B	Type B symptoms of fever, night sweats, > 10% weight loss

Platelets usually normal, but may be ↓
ESR usually raised

U + Es
Na normal
K normal
Urea and creatinine may ↑ if ureteric obstruction
from lymphadenopathy

LFTs
Bilirubin ↑
AST ↑
ALP ↑ (may ↑ due to liver or bony disease; may
also merely reflect disease activity)

Calcium ↑ if bony disease
Uric acid ↑
LDH ↑
Paraproteins may be seen (in NHL)
Ig levels may be reduced
Coombs test may be positive

Chest X-ray: hilar enlargement

DIAGNOSIS
Is made on lymph node biopsy and/or bone
marrow biopsy and trephine
CT scan of chest (Fig. 9.6), abdomen and pelvis
is useful for staging
Biopsy of other organs may be required for
diagnosis in some situations – e.g. gut biopsy,
lumbar puncture, thyroid FNA – where the
disease is localized to an organ system

DIFFERENTIAL DIAGNOSIS
Causes of lymphadenopathy include:

Lymphoma
Metastatic malignancy
Infective: bacterial (pyogenic, TB, *Brucella*),
fungal, viral (HIV, EBV, CMV) and parasitic
(syphilis, *Toxoplasma*)
Reactive: sarcoid, rheumatoid arthritis and other
connective tissue diseases, eczema, psoriasis,
drugs (phenytoin, berylliosis)
Infiltrative: lipidosis, histiocytosis

COMPLICATIONS
Complications tend to occur due to treatment:

Radiotherapy
Radiation lung fibrosis

Coronary artery disease
Hypothyroidism

Chemotherapy
Alopecia
Infertility
Neurotoxicity
Cardiomyopathy
Aseptic bone necrosis
Infections
Secondary malignancies
Progressive multifocal leukoencephalopathy
Tumour lysis syndrome

Surgery
Overwhelming sepsis postsplenectomy

TREATMENT
Hodgkin's disease
Depends on staging of disease

Early-stage disease
External-beam radiotherapy is used. All lymph
node groups are treated in the affected half of the
body and additional doses are given to node
groups known to be involved. Short courses of
chemotherapy are used in early-stage disease
to reduce the need for wide field of
radiotherapy.

Advanced disease
ABVD (Adriamycin, bleomycin, vinblastine and
dacarbazine) are used. Radiotherapy is used on
bulky mediastinal disease

Relapsed disease
Further chemotherapy with stem cell transplantation

Non-Hodgkin's lymphoma
Treatment depends on histological type:

Low-grade disease
No treatment if asymptomatic
Single-agent chemotherapy if symptoms (e.g.
chlorambucil, interferon, fludarabine)
Occasionally, surgery or radiotherapy may be
curative for very limited disease

High-grade disease
CHOP (chlorambucil, Adriamycin, vincristine
and prednisolone) is used most often in high-
grade NHL.

Irradiation of involved lymph node areas may be added

Intrathecal methotrexate may be added if CNS involvement is present or risk of CNS involvement is high (e.g. HIV, Burkitt's lymphoma)

Rituximab (anti-CD20 antibodies) is of added value in large B-cell lymphoma

Alternative regimens, together with bone marrow transplant, may be used in refractory or relapsed disease

PROGNOSIS

80% 5-year survival in HD, though this depends on the histology

NHL carries a worse overall prognosis. Low-grade disease is usually incurable but may remain in remission for several years; high-grade disease is sometimes curable, but may be more rapidly fatal. 80% show initial response to treatment, but only 35% are still disease-free at 5 years

QUESTION SPOTTING

Lymphoma may crop up in a multitude of guises – not just as the presence of lymphadenopathy – although it may easily be confused with infective or malignant causes of lymphadenopathy. Consider the diagnosis in patients with odd GI symptoms, fever of unknown origin or odd constellations of neurological symptoms.

LEUKAEMIAS

Malignant haemopoietic disorder characterized by unregulated proliferation of one stem line which is usually non-functional. These abnormal cells replace the normal bone marrow, including haemopoietic precursors, and this results in the loss of other cell lines. Usually the cause is not known, but documented aetiological factors include:

Hereditary, e.g. Down's syndrome, ataxia telangiectasia, Wiskott–Aldrich syndrome

Chemicals, e.g. benzene, alkylating agents

Radiation exposure

Myelodysplasia

Aplastic anaemia

Viral infection, e.g. HTLV-1

The leukaemias are divided into acute and chronic and they are also divided according to which cell line is affected. The classification is shown in Table 9.4

The typical age of incidence varies for each type of leukaemia. Although all types may occur at any age, the most typical presentation of ALL is at 2–10 years old, with a smaller rise in incidence over 40 years. AML increases with age: the median age is 60. Peak incidence of CML is 40–60 years and CLL almost always occurs after 60

CML is almost always caused by the presence of the *bcr-abl* gene fusion product; in 90% of

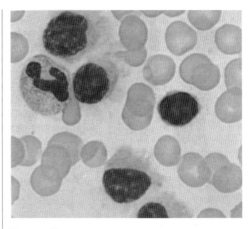

Figure 9.7 Film showing hairy-cell leukaemia – note fuzzy border of atypical lymphocytes. (Reproduced with permission from Forbes, Jackson (2003) *Colour Atlas and Text of Clinical Medicine*, 3rd edn. Mosby.)

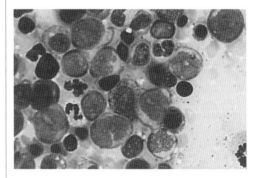

Figure 9.8 Acute myeloid leukaemia. (Reproduced with permission from Boon, Colledge, Walker et al. (2006) *Davidson's Principles and Practice of Medicine*, 20th edn. Churchill Livingstone.)

cases, this fusion is a result of the t9:22 Philadelphia chromosomal translocation, but is often present even without this translocation

SYMPTOMS

Anaemia causing tiredness, lethargy and dyspnoea

Neutropenia causing recurrent infections

Thrombocytopenia causing spontaneous bruising, menorrhagia, gingival bleeding and nose bleeds

Others: weight loss, abdominal pain and bloating, anorexia, night sweats, recurrent ulcers, bone pain and gum hyperplasia (especially in M5 AML)

Table 9.4 Classification of the leukaemias

Acute lymphoblastic leukaemia	Acute myeloid leukaemia*
Undifferentiated	M0 undifferentiated
Pre-B	M1 minimal differentiation
B-cell	M2 differentiated
T-cell	M3 promyelocytic
	M4 myelomonocytic
	M5 monocytic
	M6 erythrocytic
	M7 megakaryocytic

Chronic lymphocytic leukaemia	Chronic myeloid leukaemia
Classical B-cell	Philadelphia-positive
Prolymphocytic cell	Philadelphia-negative
Hairy cell	

*FAB (French, American, British) classification

SIGNS
Fever
Pallor
Petechial haemorrhages, purpura and fundal
  haemorrhages
Hepatomegaly
Splenomegaly
Peripheral lymphadenopathy

INVESTIGATIONS
FBC
Hb ↓ (MCV normal)
WCC may be ↓↓ or ↑↑ (range < 1.0 to > 200 ×
  10^9/L). Differential often abnormal
Platelets ↓ (often < 10 × 10^9/L)

U + Es
K ↑ especially in tumour lysis syndrome
Urea and creatinine ↑ if renal impairment

LFTs
Bilirubin may be ↑
Albumin ↓
ALP ↑
ALT ↑

Total protein ↓ in CLL
Immunoglobulins often ↓ in CLL (but may be ↑
  with a monoclonal band on electrophoresis)
Urate ↑ in acute leukaemias and occasionally in
  CML and as part of the tumour lysis syndrome
LDH ↑
Coagulation often abnormal (M3 AML is
  predisposed to DIC)
Coombs' test often positive in CLL

Chest X-ray
Mediastinal mass may occur (especially in T-cell
  ALL)
Lytic bony lesions may be seen

DIAGNOSIS
Is on the basis of blood film, and, most
importantly, bone marrow examination.
Prognostic and management information
can be obtained from cytogenetics,
cytochemistry and immunophenotyping.
Lumbar puncture may be required to detect
CNS involvement.

DIFFERENTIAL DIAGNOSIS
Lymphoma and infection for lymphadenopathy
  (e.g. glandular fever, HIV)
Myeloproliferative disorders, myelodysplasia,
  autoimmune disease and infection may all
  cause hepatosplenomegaly
Aplastic anaemia or bone marrow infiltration if
  pancytopenia
AML may be difficult to differentiate from
  polycythemia rubra vera and myelofibrosis

TREATMENT
Supportive
Transfusions of blood, platelets, FFP and
  cryoprecipitate
Antibiotics for infections – regimens vary
  from unit to unit. Multiple cultures are
  essential to target the causative organism and
  infection site
Chemotherapy support:

- Allopurinol prior to starting chemotherapy to
  prevent acute gout and renal impairment
- Intravenous hydration to prevent renal
  impairment
- Use of haemopoietic growth factors (G-CSF)
  to shorten duration of neutropenia

Barrier nursing while neutropenic
Psychological support

ALL
Combination high-dose chemotherapy, with
  intrathecal methotrexate
Cranial irradiation added if evidence of CNS
  disease
Maintenance chemotherapy is needed after
  induction of remission to reduce the chance of
  relapse
If disease relapses, or in adults with poor
  prognostic features (e.g. Philadelphia
  chromosome), allogeneic bone marrow
  transplant is used

AML
Induction of remission is with combination high-
  dose chemotherapy (anthracyclines plus
  cytarabine)
Autologous or allogeneic stem cell transplant can
  be used if patients are fit enough. An
  alternative is consolidation chemotherapy

'Mini-BMT' can be used in older people (less intensive induction chemotherapy)

Transretinoic acid can be used in AML M3 subtype to induce cell differentiation/maturation

CLL

Observation with early-stage disease (no symptoms, no anaemia or thrombocytopenia)

Single-agent chemotherapy, e.g. chlorambucil, fludarabine once disease progresses

Rituximab and other antibody-based therapies are also used in resistant or relapsed disease

CML

Imantinib (an antibody directed at the bcr-abl fusion protein)

Interferon-alpha is an alternative if imantinib not tolerated; hydroxycarbamide and busulphan are also used

Young, fit patients without comorbid disease can be treated by allogeneic bone marrow transplant

Other

Splenectomy may be useful if haemolytic anaemia (CLL) or gross splenic enlargement (CML). Leukapheresis may be needed for hyperviscosity syndrome (usually seen in CML or AML)

PROGNOSIS
ALL

70–80% cure in children. Poorer outlook seen in early relapse, CNS disease and testicular disease, high WCC at presentation, T-cell disease and < 1 year or > 10 years of age. Adults have only 30% cure rate.

AML

40–50% 5-year survival in younger patients. Poorer outlook seen in early relapse, CNS disease (rare), high WCC at presentation, > 20% blasts in bone marrow after first course of treatment, or > 60 years of age.

CLL

Median survival of 6 years. Poorer prognosis if anaemic and/or thrombocytopenic regardless of lymphoid enlargement – patients with multiple cytopenias have a median survival of 2 years; patients with lymphocytosis only have a median survival of 10 years.

CML

Median survival of 4–5 years in historical series; recent therapeutic advances appear to have considerably improved outcome.

QUESTION SPOTTING

You are unlikely to see a white count of more than 50×10^9/L – this would be too easy! This leads to diagnostic difficulty, especially if there is a possibility of chronic infection, inflammation or infarction that could give a reactive leukocytosis. However do remember that ineffective leukocytosis in leukaemic patients predisposes to recurrent infections. Questions may revolve around immunological sequelae of leukaemia (especially CLL) or choosing when to intervene in indolent or remitted disease.

MULTIPLE MYELOMA

Malignant proliferation of plasma cells (B lymphocytes). The monoclonal plasma cell line produces large quantities of immunoglobulin in most cases, and cytokine interactions between the malignant cells and the bone marrow lead to suppression of normal immunoglobulin production, enhanced osteoclastic activity and suppression of normal blood cell production. Mean age at onset is around 70 years.

SYMPTOMS
Often insidious in onset; 20% are asymptomatic
Bone pain
Tiredness
Weight loss
SOB
Fever (uncommon)
Infection, e.g. pneumonia
Thirst, polyuria

SIGNS
Pallor
Signs of infection

INVESTIGATIONS
FBC
Hb ↓ (in 60%)

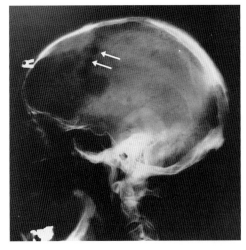

Figure 9.9 Skull X-ray showing typical lytic lesions of multiple myeloma. (Reproduced with permission from Kumar, Clarke (2001) *Clinical Medicine*, 5th edn. Saunders.)

MCV normal
WCC may be ↓
Platelets may be ↓

U + Es
Urea and creatinine raised in 20%

LFTs
Albumin often ↓ (especially in advanced disease)
Total protein usually ↑
ALP normal (unless bone fracture)

ESR ↑ in 90%
CRP often normal, but may be ↑
Calcium ↑ (in 30%)
INR, APTTR usually normal
Anion gap ↓
Blood film shows rouleaux. Plasma cells in 5%

Immunoglobulins:
Monoclonal gammopathy – IgG (60%), IgA (20–25%), IgD and non-secreting types (rare)
Light chains only in 15–20%
Other Ig levels are suppressed
Urine may show Bence–Jones proteinuria – often not detected on urine dipstix

X-rays
Lytic lesions in 60% (sclerotic lesions are rare) (Fig. 9.9). Usually in the axial skeleton
Osteoporosis (without lytic lesions in 20%)
Bone scan normal (unless fractures)
Bone marrow shows excess plasma cells, often with multiple nuclei

DIAGNOSIS
Requires monoclonal protein in serum > 30 g/L and > 10% clonal plasma cells in bone marrow (if asymptomatic)
or
Presence of monoclonal band plus clonal plasma cells in bone marrow or plasmacytoma, together with myeloma-related organ/tissue impairment (calcium > 2.75 mmol/L, new renal impairment, anaemia, lytic lesions, osteoporosis with compression fractures, hyperviscosity syndrome, amyloid, recurrent infection)

If any doubt as to whether organ dysfunction is due to myeloma, monoclonal protein should be > 30 g/L

DIFFERENTIAL DIAGNOSIS

Monoclonal gammopathy of undetermined
  significance (MGUS)
Chronic lymphocytic leukaemia
Lymphoma
Vasculitis
Primary amyloidosis
Other metastatic malignancy

COMPLICATIONS

Bone fractures
Infections, particularly pneumococcal
Hypercalcaemia
Renal failure
Amyloidosis (AL type)
Coagulopathy
Neuropathy
Hyperviscosity syndrome (usually with IgA)
Soft-tissue plasmacytoma
Spinal cord compression

PROGNOSIS

Median survival 10 months without treatment
Median survival 2–3 years with melphalan
Adverse prognostic indicators include:

Hb < 8.5 g/dL
Hypercalcaemia
Renal impairment
β_2-microglobulin > 5.5 g/L
Albumin < 35 g/L
Very high Ig levels
Advanced lytic lesions

TREATMENT

Rehydration, steroids and bisphosphonates for
  hypercalcaemia
Analgesia and radiotherapy for bone pain;
  kyphoplasty may be useful for vertebral
  collapse with refractory pain
Rehydration ± dialysis for renal impairment
Transfusion for anaemia; EPO is useful in
  anaemic patients undergoing chemotherapy
Plasma exchange for hyperviscosity syndrome
Melphalan or cyclophosphamide ± prednisolone
  can usually induce a partial remission
High-dose chemotherapy with bone marrow
  transplantation may prolong survival, but has a
  mortality of 40% and is not usually suitable for
  older, frailer patients
Newer agents, e.g. thalidomide and bortezomib,
  also appear promising, and are sometimes used
  in refractory or relapsed disease

QUESTION SPOTTING

Myeloma presents as an insidious illness with
non-specific features; suspect in anyone with
tiredness, lethargy, thirst, back pain or recurrent
infections. Osteoporosis in a man should also
alert you to this diagnosis. The following may be
clues on the blood tests:

High ESR with normal CRP
High protein gap (total protein – albumin)
High calcium plus normocytic anaemia,
  especially in the context of renal impairment

WALDENSTRÖM'S MACROGLOBULINAEMIA

Monoclonal plasma cell neoplasm, producing large quantities of monoclonal IgM. This leads to the hyperviscosity syndrome, as well as suppression of normal bone marrow activity. Unlike multiple myeloma, disruption of osteoclast activity is not usually a feature, and hypercalcaemia and renal impairment are uncommon. It is a disease of older people – mean age at onset is 70 years.

CLINICAL FEATURES
General
May be asymptomatic
Weight loss
Lethargy
Shortness of breath
Hepatomegaly
Splenomegaly
Lymphadenopathy
Mucosal bleeding

Hyperviscosity syndrome (occurs in 70%)
Visual loss or impairment
Reduced conscious level
Seizures
Ataxia, vertigo, neuropathy
Retinal vein distension ('sausage-string' appearance) and haemorrhage
Cardiac failure (due to increased plasma volume)
DVT, PE

Other features
10% show evidence of lung or skin infiltration
IgM cryoglobulinaemia
Raynaud's phenomenon
Digital gangrene
Arthralgia
Haemolytic anaemia
Vascular purpura
Amyloid (10–15%)

INVESTIGATIONS
FBC
Hb ↓
MCV normal
WCC may be ↓
Lymphocytes ↑ in late disease
Platelets may be ↓
Reticulocytes may be ↑

U + Es
Usually normal

LFTs
Bilirubin ↑ if haemolysis
Total protein ↑
Otherwise normal

Calcium normal
ESR very ↑
LDH may be ↑
Immunoglobulins show ↑ IgM; monoclonal band on electrophoresis
X-rays show no osteoporosis or lytic lesions
Urine shows Bence–Jones protein in 70%
Bone marrow shows excess numbers of lymphoplasmacytoid cells

DIAGNOSIS
Presence of IgM paraprotein (monoclonal) together with small neoplastic plasma cells in bone marrow. Lytic lesions of bone are almost always absent.

DIFFERENTIAL DIAGNOSIS
For IgM paraprotein
MGUS (see myeloma)
Non-Hodgkin's lymphoma
Chronic lymphocytic leukaemia
Primary amyloidosis

For hyperviscosity syndrome
Myeloma
Polycythaemia rubra vera
CML
AML

TREATMENT
Treatment is indicated for control of symptoms rather than solely to improve prognosis
Hyperviscosity syndrome requires plasmapheresis for treatment. It is also used for cryoglobulinaemia
Chlorambucil, melphalan, fludarabine or combination chemotherapy can be used to reduce paraprotein levels and thus improve symptoms. Rituximab and thalidomide have also been used

PROGNOSIS

Median survival is 5 years

QUESTION SPOTTING

Look for:

Normocytic anaemia

High total protein

A very high ESR (> 150 mm/h)

Symptoms of headache, coma or visual disturbance – questions may well revolve around diagnosing and managing hyperviscosity syndrome

Raynaud's phenomenon

Hepatosplenomegaly

Note that bone pain, hypercalcaemia and renal impairment suggest myeloma rather than Waldenström's disease

POLYCYTHAEMIA RUBRA VERA

A myeloproliferative disorder involving the clonal expansion of all three marrow lineages. Chromosomal abnormalities are sometimes detectable, and the disease may evolve to leukaemia. Mean age of presentation is 60 years; males and females are affected equally.

CLINICAL FEATURES
Fatigue
Plethora
Pruritus – worse in water
Splenomegaly and pain
Hepatomegaly
Arterial and venous thrombosis
GI bleeding
Skin bleeding
Gout
Hypertension

INVESTIGATIONS
FBC
Hb elevated
Haematocrit elevated
MCV usually normal (low if iron-deficient)
WCC elevated (65%)
Plts may be elevated (50%)

U + Es
Usually normal

LFTs
Usually normal

Urate: often elevated
Clotting: usually normal
Ferritin: usually low
B_{12}: usually high
Erythropoietin: usually low

DIAGNOSIS
Presence of polycythaemia is established by radiolabelled red cell mass study.
Polycythaemia rubra vera is diagnosed by:

1. Raised red cell mass and absence of secondary causes, plus:
2. Palpable spleen or abnormal marrow karyotype or two of: Plts $> 400 \times 10^9$/L, neutrophils $> 12 \times 10^9$/L; low erythropoietin/

growth of erythroid burst-forming units, splenomegaly on ultrasound

Bone marrow: hyperplasia of all three cell lineages. Iron stores often absent

DIFFERENTIAL DIAGNOSIS
Secondary polycythaemias
Due to lung disease
Smoking
Cyanotic heart disease
Living at altitude
Renal cell carcinoma
Cerebellar haemangioma
Other tumours; e.g. leiomyoma, hepatoma
Inherited erythropoietin receptor mutations; von Hippel–Lindau protein mutations
Post renal transplant

Apparent polycythaemia
Dehydration
Prolonged venous occlusion

COMPLICATIONS
15% transform into myelofibrosis by 10 years
5% transform into acute myeloid leukaemia by 10 years
Iron deficiency
Arterial and venous thrombosis

TREATMENT
Venesection – aim for a haematocrit of 0.45 and platelets of $< 400 \times 10^9$/L. This reduces thrombotic events and prolongs survival
Aspirin – low-dose aspirin reduces thrombotic events
Hydroxycarbamide is usually used if venesection fails to control red cell mass and platelet counts. Busulphan is an option in older people; interferon-alpha may be used in younger patients
Chlorambucil and ^{32}P are no longer used due to the high incidence of leukaemia
Pruritus may respond to cimetidine or SSRIs
Bone marrow transplant may be used in a few patients

PROGNOSIS

Median survival 18 months if untreated; death is
  due to thromboembolic disease
Median survival 10–15 years with treatment

QUESTION SPOTTING

Look at the haematocrit, not just the
haemoglobin level. Questions are likely to
revolve around differentiating primary from
secondary polycythaemias, or perhaps
management of a thrombotic episode in a
polycythaemic patient. Also beware leukaemic
transformation in patients with known PRV.

IRON-DEFICIENCY ANAEMIA

Iron deficiency is one of the commonest diseases on the planet; up to 2 billion people are affected, the majority due to hookworm. In western countries, peptic ulcer disease and GI malignancy are common causes. Iron deficiency is more common in older people in western countries; premenopausal women also have a high prevalence due to menstruation and pregnancy.

SYMPTOMS
Fatigue
Weakness
Breathlessness
Dizziness
Leg cramps
Dysphagia (from oesophageal web – uncommon)

SIGNS
Pallor
Glossitis
Angular cheilitis
Koilonychia
Splenomegaly (uncommon)
Signs of cardiac failure may be seen in very
  severe anaemia

INVESTIGATIONS
FBC
Hb reduced
MCV usually low, but may be normal

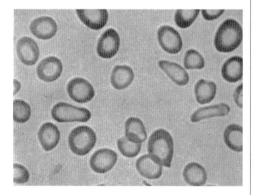

Figure 9.10 Blood film of iron-deficiency anaemia. Note hypochromic cells and the presence of a pencil cell. (Reproduced with permission from Forbes, Jackson (2003) *Colour Atlas and Text of Clinical Medicine*, 3rd edn. Mosby.)

WCC usually normal
Plts may be elevated
Reticulocytes are low

Blood film
Hypochromic, microcytic cells; pencil cells
  (Fig. 9.10)

U + Es
Normal

LFTs
Normal
Albumin: normal

ECG
May show signs of ischaemia if underlying
  coronary artery disease

DIAGNOSIS
Is usually made on iron studies. Low iron, high
  transferrin and low transferrin saturations
  suggest the diagnosis. Low ferritin is an
  alternative diagnostic marker; note that normal
  or high ferritin in no way excludes the
  diagnosis (ferritin is an acute-phase reactant)
In difficult cases, bone marrow biopsy is
  necessary; low or absent stainable iron makes
  the diagnosis
In some patients, a trial of iron is necessary; a
  brisk erythropoietic response suggests iron
  deficiency

DIFFERENTIAL DIAGNOSIS
Of microcytic anaemia
Lead poisoning
Thalassaemia
Sideroblastic anaemia
Anaemia of chronic disease

Causes of iron deficiency
Dietary deficiency
Malabsorption (gastrectomy, achlorhydria, bowel
  resection, coeliac disease)
Blood loss – urinary, vaginal, trauma,
  gastrointestinal
Haemolysis

GI causes of blood loss
Gastric duodenal ulceration
GI cancer/polyps
Angiodysplasia
Bleeding Meckel's diverticulum

Diverticular disease
Hookworm
Variceal bleeding
Note that elderly patients often have more than one source for GI blood loss

TREATMENT

Find and treat the underlying cause
Oral iron
Parenteral iron if oral iron not tolerated or malabsorption

PROGNOSIS

Depends on the underlying cause

QUESTION SPOTTING

It is highly unlikely that you will be asked to diagnose iron deficiency – this is too straightforward. However, remember that a normal MCV does not exclude the diagnosis. Questions are likely to revolve around investigating the cause of iron deficiency. Both upper and lower GI investigations are usually needed in older people.

Beware mixed deficiencies (e.g. iron and folate). These may give a normal MCV and unless both are replaced, the anaemia will not respond to iron replacement.

THERAPEUTICS AND TOXICOLOGY

10

TRICYCLIC ANTIDEPRESSANT OVERDOSE

The toxic effects of tricyclic antidepressants are myriad, due to the multiple pharmacological actions of these drugs. These actions include catecholamine uptake inhibition, anticholinergic effects and fast sodium channel blockade. Cardiac and CNS toxicity are responsible for fatalities, which currently run at 400 per year in the UK.

CLINICAL FEATURES
Cardiovascular
Tachycardia
Hypotension
SVT, VT, VF
Heart block
Pulmonary oedema

Neurological
Lethargy
Coma
Hyperreflexia
Seizures
Hallucinations
Ataxia
Loss of brainstem reflexes
Respiratory depression

Autonomic
Dry mouth
Urinary retention
Pyrexia or hypothermia
Dilated pupils
Constipation

Unusual features
Rhabdomyolysis (especially if prolonged seizures)
Skin blisters
DIC
Peripheral neuropathy

INVESTIGATIONS
FBC
Usually normal

U + Es
Sodium usually normal
Potassium may be ↓
Urea and creatinine normal

LFTs
ALT may be ↑
Otherwise normal

Clotting usually normal
CK may be ↑ (skeletal and cardiac)
ABGs show metabolic or mixed acidosis
ECG shows sinus tachycardia, ST/T-wave changes, QT prolongation, PR prolongation, QRS prolongation. QRS >100 ms carries a much higher chance of dangerous arrhythmias. RBBB, AV block, SVT, VT, torsades or VF may develop

TREATMENT
Protect airway if at risk
100% O_2
Cardiac monitoring for at least 6 hours
Gastric lavage if severe overdose within 1–2 hours
50–100 g charcoal, repeated at 2–4 hours if severe overdose
Treat convulsions with diazepam
Sodium bicarbonate if acidosis, QRS widening, low BP or arrhythmias and other signs of severe toxicity. Aim for arterial pH of 7.45–7.55
Aim for K^+ at upper end of normal
IV colloid/crystalloid for hypotension; consider glucagon in refractory cases

Arrhythmias
Sodium bicarbonate and oxygen
DC shock if refractory
Avoid antiarrhythmics if possible, but consider phenytoin, lidocaine, atenolol or esmolol
If cardiac arrest occurs, resuscitation attempts should continue for longer than usual; good recovery has been observed after 2–5 hours' CPR in tricyclic overdoses
Class Ia and Ic antiarrhythmics are contraindicated, as are physostigmine and flumazenil (in mixed overdose). Dialysis and charcoal haemoperfusion are ineffective at removing tricyclic antidepressants

PROGNOSIS
2–3% mortality rate. Serious complications usually occur within 6 hours of ingestion (peak plasma levels are usually around 4 hours). Onset of seizures or arrhythmias is extremely rare after 24 hours.

QUESTION SPOTTING

The fact that an overdose has been taken is usually obvious. The key features are usually:

Dilated pupils
Reduced level of consciousness
Tachycardia

The neurological sequelae of fits or arrhythmias can make the diagnosis more difficult, with head injury or intracranial haemorrhage entering the differential. Also consider the diagnosis in patients with unexplained acidosis.

LEAD POISONING

Acute lead poisoning is a rare event. However, chronic toxicity is more common, and is particularly seen in certain situations:

Industrial – metal workers, smelting workers

Domestic – drinking water from lead pipes, children ingesting lead-based paints

SYMPTOMS
Anorexia

Nausea and vomiting

Muscle weakness

Constipation

Abdominal colic, which may mimic an acute abdomen

Behaviour change

Seizures

Memory loss

SIGNS
Blue line around gums – due to deposition of sulphide

Peripheral neuropathy which is almost exclusively motor, and particularly affects extensors, leading to wrist and footdrop

INVESTIGATIONS
FBC
Hb normal or ↓ – may be normochromic, normocytic, sideroblastic or even haemolytic

WCC normal

Platelets normal

U + Es
Urea and creatinine ↑ if nephritis

LFTs
Normal

Blood film may show basophilic stippling

Erythrocyte protoporphyrin ↑, and ↓ ALA dehydratase activity seen

Urine
Glycosuria

Proteinuria – aminoaciduria

Long-bone X-rays
Dense metaphyseal bands, especially wrists and knees in children

DIAGNOSIS
Urine

↑ ALA and ↑ coproporphyrin

Serum lead ↑

Urine lead excretion ↑

ASSOCIATIONS
Gout

DIFFERENTIAL DIAGNOSIS
May be confused with acute intermittent porphyria

COMPLICATIONS
Interstitial nephritis – tubular dysfunction may lead to glycosuria, phosphaturia, aminoaciduria due to reduced absorption. This is reversible if caught early, but irreversible once fibrosis has occurred

TREATMENT
Remove cause

Calcium EDTA, D-penicillamine or dimercaprol to chelate the lead

Monitor U + Es

QUESTION SPOTTING
Think of this in the non-surgical causes of abdominal pain. The diagnosis is now very rare. Also consider it if glycosuria in a young patient, especially if anaemic, and occupational exposure, particularly in an unregulated industry.

DIGOXIN TOXICITY

Digoxin is thought to inhibit the action of the Na^+/K^+ ATPase of the sarcolemmal membrane. This causes sodium influx and displacement of bound intracellular calcium, giving a positive inotropic effect. Digoxin also causes an increased refractory period and slows conduction at the AV node. Other effects include mild peripheral vasoconstriction, a vagotonic effect and increased cardiac automaticity.

Because of its diversity of actions and its complicated pharmacokinetics, digoxin toxicity is a clinical diagnosis, but may often be confirmed by toxic concentrations in the blood.

FACTORS THAT INCREASE CARDIAC SENSITIVITY TO DIGOXIN

↓ K (but ↑ K may cause heart block)
↓ Mg
↑ Ca
Acidosis
Hypothyroidism
Cardiac amyloid
Chronic lung disease
Ischaemic cardiomyopathy
Renal impairment – causes increased plasma concentration

DRUGS THAT INTERACT WITH DIGOXIN

Increase

Quinidine – ↓ renal clearance
Captopril – ↓ renal clearance
Amiodarone – ↓ renal clearance
Propafenone – ↓ renal clearance
Verapamil – displaced protein binding
Nifedipine – displaced protein binding
Nitrendipine – displaced protein binding
Erythromycin – ↓ bacteria in gut which convert digoxin to inactive dihydrodigoxin
Tetracycline – ↓ bacteria in gut which convert digoxin to inactive dihydrodigoxin

Decrease

Cholestyramine – binds digoxin in resin
Phenytoin – ↑ hepatic metabolism
Rifampicin – ↑ hepatic metabolism
Sulfasalazine – delayed absorption
Neomycin – delayed absorption

CLINICAL FEATURES

Non-cardiac

Fatigue
Anorexia
Nausea and vomiting
Xanthopsia
Headaches
Abdominal pain and diarrhoea
Paraesthesia
Fits
Mental confusion
Hallucinations

Cardiac

Bradycardia – either in sinus rhythm or in AF
Second- or third-degree AV block due to increased parasympathetic and reduced sympathetic tone
Junctional bradycardias
Paroxysmal atrial tachycardia with variable block
Ventricular ectopics, bigemini and paroxysmal ventricular tachycardia
Ventricular fibrillation

INVESTIGATIONS

FBC

Normal

U + Es

Na normal
K normal or ↑. Digoxin toxicity worse if K ↓
Urea and creatinine normal or may be increased
Magnesium may be ↓
Calcium may be ↑

DIAGNOSIS

The diagnosis is clinical
Digoxin concentrations – provide a rough guide
ECG may show the features mentioned under cardiac features. See example ECG of digoxin toxicity (Figure 10.1)

DIFFERENTIAL DIAGNOSIS

Toxicity from other rate-limiting drugs – beta-blockers, calcium channel blockers
Toxicity from other antiarrhythmics
Constipation causing nausea and abdominal pain (especially in elderly)
Causes of acute abdomen

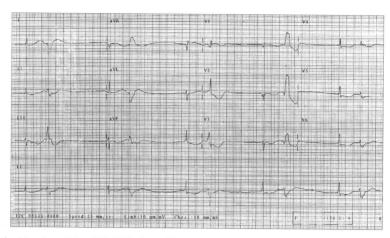

Figure 10.1 Digoxin toxicity. This ECG shows bigemini with marked bradycardia. The QRS complexes are variable in morphology and there is widespread ST segment depression with T-wave abnormality.

TREATMENT

ECG monitoring

Drug withdrawal

Treatment of electrolyte disturbances. Potassium administration may be useful for the treatment of ventricular arrhythmias, even if serum potassium levels are normal, but this requires extreme care

Atropine is useful for sinus bradycardias, AV block and sinoatrial arrest, although temporary pacing may be required

Digoxin-specific antibody fragments are used for serious arrhythmias such as VT. They give rapid and selective digoxin reversal. Improvement occurs within about 30 minutes, and toxicity is resolved within 3–4 hours. They can be used more than once in the same patient, but side-effects should be watched for. VT may also be treated with lidocaine, phenytoin, amiodarone or beta-blockers. Note that beta-blockers may lead to heart block, and

so very short-acting intravenous forms such as esmolol should be used

DC cardioversion should be avoided as it may precipitate asystole

Haemodialysis and haemoperfusion are ineffective in clearing digoxin

If toxicity is the result of overdose, then gastric lavage and activated charcoal are both useful treatments. Cholestyramine is also effective at binding digoxin and reducing serum concentrations

QUESTION SPOTTING

Suspect digoxin toxicity if unexplained nausea and vomiting, or arrhythmias, especially second- or third-degree heart block. Dimorphic VT or atrial tachycardia should also raise the suspicion of digoxin toxicity, especially in the elderly after recent introduction of a new drug – see above list. Xanthopsia is a cardinal feature, but is rare.

ETHYLENE GLYCOL POISONING

Ethylene glycol poisoning usually arises from ingestion of antifreeze, which contains > 90% ethylene glycol, often taken with ethanol. It is colourless, odourless and slightly sweet-tasting. It does not directly cause toxicity, but it is metabolized to glycolic acid by alcohol dehydrogenase. Further metabolism eventually to give calcium oxalate is slow, and so glycolic acid accumulates. Glycolate causes generalized oedema, severe acidosis, interstitial nephritis with oxalate crystal deposition and multiorgan failure.

Stages

Early (30 minutes – 12 hours)
Alcohol-like effects and effects of hypocalcaemia

Intermediate (12–48 hours)
Severe acidosis, cardiorespiratory failure with pulmonary oedema, ARDS and gastric aspiration

Late (48 + hours)
Renal failure secondary to direct toxicity and calcium oxalate deposition

SYMPTOMS
Disinhibition
Ataxia
Incoordination
Reduced conscious level
Fits

SIGNS
Tachycardia
Hypertension
Tachypnoea (Kussmaul respiration)
Hypotonia
Hyporeflexia
Myoclonic jerks
Fits
Absent pupillary reflexes
Papilloedema
Meningism
Coma
Oliguria/anuria

INVESTIGATIONS
FBC
Hb normal
WCC ↑
Platelets normal

U + Es
Na ↑
K normal or ↑
Urea ↑
Creatinine ↑

LFTs
Usually normal

Calcium ↓
Glucose normal or mildly ↑
Chloride normal
Anion gap ↑
Ethylene glycol levels ↑
Osmolar gap ↑ (calculated osmolality minus measured osmolality) – not explained by alcohol

ABGs
pH ↓↓
CO_2 ↓
O_2 ↓
HCO_3 ↓
BE ↓

Urine ketones negative (weak ketonuria may be seen in chronic alcoholics). Oxalate crystalluria from 8 hours.

Chest X-ray shows oedema or ARDS.

DIAGNOSIS
CLINICAL FEATURES
Increased anion gap and increased osmolar gap
Raised ethylene glycol levels with calcium oxalate crystalluria

DIFFERENTIAL DIAGNOSIS
Diabetic ketoacidosis
Methanol poisoning
Ethanol poisoning
Lactic acidosis
Ecstasy overdose
Amitriptyline overdose

COMPLICATIONS
Multiple organ failure
Hypocalcaemia secondary to sequestration by oxalate

TREATMENT

Airway management and resuscitation with fluids and inotropes if required

Gastric lavage and activated charcoal

Ethanol – competitively inhibits ethylene glycol metabolism with alcohol dehydrogenase (80 × the affinity). Levels should be titrated to 100 mg/dL

Sodium bicarbonate may be required for profound acidosis. Very large quantities may be required to raise pH. Note that this may increase calcium oxalate crystal deposition and renal damage

Haemodialysis is the best method of directly removing ethylene glycol and its products, but peritoneal dialysis is effective, if slower

PROGNOSIS

Renal failure is usually reversible with renal support, but may take 6–8 weeks to recover

Very high mortality rates if late presentation/ diagnosis or high doses taken

QUESTION SPOTTING

The typical patient will be young and male and will often have a history of alcohol abuse or previous psychiatric history. Watch out for severe unexplained acidosis. Ethylene glycol is a cause of a high-anion-gap metabolic acidosis.

Ethylene glycol also causes a high osmolar gap – calculate the osmolality and compare with the measured osmolality if given. Ethylene glycol poisoning often leads to renal failure, pulmonary oedema and low calcium – this can help distinguish it from methanol poisoning.

ECSTASY INGESTION

Ecstasy is the popular name for an amphetamine derivative (3,4-methylenedioxymethamphetamine or MDMA) which is increasing in popularity in the UK. It is taken for its stimulant and hallucinogenic properties which give feelings of euphoria, closeness and distorted sensory perceptions. Unfortunately ecstasy has been associated with some idiosyncratic and serious adverse reactions, even at doses previously tolerated, particularly when associated with dehydration and pyrexia from dancing.

SYMPTOMS
Excitement
Restlessness
Shortness of breath

SIGNS
Hypertension
Hyperventilation
Tachycardia
Hyperreflexia
Dilated pupils
Hyperpyrexia

INVESTIGATIONS
FBC
Hb normal
WCC may be normal or ↑
Platelets ↓ if DIC

U + Es
Na may be ↓↓
K ↑ if rhabdomyolysis and/or renal failure
Urea may be ↑
Creatinine may be ↑

LFTs
ALT may be ↑
ALP may be ↑
Bilirubin may be ↑
Albumin usually normal

Ca may be ↓
Clotting abnormal if DIC

ABGs
pH may be ↓
CK ↑↑ if rhabdomyolysis

Urine
Blood ++ to dipstix but no red cells on microscopy if myoglobinuria from rhabdomyolysis

DIAGNOSIS
MDMA levels may be taken to confirm clinical diagnosis

DIFFERENTIAL DIAGNOSIS
Cocaine overdose
Tricyclic overdose
SSRI poisoning
Intracranial bleeding or infection

COMPLICATIONS
Cardiac
Hypotension
Ventricular arrhythmias
Myocardial infarction
Aortic dissection
Shock

Respiratory
Adult respiratory distress syndrome

Renal
Acute renal failure

Hepatic
Acute hepatic necrosis

Neurological
Paranoid psychosis
Intracranial haemorrhage

Metabolic
Malignant hyperpyrexia
Hyponatraemia

Musculoskeletal
Rhabdomyolysis

Haematological
Disseminated intravascular coagulation

TREATMENT
Supportive – fluids and ECG monitoring
Diazepam if agitated or fitting
Treat complications as they arise

QUESTION SPOTTING

Ecstasy ingestion should be suspected in any young patient who presents with signs of adrenergic stimulation, especially if in multiple-organ failure. Typically, patients will be in their teens or early 20s with dilated pupils, tachycardia, hyperventilation and restlessness. Fitting, cardiac arrhythmias, rhabdomyolysis and DIC seem to be typical severe complications.

CARBON MONOXIDE POISONING

Carbon monoxide exerts its toxic effect principally by binding to haemoglobin with an avidity some 240 times that of oxygen, leading to tissue hypoxia. Secondary effects include inhibition of cytochrome oxidase activity and, possibly, peroxidation of brain lipids, which may underlie the chronic neurological sequelae of poisoning.

SYMPTOMS
Chronic or low-grade poisoning
Headache
Dizziness
Fatigue
'Flu-like' symptoms
More severe poisoning
Shortness of breath
Seizures
Coma

SIGNS
Cyanosis – may be absent
Reduced conscious level
Increased tone, hyperreflexia
Extensor plantars
Papilloedema
Hyperpyrexia
Crepitations in chest

N.B.: Cherry-red skin is very unusual

Chronic neuropsychiatric sequelae (may be delayed in onset)
Cognitive impairment
Memory problems
Cortical blindness
Peripheral neuropathy
Mutism
Parkinsonism, choreoathetosis
Personality changes
Incontinence

INVESTIGATIONS
FBC
Normal

U + Es
Normal

LFTs
Normal

ABGs
pH ↓
p_{CO_2} ↓
p_{O_2} normal, but Hb saturation on ABGs is ↓
Pulse oximetry displays normal O_2 saturation

ECG may show ST depression. Prolonged PR, QT intervals

Chest X-ray may show pulmonary oedema

DIAGNOSIS
HbCO: normal = up to 10% in smokers. Peak concentrations correlate with severity of poisoning

DIFFERENTIAL DIAGNOSIS
Drug overdose
Postictal state
Other causes of impaired consciousness
Symptoms of chronic CO poisoning may mimic influenza

COMPLICATIONS
Acute renal failure
Myocardial ischaemia, arrhythmias, infarction
Rhabdomyolysis
TTP

TREATMENT
100% O_2
Diazepam for seizures
Mannitol and dexamethasone for cerebral oedema
Dantrolene for hyperpyrexia
Avoid bicarbonate as it may further impair oxygen release

Consider hyperbaric oxygen therapy if:

Unconscious at any stage
Neurological features present
HbCO concentration > 20%
Pregnant

PROGNOSIS

1500 deaths per year in UK

80% of those developing late neurological sequelae improve by 1 year after event

QUESTION SPOTTING

You will probably not be told that the patient was found in a car with a hosepipe leading inside. Consider the diagnosis in:

Any unconscious patient

Acidosis of unknown cause

Anyone with a discrepancy between the p_{O_2} and Hb sats on the blood gases (not from a pulse oximeter)

Also consider the diagnosis in patients with headache, lethargy and non-specific symptoms

PHENYTOIN TOXICITY

Phenytoin toxicity occurs either acutely due to overdose, or chronically, in patients taking phenytoin regularly. Phenytoin has non-linear pharmacokinetics, highly variable oral absorption and a variable half-life that increases with plasma concentration, so toxic levels may result from minor changes in dose or in patient condition. Factors that may precipitate toxicity include hypoalbuminaemia, renal failure, hepatic dysfunction and concomitant administration of other drugs.

SYMPTOMS
Acute toxicity
Nausea and vomiting
Constipation
Slurred speech
Diplopia
Drowsiness
Confusion
Incoordination
Mood and behaviour change
Seizures (rare)
Hemidysaesthesia

Chronic toxicity
Gingival hyperplasia
Acne
Hirsutism
Numbness

SIGNS
Acute toxicity
Bradycardia
Nystagmus
Ophthalmoplegia
Dysarthria
Ataxia
Coarse resting tremor
Hyperreflexia with clonus
Choreoathetosis
Hepatomegaly, splenomegaly (rare)
Dyskinesia (rare)
Hemiparesis (rare)
Coma (rare)

Chronic toxicity
Lymphadenopathy
Peripheral neuropathy

INVESTIGATIONS
FBC
Usually normal
MCV may ↑ in chronic use

U + Es
Na normal or ↓
K normal
Urea and creatinine normal

LFTs
Usually normal (rarely all may be elevated if hepatic failure)
ALP may ↑ with long-term use
Glucose ↑

ECG
Bradycardia
AV block
Idioventricular rhythm

Chest X-ray
Normal but may show signs of cardiac failure

DIAGNOSIS
Phenytoin levels ↑ (toxicity rare below 20 mg/L)

DIFFERENTIAL DIAGNOSIS
Viral labyrinthitis
Posterior fossa tumour
Guillain–Barré syndrome
Botulism
Wernicke's encephalopathy
Psychological illness

COMPLICATIONS
Cardiac failure from myocardial depression
Cardiac arrest with VF or asystole
Hepatitis/hepatic failure
Coma
Death is rare and almost always from cardiac arrhythmias secondary to intravenous phenytoin administration.

TREATMENT
Supportive
ECG monitoring
Fluids for hypotension

Atropine for bradycardia/AV block. Cardiac
  pacing is occasionally required
Haemodialysis/peritoneal dialysis is of no benefit

PROGNOSIS

Very good once the phenytoin levels are reduced.
  Long-term cerebellar effects may be seen with
  chronic toxicity but are rare in acute overdose
Death is rare with levels < 70–100 mg/L

QUESTION SPOTTING

The patient may be either sex and any age, but
the typical features of ataxia, nystagmus and
drowsiness and the features of chronic use should
lead to the correct diagnosis. Watch out for
recent changes in medications with epileptic
patients.

LITHIUM TOXICITY

Lithium is a cation handled by the body like sodium and usually administered as lithium carbonate. Toxicity may occur easily, as the therapeutic window is narrow. Excretion is completely dependent on renal function. 95% of lithium is freely filtered in the glomerulus, followed by tubular reabsorption in competition with sodium. Thus during sodium depletion, lithium is preferentially reabsorbed, and in sodium excess, more lithium is lost. Therefore in situations of salt and water depletion, there is reduced lithium excretion which leads to more salt and water loss, and this sets up a vicious circle.

This cycle may be precipitated by several drugs, but especially thiazide diuretics, non-steroidal anti-inflammatory drugs, steroids and angiotensin-converting enzyme (ACE) inhibitors. Toxicity may also occur with other causes of salt loss, e.g. diarrhoea or excess sweating due to fever and thyroid dysfunction.

CLINICAL FEATURES SEEN AT THERAPEUTIC LEVELS

Symptoms
Fine tremor
Nausea
Weight gain
Skin rash
Diarrhoea
Thirst
Polyuria

Signs
Tremor
Skin rash

CLINICAL FEATURES SEEN DURING MILD TOXICITY

Symptoms
Coarse tremor
Anorexia
Tinnitus
Drowsiness

Signs
Dysarthria
Nystagmus
Hypotension

CLINICAL FEATURES SEEN DURING SEVERE TOXICITY
Severe gastrointestinal symptoms
Seizures
Hyperreflexia and hyperextension
Cardiac arrhythmias
Renal failure
Circulatory collapse
Coma

INVESTIGATIONS
FBC
Hb normal
WCC ↑
Platelets normal

U + Es
Na ↓
K normal, ↓ or ↑
Urea ↑
Creatinine ↑
Glucose ↑
Thyroid function: ↑ TSH, ↓ T_4

ECG
T-wave flattening or inversion
ST depression
Rarely conduction defects

DIAGNOSIS
Lithium levels (levels > 2.0 mmol/L are likely to be associated with toxicity)

DIFFERENTIAL DIAGNOSIS
Phenytoin overdose
Alcohol abuse
Diabetic ketoacidosis
Gastroenteritis
Other causes of diabetes insipidus
Psychogenic polydipsia

COMPLICATIONS
Nephrogenic diabetes insipidus
Hypothyroidism
Hyperglycaemia
Hyperparathyroidism

TREATMENT

Stop contributory drugs

Replace salt and water

Gastric lavage only if acute overdose

Haemodialysis is treatment of choice in severe
  intoxication with levels > 3.5 mmol/L

PROGNOSIS

Mortality rates of 25% in acute overdose and 9%
in chronic toxicity. Irreversible renal impairment
may occur

QUESTION SPOTTING

Another cause of confusion and collapse. The
patient will have a history of depression and
some precipitating event or be on diuretics or
ACE inhibitors. Look especially for the coarse
tremor; renal failure is often present – may be
cause or effect.

SALICYLATE TOXICITY

Salicylates in overdose have direct effects on the brain – especially by stimulating the respiratory centre. Salicylate also disrupts metabolism of a wide range of energy substrates, possibly by inhibiting oxidative phosphorylation. This leads to organ failure and metabolic acidosis. Although low-dose aspirin is widely used, the reduction in the use of high-dose aspirin as a painkiller has led to salicylate overdose becoming uncommon.

SYMPTOMS
Nausea and vomiting
Tinnitus and deafness
Hyperventilation and breathlessness
Confusion

SIGNS
Tachypnoea
Tachycardia
Sweating
Hypotension
Confusion
Coma
Occasionally: high temperature, tetany, bibasal
   lung crackles

INVESTIGATIONS
FBC
Usually normal

U + Es
Sodium usually normal
Potassium may be low
Urea and creatinine normal

LFTs
Usually normal
Glucose: may be low
Clotting: usually normal

ABGs
May show respiratory alkalosis in mild to moderate overdose and metabolic acidosis in more severe overdose

CXR
May show pulmonary oedema

ECG
Normal or sinus tachycardia

DIAGNOSIS
Is based on typical symptoms plus the presence of salicylates on blood testing

DIFFERENTIAL DIAGNOSIS
Other causes of metabolic acidosis, e.g. diabetic
   ketoacidosis, renal failure, methanol or
   ethylene glycol overdose, tricyclic overdose,
   lactic acidosis from severe systemic disease
Cinchonism from quinine overdose
Differential of respiratory alkalosis includes
   anxiety, pain, pulmonary embolism and other
   causes of hypoxia

COMPLICATIONS
Neurological complications (fits, coma)
Pulmonary oedema
Metabolic acidosis and circulatory collapse
Hypoglycaemia
Acute renal failure

TREATMENT
Depends on severity of symptoms and salicylate
   level. All overdoses should receive activated
   charcoal and adequate hydration.
   Hypokalaemia should be corrected. Repeat
   salicylate levels should be taken 2–4 hours after
   initial levels, as time to peak may be delayed
Moderate overdoses (> 500 mg/L) should
   receive IV bicarbonate to alkalinize the urine
   (aim for urinary pH of 8). This facilitates
   excretion. Forced alkaline diuresis (i.e. adding
   furosemide) is unnecessary and may cause
   dangerous hypokalaemia and fluid shifts
Severe overdoses (> 700 mg/L) should be
   considered for haemodialysis

PROGNOSIS
Prognosis in severe overdoses is poor, especially in cases with acidosis and coma

QUESTION SPOTTING
Consider salicylate overdose in anyone with a metabolic acidosis – look for the chloride to calculate the anion gap. Other features to look for are tinnitus and deafness. Also consider salicylates in anyone with a respiratory alkalosis.

PARACETAMOL TOXICITY

Paracetamol is metabolised to *N*-acetyl *p*-benzoquinoneimine, a toxic intermediate which is usually inactivated by conjugation with glutathione in the liver. In overdose, the liver's ability to regenerate glutathione is exhausted, and the toxic metabolite binds directly to hepatocytes, causing massive hepatocyte necrosis and consequent fulminant hepatic failure. Acute renal failure may also be precipitated by paracetamol overdose via a direct nephrotoxic effect.

SYMPTOMS

May be asymptomatic at first
Vomiting
Abdominal pain
Late symptoms are those of fulminant liver
    failure: jaundice, confusion, coma

SIGNS

Often no signs early after poisoning
If fulminant liver failure supervenes:
Right-upper-quadrant abdominal tenderness
Jaundice
Asterixis
Confusion

INVESTIGATIONS
FBC

Usually normal

U + Es

Na: May be ↓ in acute renal failure or liver
    failure
K: ↓ in acute liver failure; ↑ in acute renal failure
Urea ↑ if acute renal failure
Creatinine ↑ if acute renal failure

LFTs

Bilirubin ↑
ALT typically very high; may fall late in course
    of liver failure
ALP ↑
Phosphate: may be low
INR ↑: note that large amounts of paracetamol in
    the blood will modestly elevate the INR, even
    in the absence of liver damage
Albumin ↓

CXR

Usually normal

ECG

Normal or sinus tachycardia

DIAGNOSIS

Diagnosis is based on a history of paracetamol ingestion, a typical clinical picture and usually on the presence of paracetamol in the blood stream. Patients presenting late may not have detectable paracetamol levels however.

DIFFERENTIAL DIAGNOSIS

Other causes of fulminant liver failure, particularly hepatitis B, autoimmune hepatitis, Wilson's disease, *Amanita* poisoning, drug and traditional herbal medicine toxicity. Shock liver (liver infarction) is another cause of very high ALT (several thousand U/L)

COMPLICATIONS

Fulminant liver failure leading to hepatic
    encephalopathy, electrolyte disturbance,
    gastrointestinal bleeding, infection and
    eventual death
Acute renal failure

TREATMENT

All suspected paracetamol overdoses should have a paracetamol level checked 4 hours or more after the time of overdose. Levels taken less than 4 hours after ingestion are unreliable. If a significant overdose is suspected (> 10 g paracetamol), the patient should receive *N*-acetylcysteine as soon as possible unless a paracetamol level below the treatment line has been obtained. Those with a level above the treatment line or those where the time of ingestion is uncertain should continue therapy with *N*-acetylcysteine. Patients receiving enzyme-inducing medications, those with chronic liver disease, chronic heavy alcohol use or malnutrition are at high risk and a more conservative treatment threshold should be used.

ALT and INR are the key monitoring investigations; normal values at more than 24 hours make significant liver damage unlikely

Fulminant liver failure requires aggressive supportive care and may require liver transplantation. Involve a liver specialist early. Criteria for referral to a transplant centre include: pH < 7.3, creatinine > 300 μmol/L, INR > 2.0 at < 48 h or > 3.5 at < 72 h, grade 3 or 4 hepatic encephalopathy. Try to avoid correcting the INR with plasma products as this will obscure the underlying degree of liver function and will make decisions regarding transplantation difficult

Acute renal failure may require dialysis; tubular necrosis is often the cause and may take several weeks to recover from fully

PROGNOSIS

Excellent if *N*-acetylcysteine is instituted early after overdose. Presentation with established liver failure carries a substantial mortality rate

QUESTION SPOTTING

May occur as a management question where you are told that an overdose has occurred. Consider paracetamol overdose whenever a presentation of acute liver failure is given. The very high ALT (often several thousand) is an important clue.

ORGANOPHOSPHATE AND NERVE AGENT POISONING

Both organophosphate pesticides and nerve agents work by inhibiting acetylcholinesterase. This leads to overstimulation of nicotinic and muscarinic pathways. Nerve agents are more toxic and some rapidly cause irreversible inhibition of acetylcholinesterase. They may enter the body via inhalation, ingestion or absorption through the skin.

SYMPTOMS
Blurred vision; eye pain
Sweating
Nausea and vomiting
Abdominal pain
Diarrhoea
Cough; wheeze; breathlessness
Hypersalivation
Headache
Anxiety

SIGNS
Bradycardia
Hypotension
Sweating
Bibasal crackles
Tachypnoea
Wheeze
Small pupils
Convulsions
Fasciculations
Coma
Flaccid paralysis may also occur

INVESTIGATIONS
FBC
Usually normal

Biochemistry
Usually normal

ABGs
Hypoxia. Hypercapnoea and low pH if ventilation impaired

CXR
May show pulmonary oedema

ECG
Sinus bradycardia, tachycardia or any arrhythmia may be seen

DIAGNOSIS
Is usually on history and typical symptoms. Organophosphate pesticide poisoning can be confirmed by measuring red cell or plasma acetylcholinesterase activity; significant poisoning is associated with activity < 20% of normal

DIFFERENTIAL DIAGNOSIS
Myocardial infarction with pulmonary oedema
Other irritant gas inhalation
Acute abdomen
Intracranial bleed

COMPLICATIONS
Respiratory failure
Cardiac arrhythmias
Cardiovascular collapse
Convulsions
Coma

TREATMENT
Atropine should be administered – large and repeated doses may be required. Give repeated doses until side-effects occur (tachycardia, dry skin and mouth). Oximes (e.g. pralidoxime) should be administered as soon as possible to reverse the effect of agents before inhibition becomes irreversible.

Aggressive supportive care with artificial ventilation may be required; diazepam is a useful adjunct to treat fits and agitation.

PROGNOSIS
Highly dependent on the dose and time to treatment. Even low doses of nerve agents may be lethal within a few minutes.

QUESTION SPOTTING
Consider in any poisoning where bradycardia is a prominent feature. Another key pointer is hypersecretion – sweating, diarrhoea, hypersalivation, rhinorrhoea and pulmonary oedema.

ALCOHOL WITHDRAWAL

SYMPTOMS
Visual hallucinations
Sweating
Craving for alcohol
Agitation
Nausea and vomiting
Insomnia
Headache

SIGNS
Disorientation
Tachycardia
Hypertension
Pyrexia
Sweating
Tremor
Tonic-clonic seizures

INVESTIGATIONS
FBC
Hb usually normal (unless GI bleed)
MCV often raised
WCC may be elevated
Plts may be low

U + Es
Sodium low in chronic liver disease
Potassium often low
Urea may be low in chronic liver disease
Creatinine usually normal

LFTs
Often deranged – GGT usually elevated first
Albumin low in chronic liver disease
Clotting normal unless chronic liver disease

ECG
May show sinus tachycardia

DIAGNOSIS
Is based on the clinical history and typical examination findings, coupled with a history of not having had an alcoholic drink for a few days (typically 1–3 days)

DIFFERENTIAL DIAGNOSIS
Infection – systemic or CNS infection (e.g. encephalitis)
Hepatic failure
Alcoholic hepatitis
Wernicke's encephalopathy
Functional psychosis
Thyroid storm
Other drug side-effects
Head injury/intracranial bleed

COMPLICATIONS
Dehydration
Tonic-clonic seizures
Injury to self

TREATMENT
Diazepam (or other benzodiazepine) – usually four times per day at first, tapering over a few days to zero
Fits can be treated with antiepileptics if not responsive to benzodiazepines
Refer to alcohol counselling services

PROGNOSIS
Cognitive state usually recovers well, but the long-term outlook is less good if the patient continues to drink

QUESTION SPOTTING
Consider the diagnosis in any confused person – especially 1–3 days after admission to hospital. Also consider the diagnosis in anyone with tonic-clonic seizures. Look for signs of chronic liver disease on examination, along with blood markers (low platelets, high MCV, high GGT) that may indicate excess alcohol consumption. Lack of a history of heavy drinking does not of course exclude the diagnosis.

ABBREVIATIONS

11

5-HIAA	5-hydroxyindoleacetic acid
5-HT	5-hydroxytryptamine (serotonin)
α1AT	α_1-antitrypsin
A&E	accident and emergency
ABGs	arterial blood gases
ABPA	allergic bronchopulmonary aspergillosis
ABVD	Adriamycin, bleomycin, vinblastine and dacarbazine
ACE	angiotensin-converting enzyme
AChR	acetylcholine receptor
ACTH	adrenocorticotrophic hormone
ADH	antidiuretic hormone
AF	atrial fibrillation
AFB	acid-fast bacilli
AIDS	acquired immune deficiency syndrome
AIP	acute intermittent porphyria
ALL	acute lymphoblastic leukaemia
ALP	alkaline phosphatase
ALS	amyotrophic lateral sclerosis
ALT	alanine transaminase
AML	acute myeloid leukaemia
ANA	antinuclear antibody
ANCA	antineutrophil cytoplasmic antibody
Ao	aorta
AP	anteroposterior
APS	autoimmune polyglandular syndrome
APTT	activated partial thromboplastin time
APTTR	activated partial thromboplastin time ratio
APUD	amine precursor uptake and decarboxylation
AR	aortic regurgitation
ARDS	adult respiratory distress syndrome
ARF	acute renal failure
AS	aortic stenosis
ASD	atrial septal defect
ASOT	antistreptolysin O titre
AST	aspartate transaminase
ATP	adenosine triphosphate
ATTR	altered transthyretin receptor
AV	atrioventricular/aortic valve
AXR	abdominal X-ray
BAL	bronchoalveolar lavage

BCG	bacille Calmette-Guérin
bd	bis die (twice daily)
BE	base excess
BHL	bilateral hilar lymphadenopathy
BMI	body mass index
BMT	bone marrow transplantation
BP	blood pressure
Ca	carcinoma/calcium
cAMP	cyclic adenosine monophosphate
cANCA	cytoplasmic ANCA
CAP	community-acquired pneumonia
CCF	congestive cardiac failure
CCU	cardiac care unit
CEA	carcinoembryonic antigen
CF	cystic fibrosis
CFT	complement fixation test
CFTR	cystic fibrosis transmembrane regulator
CHOP	chlorambucil, Adriamycin, vincristine (Oncovin) and prednisolone
CK	creatine kinase
Cl	chloride
CLL	chronic lymphocytic leukaemia
CML	chronic myeloid leukaemia
CMML	chronic myelomonocytic leukaemia
CMV	cytomegalovirus
CNS	central nervous system
CO	carbon monoxide
CO_2	carbon dioxide
COMT	catechol-O-methyltransferase
COP	cryptogenic organizing pneumonia
COPD	chronic obstructive pulmonary disease
CPAP	continuous positive-airways pressure
CPR	cardiopulmonary resuscitation
Cr	chromium
CREST	calcinosis, Raynaud's, oesophageal dysmotility, sclerodactyly and telangiectasia
CRF	chronic renal failure/ corticotrophin-releasing factor
CRP	C-reactive protein
CSF	cerebrospinal fluid
CT	computed tomography
CVA	cerebrovascular accident

CVID	common variable immunodeficiency		G6PD	glucose-6-phosphate dehydrogenase
CVP	central venous pressure		GBM	glomerular basement membrane
CXR	chest X-ray		GCA	giant cell arteritis
DC	direct current		GCS	Glasgow Coma Score
DEXA	dual-energy X-ray absorption		GFR	glomerular filtration rate
DI	diabetes insipidus		GGT	gamma-glutamyltransferase
DIC	disseminated intravascular coagulation		GH	growth hormone
DIDMOAD	diabetes insipidus, diabetes mellitus, optic atrophy and deafness		GHRH	growth hormone-releasing hormone
			GI	gastrointestinal
DIF	direct immunofluorescence		GnRH	gonadotrophin-releasing hormone
DISH	diffuse idiopathic skeletal hyperostosis		GP	general practitioner
			GPI	glucosylphosphatidylinositol/ general paresis of the insane
DKA	diabetic ketoacidosis			
d-ALA	delta-aminolaevulinic acid		GTT	glucose tolerance test
DLco	carbon monoxide transfer factor		GU	genitourinary
DM	diabetes mellitus		HACEK	*Haemophilus, Actinobacillus, Cardiobacterium, Eikenella, Kingella*
DMARD	disease-modifying antirheumatic drug			
DNA	deoxyribonucleic acid		HAART	highly active antiretroviral therapy
dsDNA	double-stranded DNA		Hb	haemoglobin
DVLA	Driver and Vehicle Licensing Agency		HbCO	carboxyhaemoglobin
			HBsAg	hepatitis B surface antigen
DVT	deep-vein thrombosis		HCC	hepatocellular carcinoma
EBV	Epstein–Barr virus		HCG	human chorionic gonadotrophin
ECG	electrocardiogram		HCM	hypertrophic cardiomyopathy
EDTA	ethyldiaminetetraacetic acid		HCO$_3$	bicarbonate
EEG	electroencephalogram		HD	Hodgkin's disease
EMG	electromyography		Hct	haematocrit
ENT	ear, nose and throat		HELLP	haemolysis, elevated liver functions, low platelets
EPO	erythropoietin			
ERCP	endoscopic retrograde cholangiopancreatography		HIV	human immunodeficiency virus
			HLA	human leukocyte antigen
ESR	erythrocyte sedimentation rate		HNPCC	hereditary non-polyposis colon cancer
FAB	French–American–British			
FBC	full blood count		HP	hypersensitivity pneumonitis
FDG	18-fluorodeoxyglucose		HR	heart rate
Fe	iron		HRCT	high-resolution computed tomography
FEV$_1$	forced expiratory volume in 1 second			
			HSMN	hereditary sensorimotor neuropathy
FFP	fresh frozen plasma			
FMF	familial Mediterranean fever		HSV	herpes simplex virus
FNA	fine-needle aspiration		HTLV-1	human T lymphotrophic virus-1
FSH	follicle-stimulating hormone		HUS	haemolytic–uraemic syndrome
FTA-ABS	fluorescent treponemal antibody absorption test		ICP	intracranial pressure
			IDDM	insulin-dependent diabetes mellitus
FVC	forced vital capacity			

IF	intrinsic factor	MGUS	monoclonal gammopathy of
IGF-1	insulin-like growth factor		undetermined significance
Ig	immunoglobulin	MHC	major histocompatibility complex
IL	interleukin	MI	myocardial infarction
IM	intramuscular	MIBG	metaiodobenzylguanidine
INR	international normalized ratio	MIC	minimum inhibitory concentration
IPSS	International Prognostic Scoring	MOTT	mycobacteria other than
	System		tuberculosis
ITP	idiopathic thrombocytopenic	MR	mitral regurgitation
	purpura	MRC	Medical Research Council
ITU	intensive therapy unit	MRCP	Member of the Royal College of
IV	intravenous		Physicians/magnetic resonance
IVC	inferior vena cava		cholangiopancreatography
IVIG	intravenous immunoglobulin	MRI	magnetic resonance imaging
IVU	intravenous urography	MRSA	methicillin-resistant
JGA	juxtaglomerular apparatus		*Staphylococcus aureus*
JVP	jugular venous pressure	MS	mitral regurgitation/multiple
K	potassium		sclerosis
Kco	TLco corrected for lung volume	MSQ	mental status questionnaire
kD	kilodalton	MSU	midstream urine
LA	left atrium	MTC	medullary C cell thyroid
LACS	lacunar anterior circulation stroke		carcinoma
LAM	lymphangioleiomyomatosis	MV	mitral valve
LBBB	left bundle branch block	Na	sodium
LCH	Langerhans-cell histiocytosis	NF	neurofibromatosis
LDH	lactate dehydrogenase	NG	nasogastric
LE	lupus erythematosus	NHL	non-Hodgkin's lymphoma
LFTs	liver function tests	NIPPV	non-invasive positive-pressure
LH	luteinizing hormone		ventilation
LMN	lower motor neurone	NPH	normal-pressure hydrocephalus
LP	lumbar puncture	NSAID	non-steroidal anti-inflammatory
LRTI	lower respiratory tract infection		drug
LTOT	long-term oxygen therapy	NSCLC	non-small-cell lung cancer
LV	left ventricle	OCP	oral contraceptive pill
LVH	left ventricular hypertrophy	OCSP	Oxford Community Stroke Project
MAC	*Mycobacterium avium-*	od	omne die (every day)
	intracellulare complex	OGD	oesophagogastroduodenoscopy
MBC	minimum bactericidal	OSAS	obstructive sleep apnoea
	concentration		syndrome
MCH	mean cell haemoglobin	PA	pulmonary artery
MCHC	mean cell haemoglobin	PABA	*para*-aminobenzoic acid
	concentration	PACES	Practical Assessment of Clinical
MCP	metacarpophalangeal		Examination Skills
MCTD	mixed connective tissue disease	PACS	partial anterior circulation stroke
MCV	mean cell volume	PAN	polyarteritis nodosa
MDMA	3,4-	pANCA	perinuclear ANCA
	methylenedioxymethamphetamine	PAS	periodic acid–Schiff
MEN	multiple endocrine neoplasia	PBC	primary biliary cirrhosis
Mg	magnesium	PBG	porphobilinogen

PCP	*Pneumocystis carinii* pneumonia	RPGN	rapidly progressive
PCR	polymerase chain reaction		glomerulonephritis
PD	Parkinson's disease	RPR	rapid plasma reagin
PDA	patent ductus arteriosus	RR	respiratory rate
PE	pulmonary embolism	RSV	respiratory syncytial virus
PEFR	peak expiratory flow rate	RT	reverse transcriptase
PEG	percutaneous endoscopic	RTA	renal tubular acidosis
	gastrostomy	RUQ	right upper quadrant
PET	positron emission tomography	RV	right ventricle
PFO	patent foramen ovale	RVH	right ventricular hypertrophy
PFTs	pulmonary function tests	SBE	subacute bacterial endocarditis
PIP	proximal interphalangeal	SCC	squamous cell carcinoma
Plts	platelets	SCLC	small-cell lung cancer
PMR	polymyalgia rheumatica	sd	standard deviation
PND	paroxysmal nocturnal dyspnoea	SeHCAT	selenium homotaurocholic acid
PNH	paroxysmal nocturnal		retention test
	haemoglobinuria	SIADH	syndrome of inappropriate
pco_2	partial pressure of		antidiuretic hormone secretion
	carbon dioxide	SLE	systemic lupus erythematosus
po_2	partial pressure of oxygen	SOB	short of breath
PO$_4$	phosphate	SSRI	selective serotonin reuptake
POCS	posterior circulation stroke		inhibitor
POEMS	polyneuropathy, organomegaly,	STD	sexually transmitted disease
	endocrinopathy, M protein, skin	SVC	superior vena cava
	changes	SVT	supraventricular tachycardia
PR	per rectum	SXR	skull X-ray
PRN	pro re nata (when required)	T$_3$	triiodothyronine
PrP	prion protein	T$_4$	thyroxine
PSA	prostate-specific antigen	TACS	total anterior circulation stroke
PSC	primary sclerosing cholangitis	TB	tuberculosis
PSM	pansystolic murmur	tds	ter die sumendum (to be taken
PTH	parathyroid hormone		three times daily)
PTHrP	PTH-related peptide	TENS	transcutaneous electrical nerve
PUO	pyrexia of unknown origin		stimulation
PWP	pulmonary wedge pressure	TFTs	thyroid function tests
RA	right atrium/rheumatoid arthritis/	TIA	transient ischaemic attack
	refractory anaemia	TIBC	total iron-binding capacity
RAEB	refractory anaemia with excess	TIPSS	transjugular intrahepatic
	blasts		portasystemic stent shunting
RAEBt	refractory anaemia with excess	TLC	total lung capacity
	blasts in transformation	TLco	carbon monoxide transfer factor
RARS	refractory anaemia with ring	TNF	tumour necrosis factor
	sideroblasts	TOE	transoesophageal
RAST	radioallergosorbent test		echocardiography
RBBB	right bundle branch block	TPHA	*Treponema pallidum*
RBC	red blood cell		haemagglutination
RIF	right iliac fossa	TPN	total parenteral nutrition
RNA	ribonucleic acid	TR	tricuspid regurgitation
RNP	ribonucleoprotein	TSH	thyroid-stimulating hormone

TSS	toxic shock syndrome	VF	ventricular fibrillation
TSST 1	TSS toxin 1	VIP	vasoactive intestinal polypeptide
TTP	thrombotic thrombocytopenic	VSD	ventricular septal defect
	purpura	VT	ventricular tachycardia
U + Es	urea and electrolytes	VZV	varicella-zoster virus
UC	ulcerative colitis	WCC	white cell count
UIP	usual interstitial pneumonia	WPW	Wolff–Parkinson–White
UMN	upper motor neurone		syndrome
URTI	upper respiratory tract infection	XHM	X-linked immunodeficiency with
US	ultrasound		hyper-IgM
UTI	urinary tract infection	Zn	zinc
vCJD	variant Creutzfeldt–Jakob disease	ZN	Ziehl–Nielsen (stain)
VDRL	Venereal Diseases Research		
	Laboratory		

SELF-ASSESSMENT

QUESTION 1

A 29-year-old woman with a history of congenital heart disease attends the clinic because she wishes to become pregnant. She feels well in herself save for a moderate degree of breathlessness on climbing stairs.

On examination, she is clubbed, with marked central cyanosis and a trace of ankle oedema. She has a parasternal heave, loud second heart sound and a soft early diastolic murmur, louder in inspiration. Her lung fields are clear.

Full blood count shows Hb 19.3, WCC 6.2, Plts 384. ECG shows right axis deviation with p pulmonale, and her chest X-ray shows dark lung fields but prominent pulmonary arteries.

What will you advise her?
(a) She should be able to have a normal pregnancy and birth
(b) She will require caesarean section at term
(c) She should not become pregnant
(d) She will require a caesarean section at 34 weeks
(e) She will require antibiotic prophylaxis at delivery

QUESTION 2

A 22-year-old man with Down's syndrome presents with sudden-onset left-sided weakness. On examination, he has 3/5 power in the left arm and leg, with reduced reflexes on the left and an upgoing left plantar. He is confused. His carer tells you that he had an operation on his bowel when he was very young, and he suffers from chronic constipation, for which he takes senna. He was also diagnosed as having a 'hole in the heart' as a child, but never received any operation on his heart.

Over the next few days, he improves, and the weakness resolves. Further examination reveals that he is clubbed and is centrally cyanosed despite continuing oxygen therapy. Pulse is 70 regular, BP 110/70. JVP + 6 cm. There is a prominent parasternal heave and a loud P2. An ejection systolic murmur and soft early diastolic murmur are audible, louder on inspiration. There is marked peripheral oedema but the chest is clear. His cardiac catheter results are shown below.

	Pressure	Saturation
IVC	20	50%
High RA	26	60%
Low RA	26	56%
RV	100/20	57%
PA	100/30	56%
LV	100/10	70%
Ao	105/80	70%

What is the cardiac diagnosis?
(a) Transposition of the great arteries
(b) Fallot's tetralogy
(c) Eisenmenger's syndrome due to ASD
(d) Eisenmenger's syndrome due to VSD
(e) Patent foramen ovale with paradoxical thrombus

QUESTION 3

A 58-year-old woman with a previous history of rheumatic fever presents with a 4-week history of sweats, poor appetite and malaise. On examination, she has four splinter haemorrhages, a temperature of 37.8°C, pulse 100, BP 110/40. Auscultation reveals an ejection systolic murmur radiating to the carotids, along with an early diastolic murmur. Her JVP is raised 5 cm and she has bibasal lung crackles.

Investigations show: Hb 10.3, WCC 8.2, Plts 160, Na 132, K 5.1, urea 13.2, creatinine 251. Urinalysis shows ++ blood, +++ protein. The echocardiography report shows 'hyperkinetic undilated LV, a 1.5 cm vegetation on the non-coronary cusp of the aortic valve, together with moderately severe aortic regurgitation'.

What will you do?
(a) Commence steroids and cyclophosphamide
(b) Commence IV flucloxacillin and gentamicin
(c) Commence IV benzylpenicillin and gentamicin
(d) Refer for urgent cardiac surgery
(e) Hold off antibiotics until blood culture results are available

QUESTION 4

A 50-year-old man was admitted with a 6-day history of fever and shortness of breath. He had a history of myocardial infarction 2 years ago. He also gave a history of recent travel to Turkey.

On examination he was pyrexial at 38.2°C, pulse 104 beats/min. Blood pressure was 110/75 mmHg. The JVP was elevated 5 cm, apex beat displaced with a loud pansystolic murmur heard loudest at the apex. Respiratory examination revealed bibasal crackles and he had ankle oedema.

Investigations
Hb 10 g/dL
MCV 82 fl
WBC 16×10^9/L
Platelets 45×10^9/L
Na 135 mmol/L
K 4.1 mmol/L
Urea 13 mmol/L
Creatinine 180 μmol/L
LFTs normal
Urinalysis: blood ++, protein +++
ECG shows sinus rhythm with Q waves in the anterior leads

Which three investigations would be most important to carry out?
(a) Urine culture
(b) Blood culture
(c) *Brucella* serology
(d) Syphilis serology
(e) Antistreptolysin O titre
(f) Chest X-ray
(g) ANCA
(h) Echocardiography
(i) Renal biopsy
(j) Renal ultrasound

QUESTION 5
A 72-year-old man undergoes screening echocardiography as part of a clinical trial. This reveals moderately impaired LV function together with a heavily calcified aortic valve. The maximum gradient across the valve is 82 mmHg.

On further questioning, he denies any blackouts, breathlessness or dizzy spells. He has never had chest pain, and denies any previous heart attacks. He can walk as far as he wants. He is currently taking ramipril and bendroflumethiazide for hypertension, and he gave up smoking 15 years ago.

What will you do next?
(a) Refer for aortic valve replacement
(b) Repeat the echo in a year's time
(c) Arrange transoesophageal echocardiography
(d) Stop the bendroflumethazide
(e) Arrange an exercise test

QUESTION 6
A 72-year-old man attends for colonoscopy and polypectomy. The house officer notes a murmur and asks you to examine the patient. He gives no history of rheumatic fever or previous cardiac problems. He is allergic to penicillin. On examination, his pulse is 70 regular, BP 130/65. JVP not raised. Heart sounds I + II, late systolic murmur with a mid-systolic click. The murmur is loudest in the apical area and does not radiate. His lung fields are clear.

What will you give this man prior to his colonoscopy?
(a) Oral amoxicillin
(b) Nothing – he does not require antibiotic prophylaxis
(c) IV vancomycin and gentamicin
(d) Oral clindamycin
(e) IV clindamycin

QUESTION 7
A 29-year-old patient presents with shortness of breath, which has come on over the last 3 months. He is usually well, and has had no significant medical illnesses in the past. He drinks 30 units of alcohol per week, smokes 10 cigarettes per day, and takes no medication. He has no family history of heart disease. On direct questioning, he notes occasional episodes of palpitations but no dizziness. He is more breathless walking up hills, does not get breathless at night, and denies cough, sputum or wheeze.

On examination, he appears well, but is overweight. Pulse is 120 irregular, BP 120/65, JVP +4 cm. There is no ankle oedema. Apex is undisplaced, there is a parasternal heave, and heart sounds are difficult to hear; a soft systolic murmur is audible. His ECG shows atrial fibrillation, right bundle branch block and high-voltage complexes in V1 to V4. The data from his cardiac catheter are given below.

Site	Pressure (mmHg)	Saturation (%)
SVC	5	65
RA	6	74
RV	25/0–5	78
PA	25/10	79
LV	140/0–12	95
Ao	140/75	96

What is the most likely diagnosis?
(a) VSD
(b) Mitral valve prolapse
(c) Eisenmenger's syndrome
(d) ASD
(e) Subaortic stenosis

QUESTION 8

A 60-year-old woman presents with a progressive history of grumbling fever, weight loss, arthralgia and exertional dyspnoea. She has been previously well, except for long-standing hypertension and a small TIA 2 months previously.

Examination reveals a fever of 37.8°C, and an unwell looking woman. She has a resting tachycardia. Blood pressure is 150/90 mmHg. She has a soft late systolic murmur. Chest and abdominal examinations are normal.

Investigations

Hb 10.0 g/dL
WCC 12 × 10⁹/L
Platelets 200 × 10⁹/L
ESR 120 mm/h
Na 145 mmol/L
K 4.0 mmol/L
Urea 13.0 mmol/L
Creatinine 150 μmol/L
Urinalysis blood +, protein +
Blood cultures negative
Chest X-ray normal
ANCA, ANA negative
A transthoracic echo shows an echodense lesion
  apparently adherent to the left atrial septum

What would you do next?
(a) Anticoagulate with heparin
(b) Commence IV methylprednisolone
(c) Commence IV benzylpenicillin and
  gentamicin
(d) Refer for cardiac surgery consult
(e) Take multiple sets of blood cultures

QUESTION 9

A 24-year-old man presents having collapsed whilst playing football. On arrival, he is conscious and denies chest pain. He smokes 5 cigarettes per day, drink 40 units of alcohol per week, and has no history of heart disease, hypertension or diabetes. His uncle died of heart trouble aged 36. He has a history of asthma and uses beclometasone and salbutamol inhalers. On direct questioning, he admits to several episodes of palpitations accompanied by a dizzy feeling; he thinks he may have lost consciousness at least once before. Examination reveals a regular pulse, 68 beats/min, BP 110/75, a double apex beat and an ejection systolic murmur.

ECG shows high-voltage complexes and a PR interval of 0.08 seconds with a delta wave. Chest X-ray shows a normal heart size and clear lung fields. FBC, U + Es are all normal; troponin T is 0.02 12 hours after the collapse.

What treatment will you give?
(a) Verapamil
(b) Flecainide
(c) Aspirin and heparin
(d) Atenolol
(e) None pending echo result

QUESTION 10

A 15-year-old girl who has just returned home to the UK from a holiday visiting family in India presents with a 5-day history of sharp chest pains made worse by inspiration and lying down. She gives a history of recurrent tonsillitis. Examination reveals a fever of 38.0°C, a soft pericardial rub with a systolic murmur. She has a normal respiratory examination, but locomotor examination reveals tender and swollen joints with restricted movements in the right knee and right elbow. Some results are shown.

Hb 12.0 g/dL
WCC 12 × 10⁹/L
Platelets 200 × 10⁹/L
ESR 70 mm/h
Blood cultures negative
CXR normal
ECG shows sinus rhythm with first-degree heart
  block

Which investigation would confirm the likely diagnosis?
(a) Antistreptolysin O titre
(b) Antinuclear antibody
(c) Blood culture
(d) Aspiration of the right knee
(e) Echocardiography

QUESTION 11

A 36-year-old high-school teacher was diagnosed with testicular seminoma 4 years ago and underwent orchidectomy and radiotherapy. He has been in remission since.

His annual oncology follow-up coincided with an upper respiratory tract infection which lasted for a week. He also complained of tiredness for 3 months.

His only other symptom was pain from a minor knee injury 2 weeks ago while he was playing squash. He takes over-the-counter paracetamol, is on no other medicines and has no known drug allergies or family history of note. He has never smoked and keeps a pet dog at home. He denied any respiratory symptoms, night sweats or weight loss and did not complain of eye symptoms or skin lesions. He was unaware of any exposure to tuberculosis.

Examination of the chest, cardiovascular, abdominal and genitourinary systems was normal. There was slight tenderness on passive movement of his right knee joint.

Initial investigations revealed a normal full blood count, urea and electrolytes, liver enzymes, serum calcium and CRP. His chest X-ray showed left hilar prominence and this prompted a staging CT scan. This confirmed mediastinal and hilar adenopathy. There were no pulmonary infiltrates or para-aortic nodes seen. He had a negative antituberculin skin test and normal serum ACE levels.

Question 1
The most likely diagnosis is:
(a) Berylliosis
(b) Relapse of his seminoma
(c) Sarcoidosis
(d) Sarcoid-like reaction
(e) Lymphoma

Question 2
The most appropriate next step in his management would be:
(a) Pulmonary function tests, including transfer coefficient and, if normal, observe the patient and refer to the chest clinic for follow-up
(b) Oral prednisolone 40 mg for 4 weeks
(c) Oral prednisolone 40 mg for 4 weeks and then reduce to a maintenance dose of 5–10 mg/day or alternate days
(d) Refer to haematology to consider chemotherapy
(e) Refer for further radiotherapy in case this is disseminated seminoma

QUESTION 12

A 40-year-old man who works in a security firm presented to his general practitioner with a 1-week history of right-sided facial nerve palsy. Initially he was diagnosed with Bell's palsy but he came back 2 weeks later noting that he was more lethargic and breathless when required to exert himself, particularly on inclines. A chest X-ray was requested at the time and revealed bilateral hilar lymphadenopathy and a chest clinic referral was made.

When reviewed at the chest clinic he admitted to a dry cough over a few months. He denied any family history of lymphoma, held no other occupation in the past and his grandfather suffered from tuberculosis. He smoked 20 cigarettes per day, and has done so from his teenage years, and drank alcohol in moderation, estimating his intake at 22 units per week. He kept no pets and his most recent travel was to the USA 18 months ago to visit friends.

On examination he had no evidence of finger clubbing, jaundice or lymphadenopathy. His pulse was regular with normal heart sounds and no added sounds or murmur heard. Chest examination was unremarkable but his liver was enlarged at 2 finger-breadths. Central nervous system examination revealed mild lower motor neurone facial nerve palsy on the right and the rest of his neurological examination was deemed normal.

Blood tests showed an elevated plasma viscosity, serum calcium was also mildly elevated and his urinalysis showed a trace of protein with normal urea, creatinine and electrolytes.

Pulmonary function tests showed a mild mixed spirometry picture with slight reduction in transfer factor. High-resolution computed tomography showed mediastinal and hilar lymphadenopathy with micronodules in a subpleural and bronchovascular distribution.

Magnetic resonant brain imaging was reported as normal and his CSF examination showed an increased protein level (960 mg/L), oligoclonal bands and raised spinal fluid ACE with a corresponding normal serum ACE level. His CSF cytology result was negative and tissue obtained from endobronchial biopsy confirmed non-caseating granulomas.

What treatment would you recommend for this patient?

(a) Methotrexate 10 mg once a week increasing to 15 mg once a week in 6 weeks with folic acid cover
(b) Oral cyclophosphamide at 2 mg/kg
(c) Observe patient and consider immunosuppressive treatment if worsening respiratory symptoms, pulmonary function tests and chest X-ray in 3 months
(d) Oral prednisolone 40 mg once daily for 4 weeks followed by reducing to a maintenance dose of 5–15 mg/day for symptom control and then reducing to 5–7.5 mg over a few months with follow-up at the neurology clinic
(e) Oral azathioprine 2 mg/kg per day checking the full blood count 2-weekly for the first 3 months and then monthly and slowly increase to maximum dose of 150–200 mg/day

QUESTION 13

A 21-year-old woman who is in her third year studying accountancy at university presents to her GP with a 5-day history of feeling unwell and associated with a purulent productive cough with fevers and sweats over the past 48 hours. She has been finding it hard at university and reports at least two chest infections in the last year, one of which greatly affected her performance at university.

On examination she has mild clubbing of her fingers and coarse inspiratory crackles at the bases associated with wheeze. Urinalysis reveals glycosuria. She is commenced on a 7-day course of oral antibiotic therapy and a short-acting bronchodilator and the GP writes to you at the chest clinic for a further opinion.

This woman was reviewed at the chest clinic and underwent a battery of tests which included the CT scan pictured in Figure 12.1. What does this show?

(a) Gross emphysema
(b) Pulmonary fibrosis and traction bronchiectasis
(c) Bronchiectasis
(d) Non-specific interstitial pneumonitis
(e) Chronic hypersensitivity pneumonitis-type pattern

QUESTION 14

A 28-year-old cystic fibrosis patient has disease which mainly manifests with recurrent chest infections, pancreatic insufficiency and diabetes mellitus, which he is not keeping under good control. He has poorly attended the CF clinic in the past but this time turned up with a history of recurrent abdominal pains, suffering his fourth

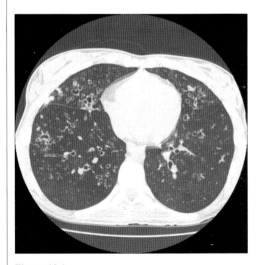

Figure 12.1

episode in 6 weeks at the time of attending the clinic.

Examination revealed a thin man who had central cyanosis and chest findings in keeping with his known bronchiectasis. His abdomen was tender to deep palpation throughout and to light palpation over the epigastrium. There were no palpable organs and bowel sounds were present. His chest plain film was similar to the one he underwent 9 months ago, which had a Northern score of 2.

Blood Tests
Hb 12.3 g/dL
WCC 13.6 $\times$ 10^9/L
Plts 403 $\times$ 10^9/L
Na 136 mmol/L
K 3.7 mmol/L
Urea 4.2 mmol/L
Creatinine 76 µmol/L
Bilirubin 37 µmol/L
ALP 110 U/L
ALT 63 U/L
Alb 33 g/L
Calcium 2.20 mmol/L
Glucose 11.1 mmol/L
CRP 76 mg/L
Amylase 78 U/L

The most likely diagnosis is:
(a) Gastro-oesophageal reflux disease
(b) Acute pancreatitis
(c) Acute upper GI bleeding ulcer
(d) Chronic peptic ulcer disease
(e) Chronic pancreatitis

QUESTION 15

A 61-year-old bus driver presents acutely with 2 days of abdominal pain, nausea and vomiting. Prior to this illness he has suffered from malaise and has been finding activities difficult in general, and getting out of his bed or off his chair is extremely difficult. He is a lifelong heavy smoker, accumulating at least 45 pack-years, drinks alcohol seldom and previously worked as a joiner.

He was cachectic on examination and had reduced skin turgor, dry mucous membranes and a postural BP drop of 20 mmHg. He had gynaecomastia but wasn't taking any causative drugs. He had previous appendicectomy and the

rest of his abdominal examination was unremarkable.

Blood results showed:
Hb 11.2 g/dL
MCV 81 fl
WCC 6.3 $\times$ 10^9/L
Plts 210 $\times$ 10^9/L
Na 146 mmol/L
K 3.3 mmol/L
Urea 15.4 mmol/L
Creatinine 166 µmol/L
Bilirubin 22 µmol/L
ALP 410 U/L
ALT 27 U/L
Albumin 39 g/L
Calcium 2.96 mmol/L
Glucose 6.3 mmol/L
CRP 9 mg/L

You commence aggressive rehydration therapy and arrange a CXR which shows a 3 cm dense round opacity of soft-tissue attenuation in the left mid-zone. In view of the raised ALP you arranged a bone scan which is normal and serum PO$_4$ is reduced from the sample sent from his admission blood tests.

Question 1
The most likely diagnosis is:
(a) Squamous cell carcinoma
(b) Small cell lung carcinoma
(c) Alveolar cell carcinoma
(d) Adenocarcinoma
(e) Carcinoid tumour

Question 2
The most useful next investigation would be:
(a) Repeat chest X-ray in 3 months and consider bronchoscopy
(b) Staging CT scan of the chest
(c) Positive emission tomography imaging
(d) Repeat chest X-ray in 4–6 weeks
(e) Sputum for cytology

QUESTION 16

A 35-year-old mother of two presents feeling unwell with fevers, sweats and diarrhoea. She had just returned from holiday in Blackpool a week ago and doesn't remember any food

281

consumption that might have triggered her symptoms. She is usually well and her only admission was following a road traffic accident 2 years ago when she sustained a head injury which was managed conservatively with 24-hour observation in the short-stay ward.

She smokes 5–10 cigarettes per day and consumes about 28 units of alcohol per week. She works as a barmaid and keeps a pet hamster.

Examination revealed reduced skin turgor, dry mucous membranes and pale conjunctivae with mild icterus. Temperature was 37.6°C, HR was 110 beats/min, RR 26/min, BP 109/45 and her oxygen saturations were 94% on 6 litres of oxygen. Heart sounds were pure with no added sounds and she had a few inspiratory crackles at the bases of her lungs. She had a palpable, tender liver edge but the abdomen was otherwise soft with active bowel sounds. She had normal rectal examination. Mental state questionnaire was 7/10.

Investigations

Hb 11.9 g/dL
MCV 93 fl
WCC 22 × 10^9/L (neutrophils 16.2 × 10^9/L)
Plts 555 × 10^9/L
Na 129 mmol/L
K 3.3 mmol/L
Urea 9.3 mmol/L
Creatinine 96 μmol/L
Bilirubin 63 μmol/L
ALP 76 U/L
ALT 110 U/L
Albumin 45 g/L
Calcium 2.56 mmol/L
Glucose 7.1 mmol/L
CRP 362 mg/L
CXR: patchy ill-defined opacification, with blunting of the left costophrenic angle

Question 1

The most likely diagnosis is:
(a) Bilateral pneumonia with alcoholic liver disease
(b) Bacterial peritonitis with haematogenous spread to the lungs
(c) Bilateral community-acquired pneumonia
(d) Bacterial gastroenteritis
(e) Empyema

Question 2

The most appropriate antibiotic regimen is:
(a) IV cefuroxime and oral erythromycin
(b) IV cefuroxime and oral clarithromycin
(c) IV co-amoxiclav and IV clarithromycin
(d) IV cefuroxime, IV metronidazole and IV thiamine
(e) IV ciprofloxacin

QUESTION 17

A 59-year-old man presents to your acute medical unit with worsening breathlessness. He has a background of Churg–Strauss vasculitis, asthma, chronic sinusitis and peripheral neuropathy and previously suffered bone marrow suppression secondary to his azathioprine therapy, which was discontinued.

He currently takes prednisolone 10 mg od, co-trimoxazole 480 mg bd, mycophenolate 500 mg tds, salmeterol/fluticasone 500 one puff twice daily, salbutamol as required which he hardly requires normally, calcium/vitamin D_3 2 tablets once daily, risedronate 5 mg once daily, omeprazole 20 mg od, carbamazapine 200 mg at night and a steroid nasal spray.

His shortness of breath had been stable up until a week ago when he noticed lethargy and a dry persistent non-productive cough. On examination he was not unduly breathless but did seem to barely manage long sentences and was really breathless walking to the male washroom on the ward. His baseline saturations at rest were 98%. Vital signs were normal but it was noted that he spiked a fever of 38.1°C in the A&E department prior to his admission on the ward. Chest auscultation revealed a few crackles at the right base and the rest of his examination was unremarkable.

His chest plain film showed some atelectasis at the left base but otherwise demonstrated no other changes to suggest acute pathology.

Bloods

Hb 12.3 g/dL
MCV 88 fl
WCC 3.1 × 10^9/L
Plts 233 × 10^9/L
Na 139 mmol/L
K 4.6 mmol/L
Urea 2.6 mmol/L

Creatinine 76 μmol/L
Bilirubin 13 μmol/L
ALP 32 U/L
ALT 74 U/L
Albumin 35 g/L
CRP 88 mg/L
d-dimer 0.36 U/L
Lung perfusion scan: normal
Spirometry at last month's clinic:
FEV$_1$ 1.99 L FVC 2.89 L

At first you suspected PCP infection and arranged induced sputum, which was negative. CT pulmonary angiogram request was declined by the duty radiologist in view of the negative perfusion scan.

The most appropriate next step in his management would be:

(a) Increase his prednisolone dose
(b) Bronchoscopy with BAL
(c) Bronchoscopy and transbronchial biopsy
(d) High-resolution CT scan of the chest
(e) Empirical antituberculous therapy

QUESTION 18

A 29-year-old mother of two presents to your general medicine clinic with a diagnosis of 'brittle asthma'. Her diagnosis was made 2 years ago as she found her exercise tolerance greatly reduced and she now gets tired on minimal exertion. At the time the diagnosis was based on obstructive spirometry figures and she has been treated with short- and long-acting beta-2 agonists, inhaled corticosteroids, leukotriene antagonist and has had at least six courses of high-dose oral prednisolone and anti-biotic courses for infective exacerbations. She does suffer from a predominantly dry cough, which becomes productive when she suffers an exacer-bation. She also complains of losing a stone (6.5 kg) in weight over the past 2–3 years but does admit that her appetite has never been great. She denies any other features on systematic enquiry. She has otherwise had no problems in the past and her second child was delivered by caesarean section. Her father smokes heavily and suffers from COPD. Her mother and two siblings keep well. She herself smokes 5–10 cigarettes per day and has done so for at least 12 years. She keeps a pet dog and her most recent travel was on holiday to Spain 3 years ago.

Examination revealed a thin woman with no clubbing, cyanosis or palpable lymphadenopathy. Heart sounds revealed a loud P2 with no murmurs heard, JVP was not elevated and she had no ankle oedema. Her trachea was central and she did have reduced cricosternal distance with resonance to percussion over the cardiac border and globally reduced breath sounds with none added. Her abdominal, musculoskeletal and central nervous systems were unremarkable.

Her initial investigations are as follows:

Hb 16.3 g/dL
MCV 83 fl
WCC 4.1 × 10^9/L
Plts 162 × 10^9/L
Na 143 mmol/L
K 4.8 mmol/L
Urea 4.1 mmol/L
Creatinine 73 μmol/L
Bilirubin 11 μmol/L
ALP 52 U/L
ALT 28 U/L
Albumin 41 g/L
Calcium 2.36 mmol/L
Glucose 5.2 mmol/L
CRP < 3 mg/L
CXR shows basal emphysema
PFTs (obstructive dynamic, static and reduced DLCO with classic flow–volume loop)

What would be the most useful next investigation?
(a) CT scan of the neck
(b) Histamine challenge
(c) Exercise testing (shuttle test)
(d) Serum electrophoresis to detect alpha-1 antitrypsin
(e) Total IgE

QUESTION 19

A 39-year-old woman with chronic asthma and allergic bronchopulmonary aspergillosis (ABPA) diagnosed 3 years ago is currently on maintenance therapy with prednisolone 10 mg od. She presented with a 1-day history of frank haemoptysis. She reports coughing up copious amounts of blood with mucus, estimating a total of 3 small cupfuls. She also complained of right-sided pleuritic chest pain which is long-standing

283

and denies any major risk factors for venous thromboembolism. Her mother suffered from pulmonary tuberculosis but there was no other family history to note. She has never smoked, seldom drinks alcohol and keeps a couple of budgerigars at home. On systematic enquiry, she denies any night sweats or weight loss and suffers from occasional indigestion.

On examination, she was comfortable at rest with no witnessed haemoptysis episodes.

RR 14/min HR 90/min BP 122/83 with no postural drop. Temp 36.5°C. Saturations 94% on room air

Hb 11.2 g/dL

MCV 87 fl

WCC 12.6 × 10^9/L (neutrophils 9.2 × 10^9/L)

Plts 410 × 10^9/L

Na 136 mmol/L

K 3.9 mmol/L

Urea 5.3 mmol/L

Creatinine 111 μmol/L

Bilirubin 7 μmol/L

ALP 31 U/L

ALT 25 U/L

Albumin 31 g/L

Calcium 2.36 mmol/L

Glucose 6.9 mmol/L

CRP 36 mg/L

D-dimer 0.06 U/L

Her recent CT scan revealed a left upper lobe cavitating lesion

No acid-fast bacilli detected from 2 sputum samples submitted

Question 1

What is the most likely cause of this woman's haemoptysis?
(a) ABPA
(b) Aspergilloma
(c) Tuberculosis
(d) Mycobacteria other than tuberculosis (MOTT)
(e) Pulmonary embolism

Question 2

The most useful next step in her management would be:
(a) Intravenous amphotericin
(b) Prednisolone increased to 20 mg od
(c) Prednisolone increased to 30 mg od
(d) Rifampicin and ethambutol
(e) None of the above

QUESTION 20

A 42-year-old obese heavy-goods vehicle driver who is a lifelong smoker presents with lethargy and low mood. This has been going on for some time and hasn't been helped by separation from his wife. On direct questioning you note that he has recently suffered interrupted sleep as he requires passing water 3–4 times during the night. He mentions that his symptoms don't really affect his driving but otherwise he spends most of his day wanting to catch up on sleep. He suffers from hypertension which is controlled on thiazide diuretics but otherwise keeps well. He doesn't go over the recommended male weekly alcohol consumption and is currently living alone.

Clinically, he is obese, weighing 115 kg with a body mass index of 36. He has a healthy oropharynx and wears a size-17-collar shirt. His blood pressure was 143/68 but the rest of his cardiovascular, respiratory and abdominal systems were unremarkable.

Hb 16.0 g/dL

MCV 86 fl

WCC 4.5 × 10^9/L

Plts 189 × 10^9/L

Na 131 mmol/L

K 3.1 mmol/L

Urea 6.2 mmol/L

Creatinine 110 μmol/L

Glucose 8.3 mmol/L

PFTs (restrictive with normal DLCO and reduced FRC N2)

Epworth Sleepiness Scale 11/24

Question 1

What would be the most useful next investigation(s)?
(a) Limited polysomnography
(b) Full polysomnography
(c) Limited polysomnography with overnight pulse oximetry
(d) Overnight pulse oximetry
(e) EEG

Question 2

As far as his livelihood is concerned:
(a) He needs to inform the DVLA immediately
(b) You give him verbal and written advice to refrain from driving if his symptoms affect his performance on the road
(c) You need to ensure that the DVLA is informed by copying his clinic letter to them
(d) OSAS is an unlikely diagnosis
(e) You need not expedite his investigation(s) as a positive diagnosis will mean that he will never hold a heavy-goods vehicle HGV licence again

QUESTION 21

A 36-year-old painter presented acutely breathless to the Accident and Emergency department and was found to be in profound type 1 respiratory failure, quickly requiring ventilatory support and transfer into the intensive care unit.

His chest X-ray was in keeping with acute lung injury, showing diffuse alveolar infiltrates and air bronchograms, and a vital collateral history was obtained from his partner. She noted that her boyfriend had only started working as a painter last week. He hadn't been well over the past 2–3 days with headaches, myalgia, fevers and breathlessness on very minimal exertion. He had never had an illness to note during his life. He only tried a few cigarettes in his teens, drinks alcohol in binges with his friends at the weekends and they were on holiday to Florida 6 months ago. They had a fish tank at home and a pet cat which they have had for a number of years.

ITU support included a course of intravenous empirical antibiotics and 10 days of high-dose steroid therapy. He made a good recovery and was discharged home. His investigations were not rewarding as far as identifying a bacterial or viral organism to explain his acute respiratory failure.

Three weeks later on the first day back to work he telephoned his partner to pick him up from work as he was feeling unwell again. He had a constant dry non-productive cough and his girlfriend took him to see his GP. His GP examined him and found him not to be distressed but did note bibasal crackles on chest auscultation and in view of his recent illness arranged his admission to hospital with a suspected diagnosis of bilateral pneumonia.

On arrival he had a mild cough but was feeling a lot better. His oxygen saturations were normal along with his vital signs. He was afebrile and chest examination revealed bibasal inspiratory crackles. Chest X-ray was unremarkable but his antibiotic therapy was continued.

Hb 14.3 g/dL
MCV 80 fl
WCC 13.2 × 10^9/L (normal differential count)
Plts 410 × 10^9/L
Na 139 mmol/L
K 3.6 mmol/L
Urea 3.6 mmol/L
Creatinine 56 µmol/L
Bilirubin 8 µmol/L
ALP 32 U/L
ALT 20 U/L
Albumin 44 g/L
Calcium 2.50 mmol/L
Glucose 6.9 mmol/L
CRP 71 mg/L

He was asymptomatic the following day with only a few faint crackles at the bases of his lung and you decided to discharge him home. He was enquiring about when he should go back to work as he is feeling fine. What would you advise him?
(a) Go back to work in 3 weeks
(b) Go back to work in 2 weeks
(c) Find an alternative career
(d) Consider using a protective facemasks
(e) Go back to work in 2 weeks and give up the cat

QUESTION 22

A 67-year-old retired joiner and lifelong smoker presents to your clinic with breathlessness. This has been going on for at least 2 years and he has finally decided to seek help now that he is struggling to complete two flights of stairs without taking a break. He also complains of a cough which mainly occurs on awakening and is often productive of white phlegm, although it was green in colour when he suffered an LRTI.

He also suffers from angina but only rarely uses his GTN spray as it gives him headaches. He is also on a tablet that lowers his cholesterol and takes low-dose prophylactic aspirin. He has struggled with his weight in recent times and takes little exercise. He continues to smoke 30 cigarettes per day as he thinks this should not be affecting his 'asthma'.

Examination revealed an obese man, weighing 110 kg with a BMI of 36 kg/m^2

He was not breathless at rest and had scattered rhonchi on auscultation with localized wheezing over the left sternal edge. Respiratory rate was 10 breaths/min and his oxygen saturations were 93% on room air. He was clubbed but had no carbon dioxide retention tremor.

Spirometry
FEV$_1$ 2.31 L (72%) FVC 3.5 L (71%) FEV$_1$/FVC 66%

Question 1
Your next investigation/management option would be:
(a) Static lung volumes and transfer factor
(b) Sputum for culture and sensitivity
(c) High-resolution CT to look for emphysema and bronchiectasis
(d) CXR
(e) Sputum cytology

Question 2
This patient's COPD is:
(a) Moderate
(b) Mild
(c) Moderately severe
(d) Severe
(e) None of the above

QUESTION 23
A 53-year-old man presents to the chest clinic after he was referred by one of the cardiologists. He initially presented to the cardiology clinic with chest tightness and they also noted that he was breathless on exertion over past 6–8 months. His CXR revealed diffuse reticular nodular shadowing; a high-resolution CT was arranged which revealed variable-thickness walled cysts with an upper- and lower-zone predominance.

He smokes 30 cigarettes per day, owns a pet shop and was recently in Florida with his family.

Examination was unremarkable.

PFTs showed an obstructive picture with preserved adjusted gas transfer.

FBC, LFTs and U + Es were normal.

Question 1
The most likely diagnosis is:
(a) Lymphangioleiomyomatosis
(b) Centrilobular emphysema
(c) Alpha$_1$-antitrypsin deficiency
(d) Langerhans-cell histiocytosis
(e) Alveolar cell carcinoma

Question 2
The most useful treatment option is:
(a) Hormone manipulation therapy
(b) Smoking cessation
(c) Smoking cessation and oral steroid therapy
(d) Immunoglobulin
(e) Long-acting bronchodilator antimuscarinic

QUESTION 24
A 39-year-old woman who works as a hairdresser presents to your clinic with breathlessness. This has been gradual in onset and slowly progressive over the past 14 months to the point that now she finds that she can only manage 2–3 flights of stairs at very slow pace and occasionally has to stop to 'catch her breath'. She initially put this down to her stressful job but her symptoms have progressed despite a couple of 3-week breaks in the past 6 months. She also complains of a dry cough which is intermittent and had asthma in her childhood years. She had a pneumothorax of the left lung 3 years ago which was aspirated in the accident and emergency department and decided to give up her 10 cigarettes-per-day smoking habit there and then. On further questioning she denies weight loss and the rest of her systematic enquiry was unremarkable apart from problems with her periods that have become less frequent: she is awaiting investigation by the gynaecologists for suspected premature menopause. There is no family history of atopy, asthma or respiratory illness to note.

On examination she was comfortable at rest with stable vital signs, including a respiratory rate of 14 breaths/min. She had pale conjunctivae but the rest of her general, cardiovascular and respiratory examinations were unremarkable. Her abdomen revealed non-tender, fixed central fullness measuring 5 × 5 cm on deep palpation.

Hb 13.5 g/dL
MCV 96 fl
WCC 3.2 × 10^9/L (lymphocytes 17%)
Plts 166 × 10^9/L
Na 139 mmol/L
K 4.9 mmol/L
Urea 2.9 mmol/L
Creatinine 100 μmol/L
Bilirubin 15 μmol/L
ALP 36 U/L
ALT 22 U/L
Albumin 33 g/L
Calcium 2.33 mmol/L
Glucose 4.3 mmol/L
TSH 1.2 mu/L
PFTs: normal spirometry and static lung volumes with mild reduction in DLCO
CXR: normal
Abdominal ultrasonography revealed a large retroperitoneal mass

Question 1
Which of the following investigations is most likely to establish the diagnosis?
(a) Staging CT scan of chest, abdomen and pelvis
(b) Peak flow rate monitoring for 2 months
(c) High-resolution CT scan of the chest
(d) Histamine challenge for bronchial hyperresponsiveness
(e) Bone marrow examination

Question 2
What is the most likely diagnosis?
(a) Langerhans-cell histiocytosis
(b) Asthma
(c) Occupation asthma
(d) Sarcoidosis
(e) Lymphangioleiomyomatosis

QUESTION 25
A 42-year-old man with a history of heavy alcohol intake for many years presents with confusion and worsening jaundice. He has also

noticed that his abdomen and ankles are swelling up. He denies vomiting, and says that his last drink was a week ago. He usually takes spironolactone, thiamine, a B-vitamin preparation and propranolol. On examination, he is icteric and apyrexial. Pulse 110 reg, BP 90/50 lying, 50/0 standing. He is drowsy with asterixis. Chest is clear, abdomen is non-tender, but demonstrates marked shifting dullness. His ankles are swollen. PR shows brown stool.

Biochemistry
Na 117 mmol/L
K 2.6 mmol/L
Urea 5.2 mmol/L
Creatinine 190 μmol/L
Bilirubin 245 μmol/L
ALT 150 U/L
ALP 265 U/L
Albumin 24 g/dL

Haematology
INR 2.6
Hb 13.4 g/dL
WCC 5.6 × 10^9/L
Plts 78 × 10^9/L
An ascitic tap reveals straw-coloured fluid with 570 white cells/mm^3 but no organisms

What three steps would you take next?
(a) Give normal saline
(b) Give blood
(c) Give colloid
(d) Give albumin
(e) Insert a central line
(f) Give broad-spectrum antibiotics
(g) Give lactulose
(h) Double the spironolactone
(i) Give diazepam
(j) Give FFP

QUESTION 26
A 68-year-old man with a 3-day history of black stools presents having vomited a large amount of fresh blood. He has a long history of heavy alcohol intake. He also has COPD and hypertension. He takes simvastatin, aspirin, thiamine, amlodipine, salbutamol and beclometasone. On examination, he is pale and sweaty. Pulse 120 reg, BP 75/40. He appears

jaundiced and tremulous. Chest is clear, but abdominal examination reveals ascites and a liver edge palpable 6 cm below the costal margin. His bloods have been sent off but are not back yet, and he has 2 bags of intravenous colloid running through large IV cannulae. What two actions will you carry out next?

(a) Insert urinary catheter
(b) Insert central venous line
(c) Give vitamin K
(d) Order FFP
(e) Alert the endoscopist
(f) Give diazepam
(g) Give terlipressin
(h) Perform ascitic tap
(i) Insert Sengstaken tube
(j) Insert a nasogastric tube

QUESTION 27

A 23-year-old waitress with Wilson's disease has been taking penicillamine for 4 years. At her routine follow-up appointment, she notes that she is feeling more tired than usual. She denies low mood, and has not noticed any abdominal pain or swelling, ankle swelling, difficulty speaking or trouble with her writing.

On examination, she has no ascites or ankle oedema. The liver is impalpable, as are the spleen and kidneys. There is no tremor, dysarthria or chorea present.

Investigations reveal the following:
Na 140 mmol/L
K 3.1 mmol/L
Bicarbonate 14 mmol/L
AST 55 U/L
Bilirubin 31 μmol/L
Glucose 4.5 mmol/L

Urinalysis

Glucose ++
Protein –
Blood –

What will you do next?
(a) Stop penicillamine
(b) Refer for renal biopsy
(c) Carry out an autoimmune screen
(d) Perform a pregnancy test
(e) Give bicarbonate and potassium

QUESTION 28

A 54-year-old accountant presents to Accident and Emergency with haematemesis and melaena. She gives a 4-month history of upper abdominal discomfort, and has recently been to her GP complaining of a persistent itch. She also complains that her eyes seem dry and sore recently. She gives no history of indigestion, drinks 7 units of alcohol per week and has never received a blood transfusion. She has taken thyroxine for 5 years, but takes no other medication.

On examination, her pulse is 120 beats/min and regular, BP 85/50 mmHg. Prominent xanthelasma are present. No palmar erythema or spider naevi are noted. She appears to be clubbed, but chest examination is unremarkable. A 4-cm smooth liver edge plus 3-cm spleen tip are palpable in the abdomen; PR examination confirms melaena.

Investigations

Hb 7.1 g/dL
WCC 13.5 × 10^9/L
Plts 540 × 10^9/L
Na 138 mmol/L
K 4.5 mmol/L
Urea 12 mmol/L
Creatinine 67 μmol/L
Cholesterol 8.7 mmol/L
Protein 81 g/L
Albumin 33 g/L
Bilirubin 28 μmol/L
ALT 41 U/L
ALP 895 U/L
INR 1.1
APTTR 1.0

Question 1

What would be the two most appropriate immediate therapies whilst you are organizing upper GI endoscopy?
(a) Intravenous albumin
(b) Intravenous terlipressin
(c) Intravenous saline
(d) Blood transfusion
(e) Intravenous vitamin K
(f) Intravenous dextrose
(g) Intravenous B-group vitamins
(h) Intravenous N-acetylcysteine

(i) Intravenous fresh frozen plasma
(j) Sengstaken–Blakemore tube

Question 2

What test would best confirm the likely underlying diagnosis?
(a) Antimitochondrial antibodies
(b) Liver biopsy
(c) Liver ultrasound
(d) Antinuclear antibody
(e) Serum ferritin level

QUESTION 29

A 60-year-old man presents with an 18-month history of abdominal pains and loose stools. He has noted 13 kg of weight loss over the past year. The patient also notes that his stool is offensive and tends to float in the pan. He admits to drinking heavily in the past, but had to give up a few months ago as alcohol made the pain worse. He takes tramadol and paracetamol, along with temazepam at night. On examination, he appears thin. There is no jaundice, anaemia or lymphadenopathy. Chest is clear, and abdominal examination reveals mild epigastric tenderness.

Initial investigation shows:

Hb 13.0 g/dL
MCV 86 fl
WCC 7.4 × 10^9/L
Platelets 250 × 10^9/L
U + Es normal
3-day faecal fat excretion: 18 g/day

What investigation will you perform next?
(a) CT pancreas
(b) Upper GI endoscopy
(c) Pancreolauryl test
(d) Antiendomysial antibody test
(e) Stool culture

QUESTION 30

A 40-year-old woman presents with acute abdominal pain. She denies excessive alcohol ingestion. She takes no regular medications except the contraceptive pill, and occasional analgesia for back pain. She has no other current illnesses, but had a deep-vein thrombosis 5 years ago following a flight from Australia. She does not smoke, and has not had any previous abdominal surgery. On examination, she was in pain. Pulse 110 reg, BP 120/85. JVP not raised, but absent hepatojugular reflex. Heart sounds were normal, with no ankle oedema. Chest was clear, and abdominal examination reveals tender hepatomegaly and ascites.

Investigations

Na 135 mmol/L
K 4.6 mmol/L
Urea 4.5 mmol/L
Creatinine 54 μmol/L
ALT 60 U/L
Bilirubin 40 μmol/L
Total protein 40 g/L
Albumin 36 g/L
ALP 300 U/L
CRP 52 mg/L
Hb 16.2 g/dL
WCC 17.5 × 10^9/L
Plts 114 × 10^9/L
INR 1.1
APTTR 1.8
HBsAg negative
Anti-smooth-muscle antibodies negative
Antimitochondrial antibodies negative
Rheumatoid factor negative

Question 1

What investigation would you do to confirm the cause of her abdominal pain?
(a) Erect abdominal radiograph
(b) Doppler ultrasound of the liver
(c) Ascitic tap
(d) Serum amylase
(e) ERCP

Question 2

What is the most likely underlying cause for her illness?
(a) Hepatic venous web
(b) Intra-abdominal malignancy
(c) Antiphospholipid syndrome
(d) Behçet's disease
(e) Polycythaemia rubra vera

QUESTION 31

A 55-year-old man presents with watery diarrhoea and abdominal pains. He has lost 13 kg

(2 stone) in weight over the last 6 months. He has a long history of Crohn's disease and has had two bowel resections for this previously; however his terminal ileum was preserved. Recently he had become so weak that he was confined to bed. He takes balsalazide, paracetamol and dihydrocodeine.

Examination reveals a cachectic man with multiple abdominal scars from previous surgery. He is mildly tender in the right and left iliac fossae. There was also marked wasting of the quadriceps muscles with weakness. Chest was clear, with no jaundice or clubbing. He looked pale.

Blood tests show:

Hb 8.2 g/dL
MCV 115 fl
WCC 4.1 × 10⁹/L
Plts 97 × 10⁹/L
Na 129 mmol/L
K 3.1 mmol/L
Urea 2.6 mmol/L
Creatinine 56 μmol/L
Bilirubin 14 μmol/L
ALT 20 U/L
ALP 186 U/L
Glucose 5.2 mmol/L
Calcium 2.24 mmol/L
Albumin 31 g/L
CRP 12 mg/L

What investigation will you carry out next?
(a) Upper GI endoscopy
(b) Barium followthrough
(c) Hydrogen breath test
(d) Plain abdominal X-ray
(e) Radiolabelled white cell scan

QUESTION 32

A 22-year-old woman presents with a 5-day history of jaundice, abdominal pain and confusion. She was unable to give any further history, but her parents denied previous ill health, medications or depression. On examination she was apyrexial. Pulse 95/reg, BP 100/50. JVP not raised and chest clear. She was jaundiced, with 5 cm tender hepatomegaly and ascites. Asterixis was present and her GCS was 13/15.

Investigations
Hb 10.1 g/dL
WCC 11.0 × 10⁹/L
Platelets 186 × 10⁹/L
INR 2.3
ESR > 100 mm/h
Na 139 mmol/L
K 4.9 mmol/L
Urea 9.1 mmol/L
Creatinine 67 μmol/L
Amylase 44 U/L
Glucose 3.0 mmol/L
Bilirubin 122 μmol/L
ALT 3565 U/L
ALP 410 U/L
Paracetamol levels undetectable
Urinary drug screen negative
Hepatitis A, B, C, E serology negative
EBV serology shows low titres of IgG. IgM negative
CMV serology negative
ANA titre 1/160
Anti-smooth-muscle antibody titre 1/320
Antimitochondrial antibody negative
Caeruloplasmin normal
Urinary copper normal

What is the most likely diagnosis?
(a) Autoimmune hepatitis
(b) *Amanita* poisioning
(c) Paracetamol overdose
(d) Acute hepatitis B infection
(e) Weil's disease

QUESTION 33

A 31-year-old woman with a 7-year history of Crohn's disease presents with persistent diarrhoea. Her bowels are opening six times per day at present, with vague lower abdominal pain. She has previously had two extensive bowel resections for Crohn's, and usually takes azathioprine and prednisolone 40 mg/day. She has previously tried methotrexate but reacted badly to this. On examination, she appears thin, with a BMI of 17. Pulse is 95/min and BP 100/50. Joint and eye examination are normal, but there is tenderness in the right and left iliac fossae.

Investigations show Hb 9.7 g/dL, WCC 4.3 × 10^9/L, Plts 359 × 10^9/L. CRP 82, ESR 57 mm/h. Na 135 mmol/L, K 3.2 mmol/L, urea 1.3 mmol/L, creatinine 76 μmol/L. Albumin is 26 g/dL. Barium follow-through shows a fistula between her jejunum and ileum. CT scanning of the abdomen confirms the fistula and the presence of extensive small-bowel inflammation, but shows no evidence of abscess formation.

What treatment will you try next?
(a) Metronidazole
(b) Infliximab
(c) Surgery to tie off the fistula
(d) IV methylprednisolone
(e) Cholestyramine

QUESTION 34

A 61-year-old woman presents with an 18-month history of pruritus. She has tried several different antihistamines with little benefit. She is otherwise well, drinks very little alcohol, has never had a blood transfusion, and her only sexual partner has been her husband. She was diagnosed with hypothyroidism 5 years ago. She is currently taking desloratidine and thyroxine. She is not allergic to anything. On examination, there are no stigmata of chronic liver disease. Abdominal examination reveals no ascites, and both liver and spleen are impalpable. Her bloods show:
Na 141 mmol/L
K 3.7 mmol/L
Urea 2.6 mmol/L
Creatinine 54 μmol/L
ALT 37 U/L
Bilirubin 17 μmol/L
Alkaline phosphatase 430 U/L
Albumin 36 g/dL
INR 1.1
Liver ultrasound is normal and her anti-mitochondrial antibody is strongly positive.

How will you treat her?
(a) Observe and do nothing
(b) Refer for liver transplant work-up
(c) Proceed to ERCP
(d) Give ursodeoxycholic acid
(e) Give ranitidine

QUESTION 35

A 57-year-old man presents with increasing abdominal girth, mild abdominal discomfort and tiredness. He was diagnosed as having haemochromatosis 3 years ago, and has a history of diabetes and hypertension. He takes gliclazide, ramipril and aspirin, and undergoes regular venesection. He has not drunk alcohol for 3 years. On examination, he is not jaundiced. Several spider naevi are present. There is no asterixis. Pulse 80 regular, BP 135/75. JVP not raised, heart sounds normal, chest clear. There is shifting dullness in the abdomen but no organs are palpable. He is mildly tender in the right hypochondrium.

Bloods
Na 129 mmol/L
K 3.6 mmol/L
Urea 2.5 mmol/L
Creatinine 75 μmol/L
Bilirubin 35 μmol/L
ALT 58 U/L
Alkaline phosphatase 430 U/L
Albumin 28 g/dL
INR 1.5
Hb 11.3 g/dL
WCC 5.8 × 10^9/L
Plts 293 × 10^9/L.
His alpha-fetoprotein level is significantly elevated

What diagnostic test would best confirm the diagnosis?
(a) Ascitic tap
(b) Ultrasound of the abdomen
(c) Percutaneous liver fine-needle aspiration
(d) CT with contrast
(e) ERCP

QUESTION 36

A 28-year-old man presents with a 1-day history of myalgia, malaise and fevers. He denies cough or sputum production, and does not complain of urinary symptoms. He passes two loose stools a day, which he has done for several years. He denies recent foreign travel or unprotected sexual intercourse. He has a past medical history of coeliac disease, diagnosed at the age of 12, and also has type 1 diabetes. He smokes 10 cigarettes per day but does not drink alcohol. He takes insulin twice a day.

On examination, he is pyrexial at 38.7°C. Pulse 120 regular, BP 70/35. He appears dehydrated. Chest is clear, respiratory rate 24 per minute. Abdominal examination shows no liver or spleen, soft, non-tender. Bowel sounds are present. There is no neck stiffness or photophobia; he is fully oriented in time and place.

Investigations
Na 132 mmol/L
K 5.2 mmol/L
Urea 9.6 mmol/L
Creatinine 156 μmol/L
LFTs are normal
Albumin 29 g/L
INR 1.4
Hb 10.7 g/dL
MCV 104 fl
WCC 35 × 10^9/L
Plts 637 × 10^9/L

Blood film shows target cells and Howell–Jolly bodies; blood cultures grow Gram-positive diplococci. He recovered fully with aggressive fluid resuscitation and intravenous antibiotics.

What would be the most important next step?
(a) Upper GI endoscopy
(b) Long-term prophylactic penicillin
(c) Splenectomy
(d) Bone marrow biopsy
(e) HIV test

QUESTION 37
A 38-year-old woman has a 5-year history of autoimmune hepatitis. She discontinued taking steroids because of side-effects a year ago, and is currently on no medication other than the oral contraceptive pill. She does not drink alcohol.

You see her in the liver clinic, where she complains of feeling tired all the time. On examination, pulse is 80 regular, BP 110/70. Several spider naevi are present and there is palmar erythema. A 4-cm liver edge is palpable and is mildly tender on inspiration. There is no splenomegaly or ascites.

Bloods
Na 136 mmol/L
K 4.1 mmol/L
Urea 2.2 mmol/L

Creatinine 68 μmol/L
Bilirubin 16 μmol/L
ALT 230 U/L
ALP 135 U/L

What will you do next?
(a) Liver biopsy
(b) Reintroduce steroids
(c) Test for viral hepatitis
(d) Test for liver autoantibodies
(e) Start ciclosporin

QUESTION 38
A 47-year-old man presents with tiredness and muscle pains. His GP tested his urine and found glycosuria and referred him to the local endocrine clinic, where routine testing revealed elevated blood sugars and deranged liver function tests. He has no history of drug abuse or blood transfusion, and is normally healthy. He does not smoke, but drinks 15 units of alcohol per week. He gives a family history of heart attacks but no other diseases.

On examination, there are no signs of chronic liver disease. Chest and abdominal examination are normal, as is neurological examination.

Bloods
Hb 13.6 g/dL
MCV 94 fl
WCC 6.7 × 10^9/L
Plts 299 × 10^9/L
INR 1.1
Na 142 mmol/L
K 4.8 mmol/L
Urea 3.4 mmol/L
Creatinine 87 μmol/L
Bilirubin 18 μmol/L
ALT 78 U/L
ALP 192 U/L
Albumin 34 g/dL
Glucose 12.2 mmol/L
X-ray knee: reported as showing
    chondrocalcinosis of the knee joint

What test would best diagnose this man's underlying condition?
(a) Serum ferritin
(b) Transferrin saturation
(c) Genotyping
(d) Liver biopsy
(e) CT of the liver

QUESTION 39

A 37-year-old woman presents to clinic feeling tired all the time. This has been going on for 4 years. She denies dizziness, chest or abdominal pain, and does not feel the cold. She has lost 4 kg in weight over the last 2 years without really trying. On direct questioning, she admits to bouts of indigestion, especially after 'rich' food. She denies change in bowel habit or rectal bleeding. She does not smoke and drinks 10 units of alcohol per week. She takes the contraceptive pill, and has taken iron for the last 3 months as her GP found her to be slightly anaemic.

On examination, pulse was 70 regular, BP 115/70. Chest and abdominal examination were normal, and the thyroid was impalpable.

Bloods

Hb 9.7 g/dL
MCV 94 fl
WCC 5.4 × 10^9/L
Plts 329 × 10^9/L
Ferritin 14 µg/L
Folate 1.7 µg/L
Na 141 mmol/L
K 4.0 mmol/L
Urea 3.7 mmol/L
Creatinine 68 µmol/L
Albumin 36 g/dL
Bilirubin < 5 µmol/L
ALT 21 U/L
ALP 139 U/L
Calcium 2.17 mmol/L
Glucose 4.6 mmol/L

She undergoes upper GI endoscopy, which appears normal, thus no biopsies are taken.

What will you do next?
(a) Lower GI endoscopy
(b) Barium followthrough
(c) Repeat upper GI endoscopy with duodenal biopsies
(d) Bone marrow biopsy
(e) Trial of folic acid supplements

QUESTION 40

A 34-year-old man presents with worsening abdominal pain and bloody diarrhoea. His bowels are open 4–5 times per day. He was diagnosed with ulcerative colitis 3 years ago, and his disease has been quiescent for several months,

with his bowels open twice a day. He rarely notices blood in his stools. He smokes 10 cigarettes per day, drinks 30 units of alcohol per week, and takes mesalazine.

On examination, he appears pale and thin. Temperature 37.4°C. Pulse 85 reg, BP 120/60. Chest is clear, and he is mildly tender in the left iliac fossa. Bowel sounds are active and there is no abdominal distension.

Bloods

Hb 11.4 g/dL
WCC 12.1 × 10^9/L
Plts 410 × 10^9/L
Na 144 mmol/L
K 3.6 mmol/L
Urea 3.5 mmol/L
Creatinine 76 µmol/L
CRP 59 mg/L
Albumin 34 g/L

What will you do?
(a) Refer for surgical opinion
(b) Take stool cultures
(c) Add in oral prednisolone
(d) Give IV methylprednisolone
(e) Continue mesalazine and add in Predfoam enemas

QUESTION 41

A 52-year-old man with a 4-year history of ulcerative colitis presents for review. He complains of intermittent abdominal pain, worse in the right upper quadrant. During the last episode of pain, he noticed that his eyes looked rather yellow. His bowels are open 2–3 times per day. They are loose, but he is not losing blood. He takes mesalazine and azathioprine, does not smoke or drink, and is otherwise well. He underwent a cholecystectomy 15 years ago.

On examination, he appears well. There is no jaundice, spider naevi or palmar erythema. Pulse 80 reg, BP 140/85. Chest is clear, heart sounds normal. Abdominal examination reveals mild right upper quadrant tenderness but no palpable liver or spleen.

Bloods

Hb 10.5 g/dL
WCC 5.1 × 10^9/L
Plts 177 × 10^9/L

Na 141 mmol/L
K 4.0 mmol/L
Urea 4.4 mmol/L
Creatinine 92 µmol/L
Bilirubin 41 µmol/L
ALT 35 U/L
ALP 371 U/L
Albumin 32 g/L

Ultrasound of the abdomen reveals normal liver parenchyma and a common bile duct diameter at the upper limit of normal.

What investigation would be most likely to confirm the diagnosis?
(a) ANCA
(b) ERCP
(c) CT of the liver and abdomen
(d) Liver biopsy
(e) Viral serology

QUESTION 42

A 61-year-old man presents with a 6-month history of dysphagia. He initially had problems swallowing meat; he now finds even porridge difficult to get down. He has lost 20 kg (3 stone) in weight over the last 6 months. He also suffers from hypertension and angina and continues to smoke 10 cigarettes per day. He takes aspirin, diltiazem and nitrates.

On examination, he appears cachectic. Pulse 70 reg, BP 150/80. His voice is hoarse. Lymph nodes are palpable in the left supraclavicular fossa. Chest examination is normal, and there is no liver or other masses palpable in the abdomen.

Endoscopy confirms an ulcerated stricture at 35 cm in the oesophagus, and CT of the chest and abdomen shows thickening of the mid-oesophagus but no liver or lung metastases.

Bloods
Na 139 mmol/L
K 4.4 mmol/L
Urea 4.7 mmol/L
Creatinine 118 µmol/L
Calcium 2.29 mmol/L
Hb 10.4 g/dL

What will you do next?
(a) Arrange for endoscopic ultrasound of the oesophagus
(b) Refer for oesophagectomy

(c) Refer for stenting of the stricture
(d) Refer for chemotherapy
(e) Arrange for lymph node biopsy

QUESTION 43

A 28-year-old woman is admitted having taken an overdose. No empty bottles were found in the house, but she told a friend what she had done prior to admission. The friend notes that the patient is known to have epilepsy but does not know what medicines she normally takes. On examination, she is drowsy. Pulse 90 reg, BP 110/60. Chest and abdominal examination are normal. Pupils are normal-size and reactive; reflexes and plantar responses are normal.

Bloods
Na 143 mmol/L
K 4.1 mmol/L
Urea 2.7 mmol/L
Creatinine 69 µmol/L
Paracetamol 55 mg/L
Salicylate not detected
Bilirubin 7 µmol/L
ALT 48 U/L
ALP 131 U/L
INR 1.2

What is the most appropriate course of action?
(a) Observe and repeat blood tests in 4 hours
(b) Start N-acetylcysteine
(c) Request anticonvulsant blood levels
(d) Give activated charcoal
(e) Send urine for a toxicology screen

QUESTION 44

A 35-year-old man is admitted 48 hours after taking a paracetamol overdose. He has vomited 2–3 times over the last 2 days and complains of mild epigastric discomfort. He is usually fit and well, with no significant past medical history. He smokes cannabis but does not drink alcohol. On examination, he is not jaundiced. Pulse 80 reg, BP 120/60. Chest and abdominal examination normal. GCS is 15, with no asterixis, and he is fully oriented.

Bloods
Na 137 mmol/L
K 4.7 mmol/L
Urea 7.2 mmol/L

Creatinine 102 μmol/L
Paracetamol not detected
Salicylate not detected
Bilirubin 7 μmol/L
ALT 81 U/L
ALP 131 U/L
INR 1.6

What will you do?
(a) Refer to liver transplant unit
(b) Repeat blood tests in 24 hours
(c) Administer *N*-acetylcysteine
(d) Discharge patient to home
(e) Arrange liver ultrasound

QUESTION 45

A 39-year-old woman with schizophrenia is admitted having swallowed all of her mother's supply of aspirin. She is drowsy on admission, but her mother tells you that she usually takes haloperidol. She does not drink alcohol but smokes 40 cigarettes per day. On examination, GCS = 10. Pulse 120 reg, BP 80/40. Chest examination reveals bibasal crackles and a respiratory rate of 28 per minute. Abdominal examination is normal.

Bloods
Na 129 mmol/L
K 3.1 mmol/L
Urea 10.1 mmol/L
Creatinine 147 μmol/L
Paracetamol not detected
Salicylate 950 mg/L
Bilirubin 12 μmol/L
ALT 23 U/L
ALP 99 U/L
INR 1.1

Arterial Blood Gases
pH 7.21
pco_2 2.5 kPa
po_2 8.7 kPa
Bicarbonate 8 mmol/L

What will you do?
(a) Administer IV sodium bicarbonate
(b) Administer IV furosemide
(c) Refer for haemodialysis
(d) Administer IV bicarbonate plus furosemide
(e) Give activated charcoal via NG tube

QUESTION 46

A 47-year-old man is admitted to the Accident and Emergency department. He was found at home by a neighbour who had not seen him for a couple of days. The neighbour noted that the patient had recently been withdrawn following the death of his wife. On examination, there was no jaundice or cyanosis. Pulse was 100 reg, BP 100/60. Chest and abdominal examination were normal, but his respiratory rate was elevated at 30/min. Pupils, reflexes and plantars were normal; his GCS was 12/15.

Bloods
Na 140 mmol/L
K 3.7 mmol/L
Urea 6.1 mmol/L
Creatinine 122 μmol/L
Chloride 87 mmol/L
Calcium 2.41 mmol/L
Albumin 36 g/L
Glucose 5.1 mmol/L
Bilirubin 10 μmol/L
ALT 39 U/L
ALP 105 U/L
Plasma osmolality 301 mOsm/kg

Urinalysis
Protein +
Blood −
Ketones −

Arterial Blood Gases
pH 7.24
pco_2 3.1 kPa
po_2 16.1 kPa
Bicarbonate 10 mmol/L

What is the most likely diagnosis?
(a) Methanol overdose
(b) Diabetic ketoacidosis
(c) Ethylene glycol overdose
(d) Salicylate overdose
(e) Amitriptyline overdose

QUESTION 47

A 19-year-old woman is admitted comatose, having been found at home by her boyfriend, with whom she had argued after a heavy night's drinking. An empty bottle of tablets was found by paramedics in the kitchen.

On examination, she was apyrexial. Pulse 130/min, BP 80/40, JVP not raised. Chest is clear to auscultation, abdomen soft. Pupils are dilated, GCS = 3/15, extensor plantars bilaterally. No neck stiffness.

Investigations
Hb 13.1 g/dL
WCC 9.0×10^9/L
Platelets 225×10^9/L
Na 138 mmol/L
K 4.0 mmol/L
Urea 3.0 mmol/L
Creatinine 59 µmol/L
Glucose 4.8 mmol/L
Bilirubin 10 µmol/L
ALT 110 U/L
ALP 92 U/L
CK 533 U/L
Osmolality 310 mOsm/kg
ECG: sinus tachycardia, 130/min
po_2 18 kPa (on 60% O_2)
pco_2 3.1 kPa
pH 7.28

What is the most likely diagnosis?
(a) Amitriptyline overdose
(b) Benzodiazepine overdose
(c) Ecstasy overdose
(d) Codeine overdose
(e) Paroxetine overdose

QUESTION 48
A 68-year-old man is admitted having taken an overdose of imipramine. The paramedics report that he sustained a tonic-clonic seizure in the ambulance. He has a past medical history of angina and sustained a small stroke last year. On examination, pulse 110 reg. BP 120/60. JVP not raised; chest is clear. Abdominal examination is normal. Pupils are dilated; GCS = 6/15. Both plantars are upgoing. As you are examining him, he has a run of broad-complex tachycardia on his cardiac monitor and he briefly loses his pulse.

12-lead ECG shows sinus tachycardia with a QRS duration of 140 ms. Arterial blood gases show:
pH 7.32
pco_2 4.1
po_2 10.6 on 40% O_2
Bicarbonate 16 mmol/L

What is the most appropriate treatment for his arrhythmia?
(a) IV phenytoin
(b) Haemodialysis
(c) IV sodium bicarbonate
(d) IV amiodarone
(e) IV lidocaine

QUESTION 49
A 70-year-old man presents with collapse to the local hospital. He has recently complained of fever, shortness of breath and cough productive of yellow sputum. The GP had started erythromycin 5 days ago to cover a presumed chest infection. For the last 2 days he has felt nauseated, and has had rather loose stools. He takes regular aspirin, bendroflumethiazide and digoxin. He has a resting heart rate of 56 beats/min irregular, and a blood pressure of 110/60 mmHg. Cardiac examination is normal. Chest examination reveals left-sided basal crackles with bronchial breathing.

Investigations
Na 135 mmol/L
K 4.3 mmol/L
Urea 5.0 mmol/L
Creatinine 110 µmol/L
Troponin T: 0.01 U/L
CXR left lower zone consolidation
ECG shows atrial fibrillation with a rate of 40 beats/min. QRS complexes are 120 ms wide. There is widespread ST depression of 2 mm and T-wave inversion in the anterior leads
Whilst on CCU, a short run of non-sustained VT is noted on his cardiac monitor

What investigation is most likely to explain his collapses?

Question 1
(a) 24-hour Holter monitoring
(b) Lying and standing blood pressure
(c) EEG
(d) Exercise ECG
(e) Digoxin level

Question 2
His digoxin level comes back at 3.6 nmol/L. What will you do next?
(a) Administer potassium
(b) Attempt DC cardioversion

(c) Give amioadarone
(d) Administer digoxin-specific antibody fragments
(e) Give magnesium

QUESTION 50

A 32-year-old man is brought to the A&E department having been found unconscious at home. He lives alone in a rented flat. On examination, pulse is 90 reg, BP 115/60. Temperature is 40.1°C and the respiratory rate is 30/min. Chest is clear, abdominal examination is normal. There are no localizing neurological signs, pupils are reactive and of normal size and there is no sign of trauma.

Investigations

Na 144 mmol/L
K 3.7 mmol/L
Urea 3.1 mmol/L
Creatinine 60 μmol/L
LFTs normal
Glucose 5.1 mmol/L
CRP 7 mg/L
Hb 15.1 g/dL
WCC 12.2 × 10^9/L
Plts 224 × 10^9/L

ABGS

po_2 21 kPa (on 60% O_2)
pco_2 3.3 kPa
pH 7.21

What is the most likely diagnosis?
(a) Subarachnoid haemorrhage
(b) Acute alcohol intoxication
(c) Heroin overdose
(d) Carbon monoxide poisoning
(e) Viral encephalitis

QUESTION 51

A 62-year-old woman moved into cheap rented accommodation following the death of her husband 4 months ago. Since then, she has felt generally unwell, with headaches and dizziness. She has not felt like eating and doesn't go out much as she feels weak. On direct questioning, she denies suicidal ideation and, although she misses her husband, she does not feel particularly tearful or low in mood. She does not drink or smoke, and takes thyroxine for hypothyroidism. On examination, pulse is 70

reg. BP 140/85 with no postural drop. JVP not raised; heart sounds normal. Chest and abdominal examination is normal. Tone, power, reflexes and coordination are normal; fundoscopy is normal.

Blood Tests

Hb 13.2 g/dL
WCC 5.2 × 10^9/L
Plts 396 × 10^9/L
U + Es normal
LFTs normal
TSH 1.87 mU/L
Thyroxine 90 nmol/L
ESR 21 mm/h
Chest X-ray: normal

What will you do next?
(a) Short Synacthen test
(b) Refer for psychiatric opinion
(c) CT brain
(d) MRI brain
(e) Carbon monoxide level

QUESTION 52

A 30-year-old man presents to the A&E department with a suspected overdose of unknown tablets with some alcohol. On examination he had a heart rate of 130 beats/min, a blood pressure of 180/110 mmHg, and he was tachypnoeic. Respiratory examination revealed bilateral basal crackles. Neurological examination showed dilated and slow-reacting pupils, hypotonia, reduced tendon reflexes and flexor plantar responses.

Initial investigations show:

Hb 15.0 g/dL
WCC 20 × 10^9/L
Platelets 300 × 10^9/L
Na 148 mmol/L
K 4.8 mmol/L
Urea 10.5 mmol/L
Creatinine 250 μmol/L
Calcium 1.86 mmol/L
Albumin 37 g/L
Chloride 85 mmol/L
pH 7.12
po_2 9.2 kPa on 60% O_2
pco_2 2.2 kPa
Bicarbonate 4.0 mmol/L
Glucose 5.0 mmol/L

297

Paracetamol not detected
Salicylate not detected

Which two of the following will you give ?
(a) IV furosemide
(b) Ethanol infusion
(c) IV bicarbonate
(d) Activated charcoal
(e) Gastric lavage
(f) Haemodialysis
(g) IV calcium
(h) IV dextrose
(i) IV naloxone
(j) Sodium nitrite

QUESTION 53

A 20-year-old man presents to the surgeons with severe abdominal pain. For several weeks he has had nausea and vomiting, and for the last 2 days he has complained of severe colicky abdominal pain. The only medication he takes is lactulose for constipation. He smokes 20 cigarettes a day, drinks 3 pints of beer a night, and works for his cousin in a paint-stripping business. His brother has noticed that he has become clumsy recently – he keeps tripping over his own feet. On examination, there is no rash, cyanosis, clubbing or lymph nodes. He is oriented in time, place and person. Cardiovascular and chest examination are normal. Abdominal examination reveals no tenderness, masses or organomegaly. Bowel sounds are normal. Neurologically, sensation is normal, reflexes are brisk save for ankle jerks, and power is normal except for reduced ankle dorsiflexion and plantarflexion strength. Coordination and cranial nerves, including fundoscopy, are normal.

Investigations
Hb 9.5 g/dL
MCV 86 fl
WCC 7.0×10^9/L
Platelets 200×10^9/L
Chest X-ray normal
Abdominal X-ray normal
ECG normal

Urinalysis
Glucose ++
Protein +
ALA positive
Coproporphyrin positive

What is the most likely diagnosis?
(a) Lead poisoning
(b) Cadmium poisoning
(c) Acute intermittent porphyria
(d) Hereditary coproporphyria
(e) Churg–Strauss syndrome

QUESTION 54

A 27-year-old man is brought in after a gas attack on the London underground. He is agitated and incoherent on arrival. On examination, pulse is 50/min. BP 60/30. Respiratory rate is 30/min, O_2 sats are 92% on air. Bibasal crackles are heard in the chest, and he is salivating profusely. His pupils are small and he is twitching in an uncoordinated fashion. GCS = 13/15.

What will you administer?
(a) Atropine
(b) Pralidoxime
(c) Atropine and pralidoxime
(d) Dicobalt edetate
(e) Atropine and dicobalt edetate

QUESTION 55

A 34-year-old farm labourer is admitted to A&E. He is unconscious on arrival, and his companion is not sure what happened. His pulse is 40 regular, BP 70/30. He has bibasal crackles in the chest, respiratory rate 30/min with oxygen sats of 84% on air. He has soiled himself with loose stool and is sweating profusely.

Bloods
Hb 16.5 g/dL
WCC 18.5×10^9/L
Plts 178×10^9/L
Na 146 mmol/L
K 4.3 mmol/L
Urea 3.4 mmol/L
Creatinine 94 µmol/L
Creatine kinase 177 U/L
LFTs: normal

Blood Gases
pH 7.31
pco_2 3.7 kPa
po_2 6.5 kPa
CXR: bilateral alveolar shadowing

What test is most likely to confirm the diagnosis?
(a) Urine toxicology screen
(b) Acetylcholinesterase assay
(c) Plasma osmolarity
(d) Carboxyhaemoglobin assay
(e) 12-lead ECG

QUESTION 56

A 70-year-old man is admitted having had a fall. He has noticed becoming increasingly clumsy over the last few weeks. His past history includes epilepsy and hiatus hernia. Cimetidine has recently been added to his medications by his GP. He is a long-term smoker of 20 cigarettes a day, and drinks alcohol regularly.

Examination shows equal and reactive pupils. He is somewhat drowsy but is apyrexial and has a heart rate of 56 beats/min with a blood pressure of 120/60 mmHg. Cardiac, respiratory and abdominal examination are otherwise normal. He has horizontal nystagmus with dysarthria and limb ataxia. He demonstrates hyperreflexia with bilateral ankle clonus. There is no asterixis.

Investigations

ECG: sinus rhythm, 70/min, T-wave inversion in V5–6
Na 127 mmol/L
K 4.5 mmol/L
Urea 2.2 mmol/L
Creatinine 87 µmol/L
Bilirubin 14 µmol/L
ALT 62 U/L
ALP 210 U/L
Calcium 2.05 mmol/L
Albumin 41 g/L
Hb 11.9 g/dL
MCV 104 fl
WCC 7.1×10^9/L
Plts 110×10^9/L

Question 1

What investigation is most likely to confirm the diagnosis?
(a) CT brain
(b) MRI brain
(c) Red-cell transketolase assay
(d) Vitamin D level
(e) Phenytoin level

Question 2

His phenytoin level comes back at 17 mg/L (normal range 10–20 mg/L). What will you do?
(a) Stop phenytoin and start valproate
(b) Continue phenytoin and proceed to MRI brain
(c) Withhold phenytoin for a few days and observe
(d) Reduce phenytoin level by half
(e) Stop cimetidine

QUESTION 57

A 40-year-old woman presents to A&E with increasing confusion. There is a preceding history of diarrhoea for 2 weeks, and she has recently started vomiting. She also has non-insulin-dependent diabetes mellitus, hypertension and depression. Her medications include gliclazide, bendroflumethiazide, lisinopril and lithium.

On examination she is drowsy and confused but apyrexial. She has a heart rate of 56 beats/min with a blood pressure of 90/50 mmHg. Her chest is clear and she has hyperreflexia with increased tone.

Investigations

Hb 13.0 g/dL
WCC 14×10^9/L
Platelets 200×10^9/L
Na 128 mmol/L
K 2.7 mmol/L
Urea 30 mmol/L
Creatinine 405 µmol/L
Lithium 5.1 mmol/L

Urinalysis

Protein +
Blood –
Glucose –
ECG: sinus bradycardia
Chest X-ray normal

What is the best treatment for this patient?
(a) Stop lithium and observe
(b) Rehydrate with 0.9% sodium chloride
(c) Rehydrate with 5% dextrose and potassium
(d) Refer for haemodialysis
(e) Rehydrate, give activated charcoal and IV potassium

QUESTION 58

A 22-year-old man is admitted unconscious and fitting. He has no other medical history of note. On examination he has a temperature of 41°C. He is cyanosed, and has a heart rate of 140 beats/min. Initial blood pressure was 80/40 mmHg. Respiratory examination revealed widespread crackles.

Investigations

Na 120 mmol/L
K 6.5 mmol/L
Urea 25 mmol/L
Creatinine 350 μmol/L
Creatine kinase 19 700 U/L
Hb 14.0 g/dL
WCC 10 × 10^9/L
Platelets 50 × 10^9/L
Prothrombin time 25 s
APTT 60 s

What is the most likely diagnosis?
(a) Ecstasy overdose
(b) Cocaine overdose
(c) Serotonin syndrome
(d) Subarachnoid haemorrhage
(e) Gamma-hydroxybutyrate overdose

QUESTION 59

You are asked to see a 71-year-old woman on the orthopaedic ward. She was admitted 3 days ago with a fractured nack of femur, which she sustained falling down the stairs. She is normally well save for diagnoses of hypertension and hypothyroidism. She takes thyroxine and amlodipine, and has been receiving morphine and paracetamol in the postoperative period. On examination, she is agitated and appears distracted. She is unable to tell you her age, the place or the day of the week. She has a marked tremor and is sweating. Temperature is 37.4°C. Pulse 120 regular, BP 170/110. Chest is clear, respiratory rate is 24 per minute, and oxygen saturations are 97% on 4 L oxygen. Abdominal examination is normal.

Investigations

Na 136 mmol/L
K 3.3 mmol/L
Urea 2.5 mmol/L
Creatinine 79 μmol/L
Bilirubin 16 μmol/L
ALT 46 U/L
ALP 176 U/L
Glucose 4.9 mmol/L
Hb 9.5 g/dL
WCC 13.0 × 10^9/L
Plts 121 × 10^9/L
Urinalysis: clear
CXR: clear lung fields. Cardiomegaly
ECG: sinus tachycardia. No ST changes

What will you do?
(a) Administer naloxone
(b) Administer diazepam
(c) Administer haloperidol
(d) Give a beta-blocker
(e) Give Lugol's iodine

QUESTION 60

A 26-year-old man is admitted unconscious late on a Saturday night. His friends say that he had been at a night club with them, and that they dragged him out of a toilet cubicle. They do not recall any other medical problems, and his wallet reveals no medical alert cards. He is not wearing a Medic-Alert bracelet.

On examination, he smells of alcohol. Pulse is 100 regular, BP 120/60. Chest and abdominal examination are normal. His GCS is 5/15. Pupils are equal and reactive, and reflexes are symmetrical. He has an upgoing plantar on the right. There is no neck stiffness and fundoscopy is normal. Whilst you examine him, he vomits copiously. His capillary blood glucose is 5.1 mmol/L, and his oxygen saturations are 99% on 35% oxygen.

What will you do next?
(a) Rehydrate with dextrose
(b) Give naloxone
(c) Request urgent CT brain
(d) Request anaesthetic opinion
(e) Order a chest X-ray

QUESTION 61

A 53-year-old woman is admitted to the intensive care unit suffering from collapse and deteriorating conscious level. She had suffered a stroke a week ago which left her with left-sided weakness but was starting to recover some of her function a couple of days ago.

She has a history of hypertension and diabetes mellitus and currently takes aspirin, metformin and perindopril. She has no significant family history, never smoked, travelled to France a year ago and keeps a garden and flower shop.

Examination revealed a pulse of 82 beats/min, respiratory rate of 22/min, fever of 38.3°C, BP 139/88 mmHg. Crackles were audible at the right lung base, there was palpable hepatomegaly and a purpuric rash over the lower extremities.

Investigations
Hb 7.3 g/dL
MCV 79 fl
WCC 14 × 10^9/L (neutrophils 10 × 10^9/L)
Plts 39 × 10^9/L
Na 139 mmol/L
K 6.3 mmol/L
Urea 15.9 mmol/L
Creatinine 369 μmol/L
Bilirubin 63 μmol/L
ALP 422 U/L
ALT 333 U/L
Albumin 40 g/L
Calcium 2.72 mmol/L
Glucose 16 mmol/L
CRP 166 mg/L
INR 1.3
APTTR 0.9
LDH 2124 U/L
CK 69 U/L
Schistocytes and anisopoikilocytosis were seen on peripheral blood film
Urinalysis revealed proteinuria + and haematuria +++
Chest X-ray showed bibasal pulmonary infiltrates
CT brain showed right lacunar infarcts

Question 1
The most appropriate management step would be:
(a) Platelet transfusion
(b) Platelet transfusion, with plasma exchange
(c) Plasma exchange against FFP
(d) Plasma exchange against FFP with high-dose steroids
(e) Intravenous metronidazole

Question 2
The most likely diagnosis is:
(a) Aspiration pneumonia
(b) Hospital-acquired pneumonia
(c) Disseminated intravascular coagulation
(d) Thrombotic thrombocytopenic purpura
(e) Haemolytic–uraemic syndrome

QUESTION 62
A 42-year-old male shopkeeper of Bangladeshi origin suffered from active pulmonary tuberculosis 15 years ago which at the time responded well to anti-TB therapy. He suffered a reactivation of this 3 years ago and again completed a 6-month course of antituberculous therapy. He presents to the chest clinic after he was referred with mild cough, lethargy, pruritus and oedema. These symptoms have been insidious in onset over the past several months and the ankle oedema was particularly troublesome over the past couple of weeks, making him change his footwear. He has had no B symptoms and is not on any current medication. He keeps budgies at home and has smoked 10 cigarettes a day since the age of 16.

Examination revealed normal vital signs apart from an elevated BP at 159/86. There was no lymphadenopathy or finger clubbing, heart sounds were quiet but pure and his chest was clear to auscultation. He had palpable splenomegaly with significant pitting oedema up to his thighs.

Investigations
Hb 15.1 g/dL
MCV 96 fl
WCC 8.0 × 10^9/L
Plts 360 × 10^9/L
Na 144 mmol/L
K 3.9 mmol/L
Urea 9.3 mmol/L
Creatinine 210 μmol/L
Bilirubin 16 μmol/L
ALP 30 U/L
ALT 35 U/L
Albumin 26 g/L
Calcium 2.43 mmol/L
Glucose 6.9 mmol/L

CRP < 3 mg/L
Cholesterol 6.9 mmol/L
TSH 1.25 mU/L
ANA, rheumatoid factor and ANCA negative
Myeloma screen negative
Urinalysis showed +++ proteinuria and ±
  haematuria
CXR: old upper zone streaky opacification
ECG: sinus rhythm with first-degree heart block
Renal biopsy was positive for Congo red staining

The most useful therapeutic option in reducing this patient's proteinuria is:
(a) Colchicine
(b) NSAIDs
(c) Cyclophosphamide
(d) No therapy indicated
(e) High-dose oral prednisolone and anti-
    tuberculous therapy

QUESTION 63

A 39-year-old hairdresser presented to her general practitioner with breathlessness on exertion. She has never smoked and complained of no other associated respiratory symptoms. She also noted 13 kg (2 stone) weight loss over the past 2 months which she thought was the result of her diet that she started a year ago. There were no other symptoms to note from systematic enquiry. She takes 3-monthly progesterone injections for contraception and has no allergies or significant past medical history. Her mother and sister both suffered from breast carcinoma. She is still able to maintain an independent existence.

Examination revealed a rather thin woman but otherwise general, cardiovascular, abdominal, respiratory systems were normal. Breast examination was also unremarkable.

Investigations
Hb 10.6 g/dL
WCC 6.5 × 10⁹/L
Plts 353 × 10⁹/L
Na 140 mmol/L
K 3.8 mmol/L
Urea 5.1 mmol/L
Creatinine 74 μmol/L
LFTs: normal
Calcium 2.89 mmol/L
Albumin 36 g/L

Urinalysis showed + blood
PFTs: mild restrictive defect
CXR showed multiple round opacities scattered
  throughout both lungs
CT abdomen showed a suspicious lesion within
  the left kidney

Question 1
The most likely histological type of this tumour is:
(a) Chromophilic
(b) Chromophobic
(c) Clear cell
(d) Oncocytic
(e) Collecting duct

Question 2
Useful management option(s) would be:
(a) Radical resection
(b) Radical resection followed by interferon-
    alpha
(c) Chest radiotherapy and interferon-alpha
(d) Chest radiotherapy and IL-2
(e) Radical resection followed by IL-2

QUESTION 64

A 35-year-old Caucasian woman was admitted to hospital with gradual generalized limb weakness. She also complained of needing to pass urine more often in recent weeks. She has been noticing that her mouth and eyes have been uncomfortably dry over the past 4 months: attempts at maintaining oral hydration have slightly helped. She complained of no other symptoms apart from the occasional chest wall pain in the past which her GP diagnosed as musculoskeletal pain and recommended paracetamol.

Examination revealed dry mucous membranes in the oral cavity but was otherwise unremarkable.

Investigations
Hb 11.5 g/dL
MCV 80 fl
WCC 6.3 × 10⁹/L
Plts 230 × 10⁹/L
Na 144 mmol
K 2.9 mmol/L
Urea 2.7 mmol/L

Creatinine 82 μmol/L
Bilirubin 11 μmol/L
ALP 31 U/L
ALT 28 U/L
Albumin 39 g/L
Calcium 2.15 mmol/L
Chloride 111 mmol/L
Venous bicarbonate 18 mmol/L
Urinalysis + leukocytes
Urinary calcium raised
Urinary pH 5.9

Question 1

The most likely diagnosis is
(a) Type 1 renal tubular acidosis
(b) Type 2 renal tubular acidosis
(c) Type 3 renal tubular acidosis
(d) Type 4 renal tubular acidosis
(e) None of the above

Question 2

The history of 'musculoskeletal chest pains' is
likely due to:
(a) Osteoporosis
(b) Sjögren's syndrome
(c) Osteopenia
(d) Osteomalacia
(e) Pleurisy

QUESTION 65

A 54-year-old man presents with a 4-week
history of malaise and breathlessness on exertion.
He has recently returned from a business trip in
Japan and was referred to hospital with two
episodes of haemoptysis.

He had an appendix removed at the age of 7
and smokes 25 cigarettes per day. He seldom
drinks alcohol and takes a beta-blocker for
hypertension diagnosed 3 years ago.

On examination he is pale, with bilateral ankle
oedema and bilateral crackles on chest
auscultation with pure heart sounds. HR 122
beats/min, BP 136/81. Respiratory rate 16
breaths/min, temperature 37.7°C and saturations
were 93% on room air.

Investigations

Hb 12.2 g/dL
WCC 5.2 × 10⁹/L

Plts 110 × 10⁹/L
CRP 79 mg/L
Na 134 mmol/L
K 5.1 mmol/L
Urea 19.3 mmol/L
Creatinine 566 μmol/L

Urinalysis

Blood ++
Protein +++
Glucose +
CXR shows airspace opacification in both mid
and lower zones with blunting of both
costophrenic angles

Question 1

What would be the most useful next test?
(a) Arterial blood gas
(b) Liver enzymes
(c) Lactate
(d) Renal ultrasound
(e) Autoantibody screen

Question 2

Which test would help most in explaining the
CXR features?
(a) Kco
(b) CT chest staging
(c) Contrast-enhanced CT
(d) CT pulmonary angiogram
(e) Echocardiography

QUESTION 66

A 31-year-old woman presents with a 4-week
history of sweats, fever and aching joints. She
had felt generally tired and unwell since
returning from a trip to Greece. She was
normally healthy, took no medications, drank 30
units of alcohol per week, and smoked 10
cigarettes per day. She reported 3 kg weight loss
since her holiday, no cough or sputum, but found
that she was breathless climbing stairs. Her
bowels were normal.

On examination, she looked pale. No rashes or
lymphadenopathy were noted. T = 37.8°C. Pulse
90 beats/min reg. BP 155/90 mmHg. JVP not
raised. Heart sounds normal. The right calf was
swollen and mildly tender below the knee. Chest
examination was normal. The spleen was just

palpable in the abdomen. Neurological examination was normal. Both knees, elbows and shoulders were tender to touch, but were not swollen.

Investigations
Hb 7.7 g/dL
MCV 103 fl
WCC 3.2 × 10⁹/L
Platelets 78 × 10⁹/L
ESR 113 mm/h
CRP 12 mg/L
INR 1.0
APTTR 1.7
Na 129 mmol/L
K 5.1 mmol/L
Urea 17.6 mmol/L
Creatinine 343 μmol/L
Bilirubin 25 μmol/L
ALT 14 U/L
ALP 93 U/L
Albumin 29 g/L
Calcium 2.21 mmol/L
CK 40 U/L
CXR: normal
Urine: blood ++, protein +++
Doppler scan of the right leg reveals a DVT

What investigation is most likely to reveal the underlying diagnosis?
(a) Ultrasound of the kidneys
(b) Antinuclear antibody
(c) ANCA
(d) Echocardiography
(e) Ham's test

QUESTION 67
A 40-year-old woman presents with a 4-month history of difficulty getting up from sitting and climbing stairs. She has also noticed aching in her arms and legs. She has a history of hypothyroidism and for this she takes thyroxine. She has had some arthritis in her hands for the past 6 months and a rash across her knuckles. She does not smoke and drinks 10 units of alcohol per week. She denies change in bowel habit, indigestion or weight loss.

On examination, she appears tired. There is no jaundice, clubbing or lymphadenopathy. Pulse is 80 reg, BP 125/75. Heart sounds are normal and chest is clear. Abdominal and breast examination are normal, as is rectal examination. Neurological examination reveals tenderness over the quadriceps and deltoids, mild proximal limb weakness, normal sensation, reflexes and cranial nerve examination.

Results
Hb 10.2 g/dL
WBC 18.0 × 10⁹/L (neutrophils 85%, lymphocytes 13%)
Platelets 300 × 10⁹/L
ESR 50 mm/h
Bilirubin 5 μmol/L
Albumin 35 g/L
Total protein 80 g/L
AST 90 U/L
ALP 120 U/L
Free T4 80 nmol/L
Muscle biopsy normal
EMG: short polyphasic potentials, with spontaneous fibrillation

Question 1
What will you do next?
(a) Request autoantibodies (ANA, ANCA, rheumatoid factor)
(b) Commence 60 mg prednisolone
(c) MRI brain
(d) Commence IV immunoglobulin
(e) Perform a tensilon test

Question 2
What further investigation will you perform?
(a) Carcinoembryonic antigen (CEA)
(b) CT chest, abdomen and pelvis
(c) Mammography
(d) Ultrasound of the abdomen
(e) None

QUESTION 68
A 40-year-old woman with long-standing seropositive arthritis returns to rheumatology outpatients with progressive shortness of breath and a dry cough. She has had several DMARDs in the past, and is currently controlled on sulfasalazine, which she has been taking for 6 months. She does not drink or smoke and is cared for by her husband. She is also taking

paracetamol, celecoxib, fluoxetine, temazepam and aspirin. She denies sputum or haemoptysis but admits to low mood.

On examination, she is cyanosed. Temperature 37.7°C. Pulse is 90 reg, BP 110/70, JVP not raised. Heart sounds are normal and her chest is clear. Her ankles are not swollen and abdominal examination is normal. Her joints appear quiescent but obvious deformities are noted in the hands, shoulders and knees.

Hb 10.2 g/dL
WCC 4.9 × 10^9/L
Plts 278 × 10^9/L
ESR 56 mm/h
CRP 192 mg/L
U + Es, LFTs normal
Lung function tests show:
FVC 3.1 L (predicted 2.4–3.6 L)
FEV$_1$ 2.5 L (predicted 1.8–2.8 L)
FEV$_1$/FVC 81%
TLC 5.2 L (predicted 5.0–7.5 L)
Kco 65% expected
Chest X-ray shows bilateral infiltrates spreading out from the hila

What will you do next?
(a) Stop sulfasalazine
(b) Give steroids
(c) Give iloprost
(d) Carry out bronchoalveolar lavage
(e) Give diuretics

QUESTION 69

A 54-year-old woman, diagnosed with Raynaud's syndrome 4 years previously, presents with a 4-week history of headaches and tiredness. She is otherwise well, takes nifedipine in the winter, and on systems review complains of mild dysphagia and stiff fingers and wrists.

On examination, pulse is 70 beats/min reg, BP 190/110 mmHg. Heart sounds are normal, there are fine paninspiratory crackles at both lung bases, and abdominal examination is normal. She has waxy, thickened skin over her fingers. She appears drowsy, with bilateral papilloedema on fundoscopy.

Investigations
Hb 10.2 g/dL
WCC 4.1 × 10^9/L
Platelets 180 × 10^9/L

MCV 85 fl
Na 130 mmol/L
K 5.9 mmol/L
Urea 40.7 mmol/L
Creatinine 604 µmol/L
LFTs normal
Urinalysis protein ++, blood –
ANA 1:160
dsDNA negative

Lung Function
FEV$_1$ 2.8 L
FVC 3.2 L
Ratio 88%
Kco 70% of predicted

Ultrasound of the kidneys: normal size, no obstruction seen

She is referred to the renal team for opinion regarding dialysis. What will you do next to treat her underlying disease process?
(a) Give a fluid challenge
(b) Start an ACE inhibitor
(c) Start a calcium-channel blocker
(d) Start IV nitroprusside
(e) Ararnge for plasmapheresis

QUESTION 70

A 32-year-old woman presents with sudden shortness of breath. She gives a history of a mild cough over the preceding few months and she had occasional nose bleeds. She had no history of asthma and took no regular medications except occasional paracetamol for 'rheumatics'.

Examination was unremarkable except for a faint macular rash on her legs which she had not noticed before. In particular, chest was clear, no liver or spleen was palpable, and heart sounds were normal. Tone, power, reflexes and sensation were normal.

Results
Hb 13.0 g/dL
WBC 10.2 × 10^9/L
Platelets 400 × 10^9/L
Na 140 mmol/L
K 5.0 mmol/L
Urea 15.4 mmol/L
Creatinine 190 µmol/L
ESR 80 mm/h

305

Urinalysis: protein ++ blood +++

Chest X-ray: several nodular shadows in both lung fields

Which two investigations would best confirm the diagnosis?

(a) ANCA
(b) Lung biopsy
(c) Renal biopsy
(d) Anti-GBM antibodies
(e) Blood cultures
(f) Echocardiography
(g) Skin biopsy
(h) CT of the chest
(i) Sputum for culture
(j) Pulmonary function tests

QUESTION 71

A 30-year-old woman presents with a 3-week history of a sore left eye. On direct questioning she admits to loose stools, cramping abdominal pains and mild dysuria. She is usually well, and her only medication is mouth gel for recurrent mouth ulcers. She drinks occasional alcohol, smokes 10 cigarettes per day and works as an air hostess on the route to Turkey, her native land. Three months ago, she had an episode where her left arm and face went numb for an hour, before slowly returning to normal.

On examination, she is apyrexial. She has a faint papular rash over her trunk, two aphthous ulcers and three small genital ulcers. Her left eye is red and inflamed. Pulse 80 beats/min irregular, BP 120/70 mmHg. Heart sounds are normal, ankles are not swollen. Chest and abdominal exam are normal. Rectal examination reveals loose stool but no blood. Examination of her joints is unremarkable, and neurological examination reveals normal tone, power, sensation, reflexes and coordination.

Investigations

Hb 10.3 g/dL
WCC 8.1 × 10^9/L
Platelets 251 × 10^9/L
ESR 71 mm/h
CRP 30 mg/L
U + Es normal
LFTs normal
Rheumatoid factor negative

Question 1

What investigation would best confirm the diagnosis?

(a) Colonoscopy
(b) Pathergy test
(c) HLA B27 haplotyping
(d) MRI brain
(e) Wardell's test

Question 2

Her pathergy test is positive, and she is started on oral steroids. Three months later, her disease is better controlled, but she has gained weight and has severe acne. What will you do?

(a) Change to balsalazide
(b) Add in thalidomide
(c) Add azathioprine and reduce the steroids
(d) Taper the steroids over 3 months
(e) Add in interferon-beta and taper the steroids

QUESTION 72

A 42-year-old man is admitted with a 3-week history of fever, joint pains and abdominal pain. He also admitted that his fingers had felt numb for the past week. He drank 50 units of alcohol per week, and smoked 20 cigarettes per day.

On examination, temperature was 38.1°C. Pulse 100 beats/min, BP 170/100 mmHg. Heart sounds were normal, JVP not elevated. All peripheral pulses were intact, but the fingertips were white bilaterally, with poor capillary return. Chest was clear, and abdominal examination revealed mild tenderness in the RUQ, but no liver edge was palpable. Sensation was diminished over all the fingers, but the rest of the neurological examination was normal. Bloods were taken for analysis.

Just before the consultant ward round, he complained of central chest pain, and collapsed. Monitoring showed pulseless VT, and he was successfully cardioverted with a 200 J DC shock.

Investigations

Hb 9.9 g/dL
WCC 16.5 × 10^9/L
Platelets 540 × 10^9/L
MCV 92 fl
ESR > 100 mm/h
CRP 79 mg/L

Na 129 mmol/L
K 6.5 mmol/L
Urea 34.2 mmol/L
Creatinine 570 μmol/L
Bilirubin 12 μmol/L
ALT 34 U/L
ALP 420 U/L

ECG (Post arrest)
ST elevation in II, III and aVF
ST depression in I and aVL. Peaked T waves in the anterior leads

He undergoes primary coronary angioplasty, at which an aneurysm of the right coronary artery is seen. He is admitted to ITU, where he undergoes haemofiltration. What will you do next?
(a) Start IV methylprednisolone
(b) Test for hepatitis B and C
(c) Start IV methylprednisolone and test for hepatitis B
(d) Start IV methylprednisolone and test for hepatitis C
(e) Start IV methylprednisolone and methotrexate

QUESTION 73
A 50-year-old man presents with a history of recurrent pleural effusions and recent-onset haemoptysis. Past medical history reveals only a mild arthritis which has been put down to osteoarthritis. He denies fever, cough, facial pain, weight loss or night sweats but does feel he is more short of breath. He also complains of a non-specific rash occurring on his legs 3 weeks ago. He lives with his wife who is well, and he gave up smoking 2 years ago.

On examination, he is overweight. There is no jaundice, anaemia, cyanosis or clubbing. A non-blanching rash is faintly visible over both lower legs. Pulse is 90 regular, BP 160/95. Heart sounds are normal, and chest examination reveals mild wheeze. Abdominal examination is normal save for obesity, and neurological examination reveals normal tone, power and reflexes, with normal sensation.

Investigations
Hb 11 g/dL
WCC 8.0 × 10^9/L

Platelets 190 × 10^9/L
Na 140 mmol/L
K 5.0 mmol/L
Urea 25 mmol/L
Creatinine 315 μmol/L
Urinalysis: protein ++ blood +++
Chest X-ray reveals patchy shadowing in both lung fields

Which two investigations are most likely to identify the underlying cause of his illness?
(a) Cryoglobulins
(b) ANCA
(c) Renal biopsy
(d) Skin biopsy
(e) Antinuclear antibody
(f) Mesenteric angiogram
(g) Anti-GBM antibody
(h) Echocardiography
(i) Blood cultures
(j) HIV test

QUESTION 74
A 45-year-old smoker with late-onset asthma presents with cough, and increasing shortness of breath. He also has intermittent chest pains. He feels non-specifically unwell, with anorexia, and weight loss. He drinks 20 units of alcohol per week, and takes beclometasone, salbutamol, aspirin and amlodipine.

On examination he has a temperature of 37.8°C and a tachycardia of 110 beats/min. He has a blood pressure of 150/100 mmHg. There is a soft pansystolic murmur, widespread polyphonic expiratory wheeze and he has bilateral basal lung crackles. He has a nodular rash on his legs.

Investigations
Hb 11.0 g/dL
WCC 15 × 10^9/L (80% neutrophils and 5% lymphocytes)
Platelets 180 × 10^9/L
ESR 80 mm/h
Na 140 mmol/L
K 4.5 mmol/L
Urea 15 mmol/L
Creatinine 160 μmol/L
Chest X-ray: widespread fluffy shadowing throughout both lung fields

307

What will you do next?
(a) Bronchoscopy and biopsy
(b) Renal biopsy
(c) Start oral steroids
(d) Double his inhaled steroid
(e) High-resolution CT chest

QUESTION 75

A 75-year-old man, who is rather hard of hearing, presents with several months of increasing pain in both legs. He is reasonably mobile in the morning, but his legs become more painful as the day goes on. He takes paracetamol and tramadol for the pain, along with aspirin, simvastatin, atenolol and ramipril for his past history of myocardial infarction and hypertension. He denies back pain, numbness or tingling in his legs. He has no bowel or bladder symptoms.

On examination, he appears well. There is no jaundice, clubbing or lymphadenopathy. Pulse 70 reg, BP 160/75. Heart sounds are normal, peripheral pulses are present, chest and abdominal examination are normal. Tone is normal, power and sensation are also normal, and he has a good range of movement at the hip and knee. Both legs are diffusely uncomfortable to move.

Investigations
Hb 13.4 g/dL
WCC 5.1 × 10⁹/L
Plts 261 × 10⁹/L
ESR 11 mm/h
Na 141 mmol/L
K 3.6 mmol/L
Urea 7.4 mmol/L
Creatinine 135 μmol/L
Bilirubin 6 μmol/L
ALT 18 U/L
ALP 590 U/L
Calcium 2.47 mmol/L
Albumin 37 g/L
Vitamin D normal
PSA 6 ng/L
X-rays show mild osteoarthritis of both hips and knees

What will you do next?
(a) Start a bisphosphonate
(b) Start oral prednisolone

(c) Arrange a bone scan
(d) Arrange for a course of physiotherapy
(e) Arrange for a liver ultrasound

QUESTION 76

A 70-year-old woman presents with headaches and joint pains. She also complains of fatigue. She is previously fit apart from mild osteoarthritis, for which she takes regular analgesics. She does not drink or smoke, and helps out at the hospital volunteer stall 3 days a week. She thinks that she has lost a few kilograms in weight recently. She denies any loss of vision, bowel symptoms or indigestion.

On examination, she appears tired. There is no jaundice, clubbing or lymphadenopathy. Chest, heart and abdominal examination are unremarkable save for a soft ejection systolic murmur radiating to the carotids. Her temporal arteries are pulsatile and there is no scalp tenderness. Tone and power are normal in all muscle groups.

Investigations
Hb 11.0 g/dL
WCC 10 × 10⁹/L
Platelets 400 × 10⁹/L
ESR 70 mm/h
CRP 40 mg/L
Bilirubin 15 mmol/L
AST 25 U/L
ALP 400 U/L
Creatine kinase 150 U/L
Temporal artery biopsy negative

Question 1
How will you treat her?
(a) Prednisolone 20 mg/day
(b) Prednisolone 60 mg/day
(c) Arrange an EMG
(d) Arrange an echo and blood cultures
(e) Arrange CT of the brain

Question 2
She is started on prednisolone 20 mg and comes back to see you in 2 weeks. She is not feeling any better. What will you do now?
(a) Increase her steroids to 60 mg/day
(b) Stop steroids

(c) Arrange CT brain

(d) Arrange a myeloma screen

(e) Start an antidepressant

QUESTION 77

A 51-year-old man with a 4-year history of Wegener's granulomatosis presents with recurrent haemoptysis. He has been free of respiratory symptoms for 9 months, and his antiproteinase 3 titre when last seen in clinic was 1:4. He has had sweats and arthralgia for 2 weeks, and has brought up two cupfuls of blood in the last 3 days. He is currently taking 10 mg prednisolone per day, together with risedronate, calcium and vitamin D, paracetamol and azathioprine.

On examination, his temperature was 37.8°C. Pulse 100/reg. BP 100/50. Heart sounds were normal, but there was an area of dullness at the left lung base. Respiratory rate 20/min. Abdominal examination was normal.

Investigations

Na 131 mmol/L

K 4.8 mmol/L

Urea 14.8 mmol/L

Creatinine 170 μmol/L (was 110 μmol/L in clinic 3 months ago)

Hb 11.6 g/dL

WCC 12.2 × 10^9/L

Plts 587 × 10^9/L

Antiproteinase 3 titre: 1:320

CRP 78 mg/L

How will you treat him?

(a) Plasmapheresis

(b) IV methylprednisolone

(c) IV methylprednisolone and cyclophosphamide

(d) Stop azathioprine and start methotrexate

(e) Add in co-trimoxazole

QUESTION 78

A 56-year-old woman with a 10-year history of rheumatoid arthritis presents with a swollen, tender shoulder to clinic. This came on suddenly 2 days ago, and she has been feeling unwell since. She has a past medical history of type 2 diabetes, hypertension, anxiety and depression, and takes methotrexate, paracetamol, dihydrocodeine, paroxetine, lisinopril and metformin. She does not drink or smoke.

On examination, the right shoulder is tender, hot and swollen. She has difficulty in moving the joint because of pain. Temperature is 37.9°C, pulse 100 reg, BP 120/70. Chest and abdominal examination are normal, and her other joints are quiescent.

Hb 9.7 g/dL

WCC 13.2 × 10^9/L

Plts 499 × 10^9/L

CRP 130 mg/L

ESR 67 mm/h

Urate 0.51 mmol/L

What will you do?

(a) Aspirate the joint and send for urgent microscopy

(b) Start NSAIDs

(c) Start colchicine

(d) Aspirate the joint and inject with steroid

(e) Change her methotrexate to an alternative DMARD

QUESTION 79

You review a 36-year-old woman with systemic sclerosis in the clinic. She complains of worsening breathlessness over the last few months, accompanied by a dry cough. She takes homeopathic remedies but no other medication and is otherwise fit and well. She drinks 5 units of alcohol per week and has never smoked. She keeps no pets.

On examination, she is of short stature, with thickened skin over both hands and forearms. Pulse 80 reg, BP 105/60. JVP is raised 2 cm and there is a loud second heart sound. Chest examination reveals no crackles and abdominal examination is normal.

Bloods

Hb 14.1 g/dL

WCC 5.1 × 10^9/L

Plts 454 × 10^9/L

U + Es normal

LFTs normal

ESR 12 mm/h

Lung Function

FEV_1 2.8 L

FVC 3.5 L

Ratio 80%

Kco 70% of predicted

High-resolution CT of the chest reveals no fibrotic change. She undergoes right heart catheterization, which reveals good RV function but a raised pulmonary artery pressure.

You offer her treatment with iloprost, but she declines this, as she has read about its side-effects. What other treatment will you offer?

(a) Nifedipine
(b) Lisinopril
(c) Bosentan
(d) Pentoxifylline
(e) Warfarin

QUESTION 80

A 37-year-old woman with a 4-year history of SLE presents to the A&E department with sudden onset of left-sided weakness. She has never had any previous episodes like this. Her disease is usually well controlled on hydroxychloroquine and occasional ibuprofen. She smokes 10 cigarettes per day and drinks 15 units of alcohol per week. She has two children under the age of 5.

On examination, she appears drowsy. Pulse 90 reg, BP 105/60. Temperature 37.6°C. Heart sounds reveal a soft pansystolic murmur at the apex; chest and abdominal examination are normal. She has 3/5 power in the left arm and leg, reduced sensation in the left arm and leg, brisk reflexes on the left and an upgoing left plantar. Cranial nerve examination is normal; fundoscopy reveals cottonwool spots. No rash or joint swelling is evident.

Bloods

Hb 9.6 g/dL

WCC 3.6 × 10⁹/L

Plts 110 × 10⁹/L

Na 138 mmol/L

K 4.4 mmol/L

Urea 3.7 mmol/L

Creatinine 92 μmol/L

Albumin 32 g/L

CRP 24 mg/L

ESR 77 mm/h

MRI brain reveals evidence of an ischaemic area in the right internal capsule, with two smaller ischaemic areas in the left frontal lobe.

Lumbar puncture reveals clear CSF, with 200 mg/L protein and 10 WCC per high-power field.

What investigation would be most useful?

(a) Antinuclear antibody titre
(b) Echocardiography
(c) Carotid Doppler
(d) Antiphospholipid antibody
(e) Serum cholesterol

QUESTION 81

A 29-year-old man was diagnosed with ankylosing spondylitis 3 months ago. Since diagnosis, he has had mild lower-back pain and stiffness, helped by ibuprofen and a series of back exercises. Over the last 2 weeks, his right hip and shoulder have become more painful, to the point where walking in the morning is difficult. He does not drink or smoke and is otherwise well.

On examination, he is apyrexial. Pulse 60/min, BP 115/60. Heart sounds are normal, chest is clear with good expansion, and abdominal examination is normal. He has a good range of movement in the lower back, but his right hip and shoulder are both painful to move with a reduced range of movement.

Bloods

Hb 15.1 g/dL

WCC 9.8 × 10⁹/L

Plts 301 × 10⁹/L

ESR 51 mm/hr

CRP 25 mg/L

U + Es, LFTs normal

Hip and shoulder X-rays: no loss of joint space. No erosions or effusions noted

How will you treat his hip and shoulder pain?

(a) Sulfasalazine
(b) Infliximab
(c) Penicillamine
(d) Prednisolone
(e) Physiotherapy

QUESTION 82

A 52-year-old man with long-standing ankylosing spondylitis is seen in clinic with progressive breathlessness. He complains of a chronic cough but denies sputum production.

He suffers from chronic back pain and takes ibuprofen and paracetamol and uses a TENS machine. He drinks 20 units of alcohol per week and has smoked 30 cigarettes/day for 30 years.

On examination he looks kyphotic. Pulse is 80/min, with no collapsing character. BP 140/70, JVP not raised. He has a soft early diastolic murmur and soft ejection systolic murmur. Chest examination reveals no crackles but reduced air entry at the bases. Abdominal examination is unremarkable, and there is mild tenderness over the sacroiliac joints and lumbar spine.

His routine FBC and biochemisty are unremarkable.

Echocardiography: normal LV function with mild to moderate aortic regurgitation. The aortic root is undilated. LV end-diastolic diameter 4.9 cm. RV function appears normal. Pulmonary artery pressure 36 mmHg

PFTS
FEV$_1$ 2.3 L
FVC 4.2 L
FEV1/FVC 55%
TLC 6.1 L
Kco: 82% of predicted
CXR: patchy fibrotic change in upper zones. Flattened diaphragms

Which pathology is contributing most to his breathlessness?
(a) Aortic regurgitation
(b) Chest wall deformity
(c) Pulmonary fibrosis
(d) Pulmonary hypertension
(e) COPD

QUESTION 83
A 31-year-old fashion advertising executive presented to her GP with a 2-month history of tiredness, dating from her recent promotion. She was under a great deal of stress and complained of low mood. She also felt light-headed on occasions. In her past medical history, she had undergone a termination of pregnancy 3 years ago, and had been treated for depression in her early 20s. She is currently taking no medication, drinks 30 units of alcohol per week and smokes 10 cigarettes per day.

On examination, she appeared tanned. Pulse 70 beats/min. BP 90/50 mmHg lying, 60/40 mmHg standing. There was no ankle oedema, chest was clear, and abdominal and neurological examination were unremarkable. The thyroid was not palpable.

Investigations
Hb 14.7 g/dL
WCC 5.3 × 10^9/L
Platelets 180 × 10^9/L
Na 122 mmol/L
K 5.9 mmol/L
Urea 10.1 mmol/L
Creatinine 60 μmol/L
BM stick 3.1 mmol/L
Urine: clear

What investigation will you perform next?
(a) 24-hour cortisol collection
(b) Short Synacthen test
(c) Water deprivation test
(d) Urinary osmolality
(e) Dexamethasone suppression test

QUESTION 84
A 22-year-old man is admitted with a 3-day history of vomiting. He has a history of Crohn's disease for which he usually takes 20 mg/day of prednisolone. He has not had any diarrhoea, but stomach cramps and vomiting have made it impossible to eat for 3 days. He also takes azathioprine. He does not drink or smoke.

On examination, he appears unwell. Pulse 100 reg, BP 90/60 lying, 60/40 standing. He appears pale and dehydrated. Chest is clear, heart sounds are normal. He has mild epigastric and right iliac fossa tenderness on palpation, with active bowel sounds. Rectal examination is normal. You commence a 0.9% saline infusion whilst awaiting bloods.

Investigations
Na 124 mmol/L
K 5.4 mmol/L
Urea 6.2 mmol/L
Creatinine 57 μmol/L
Glucose 3.3 mmol/L
CRP 57 mg/L
Hb 11.1 g/dL
WCC 13.6 × 10^9/L
Plts 490 × 10^9/L

What will you do next?
(a) Give IV hydrocortisone
(b) Change to IV colloid
(c) Give oral prednisolone
(d) Obtain an abdominal X-ray and erect chest X-ray
(e) Pass a nasogastric tube

QUESTION 85

A 48-year-old woman presents with 4 months of nausea and dizzy spells, weight loss and ankle oedema. The dizzy spells are commonly brought on by drinking sherry, which she uses to try and increase her poor appetite. She also complains of vague abdominal discomfort and loose stools. She has a past medical history of anxiety disorder for which she takes diazepam. She does not smoke.

On examination, she had a reddish face. Pulse 90 beats/min reg, BP 120/50 mmHg. Her JVP contained giant V waves, heart sounds 1 + 2 with a pansystolic murmur at the left sternal edge. Ankle oedema was present to the mid-thigh level. Examination revealed bilateral pleural effusions, a distended abdomen with shifting dullness and a 6-cm pulsatile liver edge.

Which two investigations will be most helpful in the diagnosis of this woman?
(a) Echocardiography
(b) Blood cultures
(c) Abdominal ultrasound
(d) Abdominal CT
(e) Urinary 5-HIAA levels
(f) Urinary catecholamines
(g) Colonoscopy
(h) CA-125 levels
(i) Ascitic tap
(j) Pleural tap

QUESTION 86

A 77-year-old woman is diagnosed as having carcinoid syndrome. She presented with diarrhoea and collapses, and on investigation was found to have a mass at her ileocaecal junction, with multiple liver metastases. She also has a history of two previous myocardial infarctions and left ventricular systolic dysfunction. She is currently housebound with breathlessness, but is severely troubled by dizziness, flushing and diarrhoea. She takes perindopril, spironolactone, bisoprolol, furosemide, simvastatin and aspirin.

On examination, pulse is 60 reg, BP 100/50. JVP is raised 3 cm and a pansystolic murmur is audible at the axilla. Chest is clear, she has mild bilateral ankle oedema, and abdominal examination reveals 4 cm hepatomegaly and no ascites.

ECG: poor R-wave progression, sinus rhythm

Bloods
Na 132 mmol/L
K 4.8 mmol/L
Urea 15.2 mmol/L
Creatinine 161 μmol/L
Hb 11.8 g/dL
WCC 6.1 × 10⁹/L
Plts 188 × 10⁹/L

How will you treat her?
(a) Octreotide
(b) Interferon-alpha
(c) Hepatic artery embolization
(d) Chemotherapy
(e) ^{131}I-MIBG isotope therapy

QUESTION 87

A 49-year-old woman is referred to you in the endocrine clinic. She was found to have a raised calcium as an incidental finding on attendance at her GP. She has a history of controlled hypertension for which she takes lisinopril. She does not smoke but drinks 20 units of alcohol per week. Her father had a neck operation 20 years ago, but she doesn't remember why. She denies constipation and abdominal pain and has never had renal colic. On examination, she appears well. Pulse 60 regular. BP 135/75. Chest and abdominal examination are normal, as is thyroid examination.

The following tests are available in clinic:
Na 137 mmol/L
K 5.1 mmol/L
Urea 5.9 mmol/L
Creatinine 71 μmol/L
Calcium 2.81 mmol/L
PO₄ 0.8 mmol/L
Albumin 42 mmol/L

PTH 6.9 nmol/L (normal 0–7.3)
Urinary calcium 0.5 mmol in 24 h

What will you do?
(a) Discharge her from clinic
(b) Refer for parathyroidectomy
(c) Organize a parathyroid technetium scan
(d) Organize a bone scan
(e) Request a vitamin D level

QUESTION 88

A 64-year-old woman presents with dehydration and vomiting. She has been unwell for some time, feeling under the weather, and has noted that she has been rather constipated. Whilst on holiday last year, she had an episode of left-sided abdominal pain that left her bedbound for 2 days. She is otherwise fit and well, has never smoked, takes no medications and drinks only occasional alcohol.

On examination, she appears dry. Pulse 100 reg, BP 100/50 lying, 65/30 standing. Chest examination is normal; she is mildly tender in the epigastrium and left iliac fossa. There is no rebound tenderness or guarding. Bowel sounds are normal.

Investigations
Na 148 mmol/L
K 5.3 mmol/L
Urea 15.8 mmol/L
Creatinine 212 μmol/L
Calcium 4.16 mmol/L
Phosphate 1.92 mmol/L
Abdominal X-ray: faecal loading of transverse and descending colon. No distension of bowel

She receives 3 L of 0.9% saline over the next 12 hours, along with 60 mg of pamidronate. The next morning, blood is sent for calcium and PTH. The calcium level has fallen to 3.2 mmol/L and her PTH is 10.3 nmol/L.

What test would you do next?
(a) Chest X-ray
(b) Bone scan
(c) Parathyroid technetium scan
(d) Ultrasound of the neck
(e) Colonoscopy

QUESTION 89

A 24-year-old woman is referred to clinic for investigation after removal of cataracts. She tells you that although her eyesight is now much improved, she still sufffers from twitching. This has been an intermittent problem for many years; she remembers having episodes at school. She is otherwise well, does not drink or smoke, and takes no medications. On examination, she is 148 cm tall, with a short neck. Her ring fingers are noticeably short. Chest and abdominal examination are normal, as is palpation of the thyroid.

Investigations
U + Es normal
FBC normal
LFTs normal
CK 261 U/L
Calcium 1.6 mmol/L
Albumin 38 g/L
PO$_4$ 1.51 mmol/L
Magnesium 0.77 mmol/L
PTH 22 nmol/L
B$_{12}$ + folate normal
INR 1.0
Vitamin D 61 nmol/L
ECG: prolonged QT interval (520 ms)

What investigation will you request next?
(a) Technetium scan of parathyroid glands
(b) Muller–Herzog test
(c) Chase–Auerbach test
(d) Urinary calcium levels
(e) Short Synacthen test

QUESTION 90

A 27-year-old man presents with a 6-hour history of central abdominal pain and vomiting. He has not had his bowels open for 2 days, but can pass flatus. The pain is constant, but no worse on coughing. He also complains of tingling in both legs. His only previous contact with the medical profession was a 3-month stay in a psychiatric unit for psychosis 5 years ago. He smokes 20 cigarettes per day and had an alcohol binge 2 days ago.

On examination, his temperature was 38.1°C. Pulse 110 beats/min, BP 170/100 mmHg. Chest examination was normal, and abdominal examination revealed no tenderness or guarding, normal bowel sounds and no organomegaly. Sensation was reduced in both feet. As the examination is concluded, the patient has a generalized seizure, which terminates with diazepam.

Investigations

Na 126 mmol/L
K 3.8 mmol/L
Urea 7.0 mmol/L
Creatinine 77 µmol/L
Bilirubin 4 µmol/L
ALT 51 U/L
ALP 77 U/L
Glucose 5.1 mmol/L
Hb 16.4 g/dL
WCC 17.1 $\times$ 10^9/L
Plts 410 $\times$ 10^9/L

The urine specimen that you obtain takes some time to be picked up. The nursing staff notice that the urine specimen has changed colour from yellow to brown.

Question 1

What analgesia will you give this man?
(a) Morphine and metoclopramide
(b) Paracetamol
(c) Pethidine and metoclopramide
(d) Morphine and prochlorperazine
(e) Pethidine and prochlorperazine

Question 2

Which two of the following will you select to manage him?
(a) IV saline
(b) IV dextrose
(c) IV haem arginate
(d) Whole blood
(e) IV phenytoin
(f) Oral atenolol
(g) Broad-spectrum antibiotics
(h) Urgent referral to surgeons
(i) Oral ramipril
(j) IV methylprednisolone

QUESTION 91

A 59-year-old woman presented with a 6-week history of weakness, cough and dyspnoea on exertion. She had lost 13 kg (2 stone) in weight over the last 6 months. There was no history of haemoptysis or sputum production. Her GP had recently started her on Prozac because of low mood and poor appetite. She drank alcohol socially, and smoked 20 cigarettes per day.

On examination, she appeared tanned and rather thin. She had finger clubbing. Pulse 90 beats/min regular, BP 150/100 mmHg. JVP not raised, heart sounds normal. There was dullness and reduced breath sounds at the right base, and 3 cm hepatomegaly. Neurological examination demonstrated weakness of the shoulder and hip girdles.

Investigations

pH 7.49
$p$co$_2$ 4.1 kPa
po$_2$ 10.1 kPa
Na 141 mmol/L
K 2.7 mmol/L
Urea 3.1 mmol/L
Creatinine 57 µmol/L
FBC normal
Glucose 9.1 mmol/L

What test would you do next?
(a) 24-hour urinary cortisol
(b) 9 a.m. serum cortisol
(c) Dexamethasone suppression test
(d) Bronchoscopy
(e) Serum ACTH

QUESTION 92

A 42-year-old woman was seen in the hypertension clinic. Investigations revealed a high ACTH level and an elevated 24-hour cortisol level, which failed to suppress on a low-dose dexamethasone suppression test, but which reduced to 30% of the baseline level after a high-dose dexamethasone suppression test. She denies heavy alcohol intake and is otherwise fit and well. She is taking amlodipine, hydrochlorothiazide and ramipril. On examination, she is obese (BMI 32), with prominent red striae on her abdomen. Blood pressure is 180/110. Chest and abdominal examination are normal.

Investigations

Na 133 mmol/L
K 2.8 mmol/L
Urea 8.1 mmol/L
Creatinine 115 µmol/L
Glucose 7.1 mmol/L
Chest X-ray: normal

What will you do next?
(a) Give metyrapone
(b) Organize MRI of the pituitary
(c) Organize CT chest
(d) Organize CT adrenals
(e) Prescibe spironolactone

QUESTION 93

A 52-year-old man is referred with persistent thirst. He has had the problem for over 2 years, and blames a serious car accident that left him in hospital for 3 months. He finds that he has to drink a lot of water to combat the thirst. He denies abdominal pain, weight loss or visual disturbance, but he has had persistent headaches since the accident. He does not drink and gave up smoking 2 years ago. He takes venlafaxine for depression and is not allergic to anything.

On examination, he appears well. Pulse 80 reg, BP 130/80. Chest and abdominal examination are normal. Neurological examination including fundoscopy and visual fields is also normal.

Investigations

Na 149 mmol/L
K 3.7 mmol/L
Urea 8.1 mmol/L
Creatinine 57 μmol/L
Calcium 2.41 mmol/L
Albumin 41 g/L
Hb 15.9 g/dL
WCC 4.2 × 10^9/L
Plts 418 × 10^9/L
24-hour urine collection: 4.1L

What investigation will you choose to confirm the diagnosis?
(a) Urine sodium level
(b) Urine osmolality
(c) Vasopressin levels
(d) Plasma osmolality
(e) Water deprivation test

QUESTION 94

A 22-year-old woman is undergoing investigations for excessive thirst – she reports drinking up to 5 litres of fluid per day. She recalls no serious medical conditions in her past, but she did seek treatment for an eating disorder in her teens. She smokes 20 cigarettes per day and drinks 20 units of alcohol per week. She denies recent sexual intercourse; she takes the oral contraceptive pill. Physical examination including neurological examination is unremarkable.

She undergoes a water deprivation test, with the following results:

	Plasma osmolality (mOsm/kg)	Weight (kg)	Urine osmolality (mOsm/kg)
Baseline	279	62.1	320
2 hours	282	61.5	356
4 hours	283	61.7	–
6 hours	287	61.7	712
8 hours	285	61.4	–

What will you do?
(a) Give a test dose of DDAVP
(b) Stop the test and arrange MRI of the pituitary
(c) Arrange hypertonic saline infusion test
(d) Stop the test and see patient in clinic
(e) Stop the test and refer patient for a renal opinion

QUESTION 95

A 78-year-old woman with a history of epilepsy following a stroke 3 years ago presents with pain and weakness in her legs and shoulders. She thinks that this has gradually worsened over the last few months. She denies feeling stiff in the morning, and reports no visual impairment. She takes aspirin, simvastatin, ramipril, phenytoin and amlodipine. She does not smoke or drink. Since her stroke, she has needed home help once a day and gets meals provided by the council.

On examination, she appears thin and frail. Pulse 70 reg, BP 150/80. Her weight is 45 kg. There is no rash and she does not look pale. Chest and abdominal examination are normal. She has 4/5 power at her hips and shoulders, 5/5 power elsewhere save for her left leg. Reflexes are equal bilaterally, but the left plantar is upgoing. Sensation and coordination are normal, as is cranial nerve examination. There is reduced range of movement at both hips and knees.

315

Investigations

Na 136 mmol/L
K 4.1 mmol/L
Urea 12.8 mmol/L
Creatinine 151 μmol/L
Calcium 2.04 mmol/L
Albumin 39 g/L
PO_4 1.41 mmol/L
Bilirubin 22 μmol/L
ALT 71 U/L
ALP 277 U/L
PTH 16.0 nmol/L
ESR 21 mm/h

Question 1
What test will you order next?
(a) Vitamin D level
(b) 24-hour urinary cortisol
(c) Phenytoin levels
(d) Antinuclear antibodies
(e) Urinary calcium levels

Question 2
Her vitamin D level is 15 nmol/L; 24-hour urinary cortisol is normal. Her phenytoin level is 8 mg/L and her antinuclear antibodies are negative. Urinary calcium is elevated at 10 mmol/24 hours.

Which is the most appropriate treatment?
(a) Replace phenytoin with valproate
(b) 25-hydroxyvitamin D
(c) 1,25-hydroxyvitamin D
(d) Add a thiazide diuretic
(e) Parathyroidectomy

QUESTION 96
A 57-year-old man attends diabetic clinic. He has type 2 diabetes, diagnosed 4 years ago when he had a myocardial infarction. He also suffers from hypertension, heart failure, gout and COPD. He gave up smoking 2 years ago. He is currently taking lisinopril, aspirin, spironolactone, simvastatin and allopurinol, and is on the maximum dose of gliclazide.

His most recent HbA1c reading was 9.1%; he remains overweight (BMI 31.7) and his blood pressure is 149/85. His urinalysis shows the presence of microalbuminuria. His most recent urea was 14.1 mmol/L; creatinine 165 μmol/L

What will you do?
(a) Refer him for dietetic review
(b) Add in metformin
(c) Add in a glitazone
(d) Change to insulin
(e) Add in metformin and a glitazone

QUESTION 97
A 26-year-old woman with type 1 diabetes presents with a 2-day history of nausea and vomiting. She did not take her insulin yesterday or today. She denies diarrhoea, abdominal pain, cough or sputum, and also denies urinary symptoms. She normally takes 15 units of short-acting insulin with each meal and 22 units of long-acting insulin at night. On examination, she is dehydrated. Pulse 120 reg, BP 80/40. Respiratory rate 28/min. Heart sounds normal, chest clear and abdominal examination reveals no tenderness or masses. Bowel sounds are sparse.

She is started on an insulin infusion (6 U/hour) and rapid IV saline infusion with potassium, and a urinary catheter is placed. Initial bloods show:

Na 129 mmol/L
K 4.4 mmol/L
Urea 12.4 mmol/L
Creatinine 125 μmol/L
Calcium 2.19 mmol/L
Albumin 49 g/L
Amylase 140 U/L
Glucose 56 mmol/L
Hb 15.7 g/dL
WCC 17.0×10^9/L
Plts 515×10^9/L

Arterial Blood Gases
pH 7.14
po_2 11.5 kPa
pco_2 2.6 kPa
Bicarbonate 9 mmol/L
Urinalysis: glucose ++++; ketones ++++

After 8 hours, she has received 4 litres of saline. Her glucose level has fallen to 7 mmol/L; she is passing 60 mL of urine per hour. Pulse is 100/min, BP 110/60. Urinalysis: ketones +++. Repeat blood gases show pH 7.24, pco_2 3.1, po_2 10.8.

What will you do next?
(a) Continue IV saline and 6 U/hour insulin
(b) Continue IV saline and reduce insulin to 3 U/hour
(c) Change to 5% IV dextrose and continue insulin 6 U/hour
(d) Change to 10% IV dextrose and increase insulin to 8U/hour
(e) Request plasma lactate estimation

QUESTION 98

A 22-year-old secretary presents with faintness, sweating and shaking, worse in the morning and relieved by chocolate. She has blacked out twice in the last 4 months. She has gained 9 kg in weight over that period. She complains of no abdominal pain, diarrhoea, respiratory or GU symptoms. She has no history of epilepsy or head injury, smokes 20 cigarettes per day, drinks occasional alcohol and takes the oral contraceptive pill.

She appears mildly obese with a BP of 120/70 mmHg and no postural drop. Cardiovascular, respiratory, abdominal and neurological examination are normal, as is examination of the thyroid gland.

Investigations
FBC normal
U + Es normal
LFTs normal
Calcium 3.04 mmol/L
Albumin 36 g/L
An 8-hour fast was performed, after which she felt sweaty and faint.
Glucose 1.7 mmol/L
Insulin raised
C-peptide raised
A technetium parathyroid scan shows avid uptake in all four parathyroid glands.

What two further investigations would be most useful?
(a) Pentagastrin stimulation test
(b) Short Synacthen test
(c) CT of the pancreas
(d) Urinary catecholamine levels
(e) Prolactin levels
(f) MRI pituitary
(g) Urinary 5-HIAA levels
(h) CT of the chest
(i) Serum amylase levels
(j) PTH levels

QUESTION 99

A 31-year-old Indian woman presents with lethargy and dizziness for 2 years. She believed that her husband had put a spell on her. She also noted that her periods had stopped and that she had recently begun to feel thirsty. She does not drink or smoke and has been unable to have children despite trying for a number of years.

On examination, she had a small goitre. Pulse was 48 beats/min regular, BP 90/50 mmHg lying, 65/30 mmHg standing. Chest and abdominal examination were normal.

Investigations
Hb 9.2 g/dL
WCC 4.1 × 10^9/L
Plts 199 × 10^9/L
MCV 102 fl
Na 129 mmol/L
K 5.8 mmol/L
Urea 8.1 mmol/L
Creatinine 60 μmol/L
Glucose 19.5 mmol/L
B_{12} 510 pg/L
Folate 9.7 μg/L

A short Synacthen test showed a baseline of 76 nmol/L, rising to 150 nmol/L at 60 minutes.

What other test will you perform?
(a) Antinuclear antibody
(b) Calcium and PTH
(c) Thyroid function tests
(d) Antitissue transglutaminase antibodies
(e) CT of pancreas

QUESTION 100

A 14-year-old boy presents in clinic for follow-up of his autoimmune polyglandular syndrome type 1. He suffers from recurrent candidal infections and takes calcium and vitamin D supplements for hypoparathyroidism, diagnosed aged 10.

On examination, he has nail dystrophy and enamel hypoplasia of his teeth. Pulse is 70 regular. His testes are small for age and he lacks pubic hair. Chest and abdominal examination are normal.

Hb 12.5 g/dL
WCC 7.0×10^9/L
Plts 373×10^9/L

Apart from testing testosterone, FSH and LH at this clinic visit, what other test should be done on an annual basis?
(a) Antiparietal cell antibodies
(b) Short Synacthen test
(c) Liver function tests
(d) HbA1c
(e) Thyroid peroxidase antibodies

QUESTION 101

You are called to see a 37-year-old man on the neurosurgery ward who has become unwell 3 days after transsphenoidal resection of a non-functioning pituitary adenoma. He was previously fit and well; progressive visual loss and headache had led to the detection of a 2-cm pituitary mass on MRI with suprasellar extension. Since surgery, he was on IV saline which was stopped 48 hours ago.

On examination, he appears unwell. He is apyrexial. Pulse 90 reg, BP 80/50. Heart sounds are normal, chest is clear and abdominal examination is normal. His skin is dry. GCS = 10/15. Eye movements are normal, there is no neck stiffness or photophobia, and plantars are upgoing.

Initial Tests

Na 130 mmol/L
K 3.7 mmol/L
Urea 7.9 mmol/L
Creatinine 82 µmol/L
Hb 10.2 g/dL
WCC 12.1×10^9/L
Plts 202×10^9/L
Chest X-ray clear
Urinalysis – no blood, protein or leukocytes

You diagnose cortisol insufficiency and give IV saline 3 L/24 hours and IV hydrocortisone. He improves rapidly, and by the next day he is alert and oriented. The IV fluids are stopped and he is given 40 mg hydrocortisone in the morning, 20 mg hydrocortisone in the evening.

Two days later, you are asked to see him again. He is again unwell, pulse 110 reg, BP 85/45. Repeat biochemistry shows:

Na 151 mmol/L
K 4.4 mmol/L
Urea 17.1 mmol/L
Creatinine 140 µmol/L

What therapy will you give?
(a) IV saline and IV antibiotics
(b) IV saline and IV hydrocortisone
(c) Beta-blockers and Lugol's iodine
(d) IV dextrose
(e) IV dextrose and DDAVP

QUESTION 102

A 35-year-old man presents to his GP with lethargy, tiredness and myalgia. On closer questioning he admits to intolerance of cold weather, low mood and constipation. Apart from being involved in a car crash 6 months earlier; he has no past medical history. He takes regular painkillers for the myalgia, and lactulose for the constipation. On examination, he is pale and has coarse skin. He has thinned frontal hair. His heart rate is 56 beats/min, with a blood pressure of 130/80 mmHg lying and 110/75 mmHg standing.

Investigations

Hb 11.0 g/dL
WCC 6.8×10^9/L
Platelets 190×10^9/L
Na 130 mmol/L
K 4.5 mmol/L
Urea 7.0 mmol/L
Creatinine 100 µmol/L
TSH 1.0 mU/L
T_4 40 nmol/L

What will you do next?
(a) Arrange pituitary MRI
(b) Start thyroxine
(c) Give hydrocortisone
(d) Arrange pituitary stress testing
(e) Start testosterone

QUESTION 103

A 63-year-old man attends for a glucose tolerance test. His GP found glycosuria on routine testing, with a fasting glucose level of 6.8 mmol/L. He was diagnosed with hypertension 5 years ago, and has been steadily gaining weight for several years. He is taking lisinopril, amlodipine and bendroflumethiazide. On direct questioning, he admits to sweating a lot. On examination, he is obese, with a BMI of 33.5 kg/m^2. BP is 164/92. He has large hands and feet. Visual fields are normal on confrontation testing.

His glucose tolerance test shows:

Time (min)	Glucose (mmol/L)	GH (mU/L)
0	5	3
30	8	<1
60	14	<1
90	12	1
120	8	

What will you do next?
(a) Check IGF-1 levels
(b) Arrange pituitary MRI
(c) Check 24-hour urinary cortisol
(d) Refer for dietetic opinion
(e) Arrange visual field testing

QUESTION 104

A 58-year-old woman was diagnosed as having acromegaly after investigation for sweats and new-onset diabetes. She denies headache or visual disturbance, and her MRI scan shows a 4-mm pituitary adenoma with no mass effect. She has a history of hypertension, previous transient ischaemic attack, and chronic lower back pain. She takes aspirin, dipyridamole, amitriptyline, co-codamol, amlodipine and perindopril. She smokes 20 cigarettes per day but does not drink.

On examination, she has acromegalic facies and large hands. She has oily skin, pulse 80, BP 175/95. Chest examination reveals mild bilateral wheeze, and abdominal examination reveals a palpable liver and kidneys. Blood tests reveal a normal FBC, U + Es and liver function tests. Fasting glucose is 9.3 mmol/L.

What treatment will you recommend?
(a) None pending investigation of her organomegaly
(b) Cabergoline
(c) Pituitary radiotherapy
(d) Pituitary surgery
(e) Octreotide

QUESTION 105

A 41-year-old woman presents having been found unwell at home. She was recently diagnosed with hyperthyroidism and given a prescription for carbimazole; her partner reports that he has not seen any tablets in the house. He also reports that she has felt unwell with cough and sputum for 2 days. She does not smoke, drinks 10 units of alcohol per week, and works as an aromatherapist.

On examination, she is agitated and confused. She is sweating profusely and is shaking. Temperature is 40.5°C. Pulse 160 reg, BP 170/110. JVP not raised, heart sounds are normal. Chest is clear, respiratory rate 28 per minute. Abdominal examination reveals mild left-sided discomfort, active bowel sounds. Her reflexes are brisk, pupils are equal, but she is not oriented in time or place.

Blood tests show:

Na 147 mmol/L
K 4.9 mmol/L
Urea 16.1 mmol/L
Creatinine 180 μmol/L
Glucose 3.8 mmol/L
CRP 15 mg/L
Creatine kinase 115 U/L
Hb 10.5 g/dL
WCC 17.7 × 10^9/L
Plts 490 × 10^9/L
Chest X-ray is normal
ECG shows sinus tachycardia
She has IV dextrose running and has received IV hydrocortisone

What will you do next?
(a) Request thyroid function tests
(b) Give Lugol's iodine
(c) Give broad-spectrum antibiotics
(d) Give propylthiouracil
(e) Give diazepam

QUESTION 106

A 32-year-old woman with Graves disease attends clinic 6 months after her diagnosis. She has been on carbimazole for several months

319

without any ill-effects; she was able to discontinue beta-blockers 3 months ago. Her weight is currently stable at 51 kg, pulse 70 regular, BP 115/60. She has mild proptosis but does not complain of eye irritation, and her eye movements are normal. There is no tremor.

Her most recent thyroid function tests show:
TSH < 0.05 mU/L
Free T$_4$ 14.2 nmol/L

What will you do?
(a) Withdraw her carbimazole
(b) Continue with current dose of carbimazole
(c) Increase carbimazole dose
(d) Suggest radioiodine therapy
(e) Suggest subtotal thyroidectomy

QUESTION 107

A 23-year-old man attends clinic with gynaecomastia, which was noticed at a health-screening check. On close questioning, the gynaecomastia has been present since puberty. He is otherwise fit and well, does not drink or smoke, and takes no medications. On examination, he is tall and thin, with little body hair. A late systolic murmur is audible at the apex. Chest and abdominal examination are normal; the testes are small but palpable within the scrotum.

What test is most likely to confirm the clinical diagnosis?
(a) Karyotyping
(b) GnRH levels
(c) FSH and LH levels
(d) Testosterone levels
(e) MRI of pituitary

QUESTION 108

As a result of taking part in a genetics study a 42-year-old woman is discovered to have Turner's syndrome. She is single and has previously enjoyed good health. She does not drink or smoke and takes no medications. She was treated for pneumonia at the age of 22, but has remained well since. On examination, she is short, with a BMI of 29.6 kg/m^2. Pulse 80 regular, BP 164/96 right arm, 162/90 left arm, 172/96 right leg. There is no radiofemoral delay. Heart sounds are

normal. Chest examination reveals rudimentary breasts; abdominal examination is normal.

Blood tests show:
Na 134 mmol/L
K 4.6 mmol/L
Urea 10.1 mmol/L
Creatinine 130 µmol/L
Glucose 5.9 mmol/L

What will you do next?
(a) Ultrasound of the kidneys
(b) MRI angiogram of the aorta
(c) Glucose tolerance test
(d) Thyroid function tests
(e) Start amlodipine

QUESTION 109

A 76-year-old man is admitted with left-sided weakness which had become apparent over the last 24 hours. One week prior to admission, he had sustained a fall in the kitchen with transient loss of consciousness. Past medical history included hypertension and atrial fibrillation. No record of his medications was available.

On examination, he was apyrexial. No anaemia, clubbing or jaundice noted. Pulse was 80 irregular. BP 190/100. Cardiovascular and respiratory examination was normal. Neurologically, GCS was 14, with reduced power in the left arm and leg. Both plantars were downgoing. There was no papilloedema, and cranial nerve examination was normal.

Investigations
Na 129 mmol/L
K 3.2 mmol/L
Urea 6.1 mmol/L
Creatinine 90 µmol/L
Glucose 8.1 mmol/L
FBC normal
INR 2.7
Bilirubin 14 µmol/L
ALT 20 U/L
ALP 81 U/L
ECG AF, 90/min. Normal ST segments
CXR shows cardiomegaly

What investigation will you do next?
(a) CT brain
(b) MRI brain
(c) Lumbar puncture

(d) Blood alcohol levels

(e) Cardiac troponins

QUESTION 110

An 87-year-old woman is admitted with a history of confusion. She had an MSQ of 4/10 when she was seen in clinic 6 months ago; her MSQ is now 2/10. She lives in sheltered housing and receives home help twice a day; she is needing increasing amounts of help to wash and dress. She takes aspirin, perindopril, lactulose, tolterodine, diazepam and haloperidol. On examination, her pulse is 70 regular. BP 145/90. JVP is not raised, and a pansystolic murmur is audible at the apex. Chest and abdominal examination are normal. She has normal tone and power in all limbs, impaired righting reflexes, and impaired proprioception at her ankles. Plantars are downgoing and cranial nerve examination is normal. There is no papilloedema.

CT of the brain shows bilateral 3-mm chronic subdural haematomas, together with cerebral atrophy.

What will you do?

(a) Stop aspirin

(b) Refer for neurosurgical evacuation

(c) Repeat CT scan in 6 weeks

(d) Stop perindopril

(e) Request MRI of the brain

QUESTION 111

A 31-year-old woman is seen in outpatients prior to removal of a recently diagnosed phaeochromocytoma. You are given the following pulmonary function tests as part of her preoperative workup. Whilst in the consultation, she also mentions that she has become hard of hearing in her right ear. She is otherwise fit and well, save for a degree of breathlessness. She is taking phentolamine and propranolol.

On examination, chest and abdominal examination are normal. Her BP is 145/70. She has reduced hearing in the right ear; Weber's test localizes to the left.

PFTS

FEV$_1$ 4.7 L

FVC 5.5 L

Kco 42% of predicted

What test is most likely to diagnose the cause of her hearing loss?

(a) Pure-tone audiogram

(b) MRI of the brain

(c) High-resolution CT of the chest

(d) Arch aortogram

(e) Auditory evoked potentials

QUESTION 112

A 30-year-old woman presents with headaches occurring in the morning and of several weeks' duration. More recently she has noticed intermittent blurring of vision. She does not take any medicines and is not allergic to anything. She lives with her two children and works as a cleaner.

On examination she is 96 kg, and has bilateral papilloedema. Cranial nerve examination is normal, and she has normal tone, power, reflexes, coordination and sensation peripherally. MRI of the head is reported as being normal. Lumbar puncture reveals an opening pressure of 34 cm water, 3 white cells and protein of 120 mg/L.

Which treatment is most likely to improve her condition?

(a) Repeated lumbar puncture

(b) Steroids

(c) Thiazide diuretics

(d) Weight loss

(e) Nalidixic acid

QUESTION 113

A 42-year-old woman presents with a 6-week history of headaches. They are worse in the morning and on moving around. She has noticed flashing lights and double vision at times over the last week. She has a past history of DVT. She takes aspirin and paracetamol, smokes 10 cigarettes per day but does not drink alcohol.

On examination, she is overweight. Chest, heart and abdominal examination are normal. Eye movements are normal, as are visual fields to confrontation testing, but she has biateral papilloedema.

What test will you carry out next?

(a) MRI brain

(b) CT brain

(c) Lumbar puncture
(d) Sinus venography
(e) Antiphospholipid antibody titres

QUESTION 114

A 20-year-old man presents with weakness of his hands and difficulty walking over a period of several months. He denies any sensory symptoms. He had recurrent chest infections as a child but no recent medical problems. He smokes 20 cigarettes per day and drinks roughly 20 units alcohol per week.

On examination, he looks rather wasted. He has weakness in his hand and clings on to your hand for a long period of time. He also has weakness of his wrist flexors and he has a bilateral footdrop. Reflexes are reduced. There is no sensory loss. Chest examination is normal; heart sounds are normal and the apex is undisplaced. There is no organomegaly or ascites.

Investigations
Na 144 mmol/L
K 4.6 mmol/L
Urea 5.2 mmol/L
Creatinine 87 µmol/L
Bilirubin 16 µmol/L
ALT 40 U/L
ALP 181 U/L
Glucose 13.6 mmol/L
Creatine kinase 150 U/L
ECG: long PR interval and RBBB

What investigation would best confirm the diagnosis?
(a) Tensilon test
(b) EMG
(c) MRI brain
(d) Muscle biopsy
(e) Echocardiography

QUESTION 115

An 80-year-old man is referred with a history of confusion. He has been living alone, and was found by neighbours in a state of self-neglect and smelling of urine. He is diabetic, hypertensive and has emphysema. He still smokes 20 cigarettes a day but does not drink alcohol. His medications include gliclazide, bendroflumethiazide and lactulose. On examination, he has a mental test score of 14/30. He is apyrexial, and has a resting heart rate of 80 beats/min in atrial fibrillation. His blood pressure is 150/80 mmHg. Respiratory and abdominal examinations are normal. Neurological examination reveals a fine intention tremor. Tone, power, reflexes and coordination are all normal in the arms, but there is hyperreflexia, increased tone and ataxia of the legs. He is unable to walk unaided.

Investigations
Hb 12.0 g/dL
WCC 7.0 × 10^9/L
Plts 200 × 10^9/L
Na 135 mmol/L
K 4.5 mmol/L
Urea 12 mmol/L
Creatinine 140 µmol/L
ESR 20 mm/h
LFTs normal
TSH 2.0 mU/L
CXR normal
Urinalysis: protein +, culture negative

Question 1
What investigation will you perform next?
(a) CT brain
(b) CT chest
(c) Urine microscopy and culture
(d) Lumbar puncture
(e) Alcohol levels

His CT report notes grossly enlarged ventricles with no evidence of sulcal widening and no obstruction to CSF flow. He undergoes lumbar puncture, which shows no white cells, protein of 150 mg/L and opening pressure of 15 cm H$_2$O.

Question 2
What will you do next?
(a) Arrange an EEG
(b) Arrange MRI brain
(c) Await CSF culture
(d) Refer for ventriculoperitoneal shunt
(e) Retest his walking ability

QUESTION 116

A 57-year-old woman with motor neurone disease presents with worsening breathlessness. She is confined to a wheelchair and is fed via a

PEG tube. She is looked after at home by her husband, who attends to all of her washing, dressing and toileting. She has a weak cough. On examination, her pulse is 100 regular, BP 90/40. Temperature is 38.1°C. Oxygen saturations are 87% on air and she has reduced air entry and crackles at the left base. Abdominal examination is normal. Her MSQ is 8/10.

The patient indicates to you that she does not want antibiotics, but the husband insists that everything be done to save her.

What will you do?
(a) Give IV antibiotics
(b) Give antibiotics via the PEG tube
(c) Withhold antibiotics
(d) Test for depression
(e) Seek an injunction to bar the husband from visiting

QUESTION 117

A 38-year-old man presents with problems swallowing. He first noticed these a few months ago, and the other day he choked on his beer in the pub. He has no problems swallowing food, but he has also noticed that his voice becomes slurred when he is tired. He is usually fit and well, drinks 20 units of alcohol per week but does not smoke. He takes no medications.

On examination, tone, power, reflexes and sensation are normal in all limbs. Plantars are downgoing. There is no ptosis and eye movements are normal. Ptosis does not occur on sustained upward gaze. Facial sensation and muscle function are normal. Tongue movement is slow, with occasional fasciculations.

MRI of the brain is normal, and chest X-ray is also normal. FBC, U + Es and LFTs are also normal.

What investigation will you do next?
(a) Upper GI endoscopy
(b) MRI spine
(c) EMG
(d) Video fluoroscopy
(e) Tensilon test

QUESTION 118

A 79-year-old man with idiopathic Parkinson's disease attends clinic. He was diagnosed 6 years ago, but over the last few months, he has noticed that he becomes much slower and more rigid an hour before his next dose is due. He does not suffer from any involuntary movements. He is currently taking 125 mg of l-dopa/benserazide at 6 a.m., 10 a.m., 2 p.m. and 6 p.m., with 250 mg of a slow release preparation at 10 p.m.

On examination, he has increased tone in both arms with a resting tremor. His face is expressionless. He is due his next dose in 20 minutes. He has considerable difficulty getting out of the chair to try and walk across the room.

What will you do?
(a) Increase his daytime doses to 250 mg four times per day
(b) Reduce the time between doses to 3 hours
(c) Add in a dopamine agonist
(d) Add in a COMT inhibitor
(e) Change all the doses to the slow-release preparation

QUESTION 119

An 87-year-old woman is referred with a tremor. It is noticeable at rest but does not bother her; her daughter suggested that she attend the clinic for investigation. She does not drink alcohol, and takes bendroflumethiazide for hypertension. She lives in sheltered housing but still does her own cooking and cleaning.

On examination, she has a slow gait with good stride length. Her righting reflexes are preserved and there is no rigidity. She is slow to get out of a chair. Power, reflexes and sensation are normal.

What will you do?
(a) Review in 6 months' time
(b) Start l-dopa
(c) Start a dopamine agonist
(d) Give a beta-blocker
(e) Arrange MRI of the brain

QUESTION 120

A 32-year-old woman with myasthenia gravis attends the hospital with fever, dysuria and loin pain. Urine microscopy reveals Gram-negative bacilli and she is given gentamicin. She usually takes prednisolone and pyridostigmine, smokes 10 cigarettes per day, and drinks 30 units of alcohol per week.

You are called to see her 6 hours later as she has become confused and drowsy. On examination, pulse is 90 reg. BP 105/50. Respiratory rate is 16 per minute; chest is clear and she is tender in the left loin. Her GCS is 13/15 and she has decreased tone and power in all limbs. There is no neck stiffness or photophobia, fundoscopy is normal.

Bloods
Na 145 mmol/L
K 4.8 mmol/L
Urea 9.9 mmol/L
Creatinine 120 µmol/L
Hb 12.8 g/dL
WCC 17.8 × 10⁹/L
Plts 561 × 10⁹/L

ABGS on 10 L Oxygen
pH 7.24
po₂ 9.7 kPa
$p$co₂ 8.9 kPa

She is intubated and ventilated. What will you do next?
(a) Perform urgent CT brain
(b) Perform lumbar puncture
(c) Arrange plasmapheresis
(d) Give high-dose steroids
(e) Give IV aminophylline

QUESTION 121

A 45-year-old woman presents with double vision. It is not present all the time; she thinks that it is worse when she is tired. It is not worse when she looks in any particular direction. She had a flu-like illness 4 weeks ago, but has now recovered. She has rheumatoid arthritis treated with penicillamine, and a past history of hyperthyroidism. She does not drink or smoke.

Examination reveals normal eye movements, limb power and reflexes. She has no proptosis or lid lag. There is no evidence of active synovitis, and chest and abdominal examination are normal.

What investigation is most likely to confirm the diagnosis?
(a) MRI orbits
(b) Anti AChR antibodies
(c) Thyroid function tests
(d) Chest X-ray
(e) Lumbar puncture

QUESTION 122

A 17-year-old girl is referred for assessment. She has had sensory loss with pins and needles in both her legs for the last 3 months, and more recently she has noticed that she is becoming more clumsy and is tripping over more. She has been on fluoxetine for 9 months for depression. She is still low in mood, and is causing trouble at school. She is not sleeping or eating well. There is no other medical history of note.

On examination, she has ataxia when walking, but neurological examination is otherwise normal.

Investigations
Hb 14.7 g/dL
WCC 5.5 × 10⁹/L
Plts 190 × 10⁹/L
U + Es normal
LFTs normal
MRI head: mild cerebral atrophy
Lumbar puncture: no oligoclonal bands seen
CSF protein 400 mg/L
VDRL negative
Nerve conduction studies normal
EEG normal

What is the most likely diagnosis?
(a) Friedreich's ataxia
(b) Motor neurone disease
(c) Hereditary spinocerebellar ataxia
(d) Wilson's disease
(e) Variant Creutzfeldt–Jakob disease

QUESTION 123

A 20-year-old man presents with progressive clumsiness and loss of balance. He has not noticed any sensory or visual disturbances. His mother died when he was 5 years old and had similar symptoms.

Examination shows nystagmus and ataxia. He has reduced reflexes in his knees and ankles and upgoing plantar reflexes. There is some wasting of his quadriceps but muscle power is normal. Pes cavus is present. He has a kyphoscoliosis, but cardiac, respiratory and abdominal examinations are normal.

Investigations
U + Es normal
FBC normal

Glucose 10.5 mmol/L

ECG: T-wave inversion anteriorly

What investigation would assist your efforts to prolong this man's life?

(a) Echocardiography

(b) MRI brain

(c) Nerve conduction studies

(d) Pulmonary function tests

(e) Genotyping

QUESTION 124

A 72-year-old woman presents with tingling and weakness in her legs. This started a few days ago when she noticed her feet tripping up whilst walking. The weakness has now spread to her thighs and hips over the last 4 days. For the last 12 hours she has been unable to walk. She had a bout of diarrhoea a week ago, but is usually well. She complains of no cough, sputum, weight loss or abdominal pain. She takes no medication and does not drink alcohol or smoke.

On examination, she is apyrexial. Pulse 70 beats/min reg, BP 90/40 mmHg lying, 70/40 mmHg sitting. JVP not raised. Heart sounds are normal with no ankle oedema. Chest and abdominal examination are normal and she has no back tenderness. Sensation is normal in her legs, power in her arms is normal, but power in her hip muscles is 4/5 and only 2/5 at her knees and ankles. Arm reflexes are normal, but leg reflexes are absent. Plantars are normal.

Investigations

FBC normal

U + Es normal

Calcium 2.21 mmol/L

LFTs normal

Glucose 5.0 mmol/L

CSF: glucose 4.1, protein 2.1 g/dL, WBC 4, RBC 0. No growth

PFTs: FEV_1 0.8 L, FVC 1.0 L

What will you do next?

(a) Administer IV immunoglobulin

(b) Arrange for plasmapheresis

(c) Transfer to ITU

(d) Give antibotulism antitoxin

(e) Give high-dose corticosteroids

QUESTION 125

A 47-year-old woman presents with a 1-week history of blurred vision. Over the last 2 days she has found it difficult to walk, as she staggers a lot. She is normally fit and well, but had a cold a couple of weeks ago. She does not drink or smoke, lives with her partner and three children who are all well, and takes no medications.

On examination, pulse is 72 reg. BP 150/90. Chest, heart and abdominal examination are normal. Cranial nerve examination reveals severely reduced movement of the right eye in all directions, and reduced lateral gaze in the left eye. Horizontal nystagmus is present in the left eye. Finger–nose pointing is impaired, and dysdiadochokinesis is present. Tone and power are normal in arms and legs, but knee and ankle jerks are absent.

Which two investigations would best confirm the diagnosis?

(a) CT brain

(b) MRI brain

(c) Tensilon test

(d) EMG studies

(e) Antiganglioside GQ1b antibodies

(f) Anti-Hu antibodies

(g) Visual evoked potentials

(h) Mouse bioassay for toxin

(i) EEG

(j) Lumbar puncture

QUESTION 126

A 68-year-old man presents with sudden onset of left-sided weakness. He noticed it came on an hour ago at breakfast, and his wife immediately called the ambulance. He has a past history of hypertension, diabetes and myocardial infarction, and he usually takes aspirin, simvastatin, ramipril, gliclazide and amlodipine. He smokes 10 cigarettes per day.

On examination, he has a GCS of 11/15. He is making snoring sounds. Oxygen saturations are 93% on air; respiratory rate is 16 per minute. Pulse is 80 regular, BP 180/110. Heart sounds are normal and chest is clear. He has reduced tone and 0/5 power in his left arm and leg. His left plantar is upgoing and he has a left-sided facial droop. His tongue deviates to the left. Blood glucose on stix test is 18.2 mmol/L.

What will you do first?
(a) Arrange for urgent CT brain
(b) Give insulin
(c) Give oxygen
(d) Transfer to an acute stroke unit
(e) Insert a Guedel airway

QUESTION 127

A 42-year-old woman presents with sudden onset of right arm and leg weakness, accompanied by difficulty speaking. She denies headache, visual disturbance or neck stiffness. She does not suffer from migraine and has never had symptoms like this before. She is usually fit and well save for Raynaud's syndrome, which affects her during the winter. She does not smoke, and drinks 20 units of alcohol per week.

On examination, she has 3/5 power in her right arm and leg, plus an expressive dysphasia. Heart, chest and abdominal examination are normal. Pulse is 60 regular, BP 135/70.

A CT of the brain reveals no abnormality, and her symptoms resolve completely over the next 24 hours.
Which one of the following tests would be least helpful in investigating her further?
(a) ESR
(b) MRI brain
(c) Carotid ultrasound
(d) Echocardiography
(e) Lumbar puncture

QUESTION 128

A 25-year-old woman is seen in outpatients. She has noticed blurring of vision in her left eye, which was associated with pain. Two years ago she had an episode of vertigo which was put down to a labyrinthitis and which resolved spontaneously. She has a mechanical aortic valve which was inserted as part of a series of operations for congenial cardiac problems. She takes warfarin but does not drink or smoke. She has not noticed any joint pains, rashes, sweats or fever.

On examination, pulse is 80 regular. BP 115/50. She has no lymphadenopathy and there are no splinter haemorrhages. Her JVP is not raised; prosthetic heart sounds plus a soft ejection systolic murmur are audible on auscultation. Lung examination is normal, as is abdominal examination. Peripheral neurological examination is normal; cranial nerve examination reveals a blurred optic disc on the left.

Blood tests show normal FBC, normal U + Es. Glucose 4.7 mmol/L. ESR is 14 mm/h; CRP 8 mg/L. INR 3.1. What investigation will you do next?
(a) Antinuclear antibodies
(b) Echocardiography
(c) MRI brain
(d) Formal perimetry
(e) Visual evoked potentials

QUESTION 129

A 31-year-old woman with a 3-year history of multiple sclerosis is admitted to hospital unable to walk. She has noticed rapidly progressive weakness of both legs over the last 2 days, and now cannot stand. There is no history of trauma. She has had six exacerbations of her MS since diagnosis. She drinks 10 units of alcohol per week and smokes cannabis. She works as a pharmacist but takes no medications besides occasional paracetamol.

On examination, pulse is 70 reg. BP 125/70. Chest, heart and abdominal examination are normal. She has normal tone, power and reflexes in her upper limbs, but mildly impaired coordination in the left arm. There is reduced sensation below her umbilicus, reduced tone in the legs and 2/5 power in both legs. Plantars are equivocal. Her visual acuity is normal, but the optic disc on the left is pale.

What will you do next?
(a) Start interferon-beta
(b) Give high-dose steroids
(c) Start glatiramer
(d) Request MRI spine
(e) Request MRI brain

QUESTION 130

A 57-year-old woman presents with a 3-month history of weakness and tingling in her arms and legs. The tingling affects her feet and hands; she has noticed that she trips over things and that her hands get tired. She denies any visual problems or swallowing problems. She does not drink or smoke, lives alone and has been celibate since her divorce 15 years ago. No one in her family has had similar symptoms.

On examination, heart, chest and abdominal examination are normal. She has no joint swelling or rashes. Tone is normal in all limbs, but she has weakness of the small hand muscles and bilateral weakness of foot dorsiflexion. Sensation to light touch is diminished in the legs below mid-calf and in the hands. Proprioception is reduced in the fingers and toes. Her ankle jerks are absent; plantars are downgoing.

Investigations
Hb 15.0 g/dL
WCC 4.5 × 10^9/L
Plts 227 × 10^9/L
MCV 85 fl
U + Es normal
LFTs normal
Glucose 5.0 mmol/L
ESR 20 mm/h
Antinuclear antibody negative
Rheumatoid factor negative
Nerve conduction studies show a demyelinating
    polyneuropathy
Lumbar puncture reveals normal opening
    pressure, glucose 2.8 mmol/L, 1 WCC, protein
    1250 mg/L

How will you treat her?
(a) Multivitamins
(b) Steroids
(c) Plasmapheresis
(d) Undertake genetic analysis
(e) Undertake nerve biopsy

QUESTION 131
A 66-year-old woman complains of tingling and numbness in her legs. The feeling started in her feet a few months ago and has slowly progressed to involve her legs below the knees. She has not noticed any weakness, but does tend to trip over things. She takes bendroflumethiazide for hypertension. She does not smoke and drinks 10 units of alcohol per week. No one in her family has had similar symptoms.

On examination, there was no jaundice, anaemia, cyanosis, clubbing or lymphadenopathy.

Cardiac, chest and abdominal examination were normal. Cranial nerve and fundoscopic examinations were normal, and she had normal tone, power, reflexes and sensation in both arms. Lower-limb examination revealed normal tone and power, absent ankle jerks, downgoing plantars and reduced sensation to light touch below the knees. Romberg's sign was positive.

Investigations
Hb 11.9 g/dL
WCC 6.6 × 10^9/L
Plts 323 × 10^9/L
MCV 98 fl
Na 139 mmol/L
K 3.9 mmol/L
Urea 6.1 mmol/L
Creatinine 70 µmol/L
LFTs normal
Glucose 4.7 mmol/L
ESR 14 mm/h
Nerve conduction studies show a severe axonal
    polyneuropathy.

Which investigation would you do next?
(a) Lead levels
(b) Lumbar puncture
(c) MRI spine
(d) B$_{12}$ levels
(e) Sural nerve biopsy

QUESTION 132
A 39-year-old businessman presents to the Accident and Emergency department with suspected meningitis. He has been unwell for at least 2 months but has found that over the past 2 weeks he has had a headache, neck stiffness and slight photophobia.

Apart from mumps in his late teens, he has been well and suffers from no medical illness, takes no regular prescribed medication and has had no recent contact with anyone who is unwell. He smokes 20 cigarettes per day, consumes 30 units of alcohol per week and enjoys travelling, which is also part of his occupation, mostly in the Far East.

On examination, he was alert and oriented in time, place and person. He was of tall stature and had a high arched palate. He was afebrile, HR 76, RR 16, BP 177/57 with a collapsing pulse. Heart sounds were pure and there was an audible early diastolic murmur at the left sternal edge, loudest on expiration. Chest was clear to auscultation, abdomen was unremarkable and his genitals were not examined. There was no papilloedema on fundoscopy, the rest of his cranial nerves were intact and he had extensor plantars with absent ankle jerks and reduced knee reflex.

You suspect meningitis, commence him on intravenous penicillin and arrange the following investigations:

Hb 15.1 g/dL
MCV 98 fl
WCC 9.3 × 10⁹/L (neutrophils 7.3 × 10⁹/L, lymphocytes 0.9 × 10⁹/L)
Plts 130 × 10⁹/L
Na 144 mmol/L
K 3.9 mmol/L
Urea 3.5 mmol/L
Creatinine 97 µmol/L
Bilirubin 15 µmol/L
ALP 162 U/L
ALT 52 U/L
Albumin 44 g/L
Calcium 2.55 mmol/L
Glucose 5.3 mmol/L
CXR: normal
CT brain: normal
CSF: opening pressure 26 cm, white cells 7, red cells 13, no organisms seen. Protein 536 mg/L, glucose 3.9 mmol/L

Question 1
The most useful diagnostic investigation would be
(a) FTA-ABS test
(b) Cerebral angiogram and CT chest
(c) MRI scan of the brain
(d) VDRL
(e) Blood culture

The following day, he becomes very unwell, with fever and hypotension and generalized polymyalgia. What complication has occurred?

Question 2
(a) Cerebral coning
(b) Anaphylaxis to penicillin
(c) Necrotizing fasciitis
(d) Aortic dissection
(e) Jarisch–Herxheimer reaction

QUESTION 133
A 22-year-old female veterinary science student attended her GP practice complaining of lethargy and general arthropathy. These symptoms had been particularly troublesome over the past 2 months and were now affecting her course studies. She complained of back pain and pain affecting her hips and knees with occasional sweats at night. She otherwise keeps well, doesn't smoke and occasionally has a binge drink at the weekend with her friends at the union. She suffers from no past medical history and has a steady relationship with her boyfriend who she has known for 3 years. Neither have had any problems from genitourinary disease apart one episode of vaginal thrush last year that she recalls. She uses barrier contraception, takes no regular medication and keeps a pet dog which she has had for years.

On examination, she was a thin healthy-looking female. She had no clubbing or jaundice but had palpable soft lymph glands in the groin region. Heart sounds were normal and her chest was clear. She had a palpable spleen and tenderness over the thoracic and lumbar spines with slight pain on passive movement of both hip joints. Vital signs were normal and her temperature was 36.5°C.

Investigations
Hb 11.2 g/dL
MCV 87 fl
WCC 3.9 × 10⁹/L (neutrophils 30%)
Plts 410 × 10⁹/L
Na 139 mmol/L
K 5.1 mmol/L
Urea 2.6 mmol/L
Creatinine 76 µmol/L
Bilirubin 31 µmol/L
ALP 66 U/L
ALT 61 U/L
Albumin 38 g/L
Calcium 2.43 mmol/L
Glucose 6.3 mmol/L
CRP 32 mg/L
CK 66 U/L
TSH 1.3 mU/L

Which of the following tests is likely to clinch the diagnosis?
(a) Abdominal ultrasound
(b) Renal ultrasound

(c) IgG and IgM *Brucella* serology

(d) Bone scan

(e) High vaginal swab

QUESTION 134

A 41-year-old postgraduate student presents with a 10-day history of headache, anorexia, abdominal pain, fevers and mild diarrhoea. He normally keeps well and has recently returned from visiting his family in the Ahvaz district, west of Iran. He gave up smoking 5 years ago, doesn't drink alcohol and is currently studying for a Masters degree in political sciences at a UK university. He keeps no pets and took no malaria prophylaxis on his recent trip home.

Examination revealed slight icterus with cervical lymphadenopathy. His temperature was 39.9°C, heart rate was 52 beats/minute and respiratory rate was 18 breaths/minute. BP was 123/58 and the rest of his cardiovascular, respiratory and abdominal examinations were unremarkable.

Investigations

Hb 14.2 g/dL
MCV 89 fl
WCC 9.8×10^9/L
Plts 65×10^9/L
Na 133 mmol/L
K 3.6 mmol/L
Urea 3.5 mmol/L
Creatinine 93 μmol/L
Bilirubin 61 μmol/L
ALP 98 U/L
ALT 189 U/L
Albumin 39 mmol/L
Calcium 2.56 mmol/L
Glucose 6.9 mmol/L
CRP 96 mg/L
Thick and thin blood films normal
CXR normal
ECG sinus bradycardia 50 beats/min with first-degree heart block

Question 1

What is the most likely diagnosis?

(a) Legionnaire's disease

(b) Paratyphoid

(c) Vivax malaria

(d) Falciparum malaria

(e) Typhoid

Question 2

Which of the following tests is most likely to be diagnostic?

(a) Bone marrow culture

(b) Blood culture

(c) Stool culture

(d) Widal test

(e) Urine culture

QUESTION 135

A 25-year-old Iraqi Kurdish woman presents with malaise and weight loss. She denies night sweats but does admit to going to the toilet more frequently to pass large volumes of urine. Her symptoms have been insidious in onset and have been present for about 4 months. She was well prior to this and able to look after her two children aged 4 and 2.

All her family members are well and the last time she was abroad was 6 years ago. She doesn't smoke and hasn't drunk alcohol since the birth of her first child. Her mother suffers from angina and stroke disease and stays with her sister in Iraq. Her father died from pulmonary tuberculosis.

Examination revealed a thin woman. There was no clubbing or lymphadenopathy and her conjunctivae were pale. Temperature was 36.8°C. Heart sounds were normal with no murmurs. Heart rate was 86 beats/minute with a BP of 101/48. Her chest was clear and her oxygen saturations were 99% on room air with a respiratory rate of 18 breaths/minute. She had slight discomfort over the left flank but abdominal examination was otherwise unremarkable.

Hb 10.3 g/dL
MCV 79 fl
WCC 3.6×10^9/L
Plts 212×10^9/L
Na 126 mmol/L
K 4.3 mmol/L
Urea 7.3 mmol/L
Creatinine 110 μmol/L
Bilirubin 9 μmol/L
ALP 36 U/L
ALT 32 U/L
Albumin 30 g/L

Calcium 2.66 mmol/L
Glucose 6.9 mmol/L
CRP 46 mg/L
TSH 1.36 mU/L
ECG sinus rhythm
CXR streaky right upper zone scarring
Urinary Na excretion 395 (40–220 mmol/24 hours)
Recent MSU × 3 showed no growth

Question 1

The cause of the electrolyte disturbance is most likely due to:
(a) Salt-losing nephropathy
(b) Acute tubular necrosis
(c) SIADH
(d) Pyelonephritis
(e) Addison's disease

Question 2

The most likely diagnosis is:
(a) *Chlamydia* infection
(b) *Proteus* urinary tract infection
(c) Renal tubular acidosis type 2
(d) Renal tuberculosis
(e) Myeloma

QUESTION 136

A 32-year-old male hairdresser presents with breathlessness and cough productive of purulent sputum associated with fevers and sweats over the past 3 days. His chest X-ray, other clinical findings and raised inflammatory markers were in keeping with right-upper-lobe pneumonia which responded very well to antibiotic therapy.

He denies any chronic medical illnesses but this was his third episode of pneumonia over the last 14 months. He is on no regular medicines, has no allergies and his father died from alcoholic liver disease. His mother and two siblings are alive and well. He has never smoked, binge-drinks alcohol at the weekends on occasions and keeps two pet cats at home which he shares with his colleague from work.

He returns to clinic for review 6 weeks postdischarge and you find him to be symptom-free. The repeat chest X-ray that he had a week ago shows near-complete resolution of his RUL consolidation.

Examination reveals a generally fit healthy young man of reasonable build. A few palpable non-tender cervical lymph glands and a scaly erythematous rash over his forehead are noted on examination.

Hb 14.6 g/dL
MCV 89 fl
WCC 3.6 × 10^9/L (neutrophils 86%, lymphocytes 5%)
Plts 159 × 10^9/L
Na 139 mmol/L
K 4.5 mmol/L
Urea 3.9 mmol/L
Creatinine 71 μmol/L
Bilirubin 13 μmol/L
ALP 50 U/L
ALT 22 U/L
Albumin 39 g/L

You suspect HIV infection and obtain a sample after counselling the patient. The diagnosis is confirmed and you break this to him. His CD4 count is 205 × 10^6/L

The most appropriate next management step would be:
(a) Commence highly active antiretroviral therapy (HAART)
(b) Commence HAART after CD4 count falls below 200 × 10^6/L
(c) Commence HAART after CD4 count falls below 150 × 10^6/L
(d) Repeat CXR in 3 months and consider HAART
(e) None of the above

QUESTION 137

A 29-year-old woman presents to the surgical unit with right upper quadrant pain, jaundice, nausea and mild peritonism. These symptoms developed over a period of 3–4 days. Her appetite has been poor over the past 2 months and as a consequence she had lost 2.5 kg (half a stone) in weight. Bowel habit is regular and she denies any dysphagia or acid reflux. She has suffered from pelvic inflammatory disease over the past 2 years and had attended the genitourinary clinic.

There are no other features from systemic enquiry; she takes no regular medicines or recreational drugs. She only drinks alcohol on special occasions and has not been abroad. She smokes 15 cigarettes per day and currently lives with her teenage daughter.

Clinically she was icteric and febrile with a temperature of 37.9°C. Heart rate 90 beats/minute, respiratory rate 18 breaths/minute, oxygen sats 95% on air and BP 113/63. Abdomen was tender but soft in the epigastrium and the right upper quadrant and there were no stigmata of chronic liver disease. There were some palpable inguinal lymph nodes and slight dullness at the right lung base.

Investigations

Hb 13.6 g/dL
MCV 82 fl
WCC 14.3 × 10^9/L (neutrophils 88%)
Plts 503 × 10^9/L
Na 133 mmol/L
K 3.6 mmol/L
Urea 5.6 mmol/L
Creatinine 113 μmol/L
Bilirubin 71 μmol/L
ALP 171 U/L
ALT 43 U/L
Albumin 33 g/L
Calcium 2.53 mmol/L
Glucose 5.7 mmol/L
CRP 89 mg/L
Amylase 46 U/L
CXR small right pleural effusion
Urinalysis: leucocytes and trace of protein
CT abdomen: liver enhancement, small inguinal lymph nodes and small right pleural effusion

The most likely diagnosis is:
(a) Community-acquired pneumonia
(b) Atypical pneumonia
(c) Biliary sepsis
(d) Fitz-Hugh–Curtis syndrome
(e) Hepatitis A infection

QUESTION 138

A 42-year-old male teacher presents with a 6-week history of aches and pains, which have made him take time off work. He is a father of 3 children and had taken them on a camping holiday 3 months ago. He recalls developing flu-like symptoms and a rash soon after their return and, although improved, he doesn't feel that he has made a full recovery.

Examination was unremarkable apart from a right facial droop.

Investigations

FBC normal
U + Es normal
LFTs normal
Urinalyisis normal
CRP 13 mg/L
ECG first-degree heart block

Question 1

What is the most useful next investigation?
(a) Carotid Doppler
(b) CT brain
(c) MRI brain
(d) Syphilis serology
(e) *Borrelia* serology

Question 2

The most likely diagnosis is:
(a) Demyelination
(b) Lyme disease
(c) HIV
(d) Space-occupying lesion
(e) Tertiary syphilis

QUESTION 139

A 23-year-old international journalist presents with flu-like symptoms over the past week. He generally keeps well and was working on a tsunami assignment over in Sri Lanka 4 months ago. He reports completing a prophylactic course of mefloquine at the time. He had suffered from mild asthma as a child but hasn't used his inhalers for years. He doesn't smoke, drinks 30 units of alcohol per week and has the occasional cannabis joint. He also admits to having had protected sex on two occasions while he was in Sri Lanka.

Clinically, he was pale and mildly jaundiced. There was palpable hepatosplenomegaly but no rash or lymphadenopathy. His temperature was 36.6°C and other examination features were unremarkable.

Investigations

Hb 11.3 g/dL
MCV 95 fl
WCC 11.2 × 10^9/L

Plts 96 × 10⁹/L

Na 136 mmol/L

K 4.9 mmol/L

Urea 3.6 mmol/L

Creatinine 133 μmol/L

Bilirubin 18 μmol/L

ALP 35 U/L

ALT 32 U/L

Albumin 45 g/L

Calcium 2.33 mmol/L

Glucose 3.9 mmol/L

CRP < 3 mg/L

Clotting normal

Urinalysis: trace protein and ++ of blood

CXR normal

Thick and thin blood films × 1: normal

What would you do next?
(a) Abdominal US scan
(b) Repeat blood films
(c) Blood culture
(d) CT abdomen
(e) *Borrelia* serology

QUESTION 140

An 18-year-old woman in her first year at university presents unwell to the acute medical unit. She gives a history of lethargy, breathlessness, fevers and shakes over the past 3 days. She normally keeps well and her only visit to her GP was to get a coil inserted a few weeks ago. She doesn't smoke, consumes alcohol mainly at the weekends with friends but doesn't binge-drink. She is currently resident at the student halls of residence and doesn't recall anyone else being unwell.

Clinically, she had a widespread macular rash, dry mucous membranes and reduced skin turgor. Heart rate 110/min, BP 87/52, respiratory rate 24/min. Oxygen saturation 93% on air and her temperature was 39.6°C. Heart sounds were normal, chest was clear to auscultation, calves were soft and non-tender and abdominal examination revealed mild tenderness suprapubically.

You commence her on intravenous fluid resuscitation and oxygen and ask the nurses to give her antipyretics. Urinalysis shows a trace of leukocytes and you arrange a number of blood tests and send off blood cultures.

Your immediate next step in her management should be:
(a) Gynaecology review and IV flucloxacillin
(b) Gynaecology review and oral ciprofloxacin
(c) IV co-amoxiclav
(d) Decide on antibiotic therapy after review of her blood results
(e) IV flucloxacillin

QUESTION 141

A 44-year-old man who had been a veterinarian for 16 years presents with fever, headache and myalgia. He had been feeling unwell for about 10 days and went to see his referring GP with deepening jaundice. He also mentioned neck stiffness but no photophobia. He had a history of mild hypertension for which he took atenolol 50 mg once daily. He has no allergies and was on holiday in Greece 2 months ago with his young family. He smokes cigars and drinks alcohol in moderation.

On examination he was jaundiced and had palpable cervical and axillary lymphadenopathy. His heart rate was 88 beats/min and respiratory rate of 16 breaths/min. Blood pressure was 126/58 and his temperature was 38.1°C.

He had a palpable apex beat in the fifth intercostal space, mid-clavicular line and an audible fourth heart sound. JVP was not raised and there was no ankle oedema. Chest examination revealed a few audible crackles and his abdomen revealed palpable mildly tender liver extending 6 cm below the costal margin. There were no associated features of chronic liver disease. There was no objective evidence of meningism on neurological examination; tone, power, reflexes, plantars, fundoscopy and cognitive function were normal.

Investigations

Hb 12.2 g/dL

MCV 93 fl

WCC 16.2 × 10⁹/L (neutrophils 92%)

Plts 91 × 10⁹/L

INR 1.6

Na 144 mmol/L

K 5.9 mmol/L

Urea 19.3 mmol/L

Creatinine 198 μmol/L

Bilirubin 101 μmol/L
ALP 163 U/L
ALT 62 U/L
Albumin 31 g/L
Calcium 2.69 mmol/L
Glucose 7.2 mmol/L
CRP 196 mg/L
CXR: patchy opacification in the left lower zone
CSF proteins 510 mg/L (150–450). White cells 3, red cells 2, no organisms
Urinalysis positive for blood, protein and bilirubin

Question 1
The most useful investigation(s) would be:
(a) Urinary antibody and blood cultures
(b) Viral serology
(c) Thick and thin blood films
(d) Paracetamol levels
(e) Renal biopsy

Question 2
The most likely diagnosis is:
(a) Falciparum malaria
(b) Weil's disease
(c) Brucellosis
(d) Inhalational anthrax
(e) Viral meningitis

QUESTION 142
A 22-year-old art student presents with a 36-hour history of blurred vision, breathlessness and muscle weakness. This was preceded by mild diarrhoea. He is usually well and takes no prescribed or over-the-counter medication and only tried some recreational drugs 3 years ago. He keeps no pets and has not been abroad for some time in view of financial difficulties.

He was oriented in time, place and person and was afebrile with a temperature of 36.5°C. He had mild ptosis bilaterally with sluggish dilated pupils and worsening diplopia on extremes of gaze on visual pursuit. Power in the arms was reduced to 4 on the MRC grading and 4+ in the lower limbs. Tone, reflexes, coordination and sensation were otherwise intact. He was breathless and needing to use his accessory muscles with a respiratory rate of 28/min. Heart rate 76/min, BP 100/56 and oxygen saturations of 96% on room air. Chest,

cardiovascular and abdominal systems were otherwise unremarkable.

Investigations
Hb 15.2 g/dL
MCV 83 fl
WCC 6.9 × 10⁹/L
Plts 333 × 10⁹/L
Na 141 mmol/L
K 5.0 mmol/L
Urea 3.6 mmol/L
Creatinine 96 μmol/L
Bilirubin 11 μmol/L
ALP 31 U/L
ALT 26 U/L
Albumin 46 g/L
Calcium 2.55 mmol/L
Glucose 5.8 mmol/L
CRP 4 mg/L
ECG: T-wave inversion V5 and V6
CXR normal
PEFR 42% predicted

Question 1
Your next step should be:
(a) Blood culture
(b) Urine culture
(c) Inform public health
(d) Refer to coronary care
(e) Arterial blood gases

Question 2
Which drug should you administer next?
(a) Low-molecular-weight heparin
(b) Amiodarone
(c) IV benzylpenicillin
(d) IV cephalosporin
(e) Antitoxin

QUESTION 143
A 26-year-old man who suffers from haemophilia was recovering from an episode of haematoma of the left elbow. He was diagnosed with haemophilia A at the age of 3 and this has rendered him with advanced secondary degenerative hip, knee and elbow joints. There is no other past medical history; he doesn't smoke or drink alcohol.

On examination he had a haematoma of the left elbow and pain on restricted passive and active movements of both hips and knees.

Temperature was 35.6°C and vital signs were unremarkable. Heart sounds were normal with a quiet pansystolic murmur over the apex and his chest was clear to auscultation. Abdominal examination revealed no masses or organomegaly but he did have spider naevi and palmar erythema. There was no jaundice or ascites detectable.

Investigations
Hb 9.8 g/dL
MCV 74 fl
WCC 7.9×10^9/L
Plts 200×10^9/L
Na 130 mmol/L
K 4.5 mmol/L
Urea 4.5 mmol/L
Creatinine 109 μmol/L
Bilirubin 23 μmol/L
ALP 64 U/L
ALT 543 U/L
Albumin 29 g/L
INR 1.8
APTTR 3.1

Question 1
What is the most likely cause of this patient's deranged liver enzymes?
(a) Portal vein thrombosis
(b) Haemolytic anaemia
(c) Liver cirrhosis
(d) Acute hepatitis E
(e) Hepatoma

Question 2
He undergoes a liver biopsy, which confirms cirrhosis. What is the most likely cause?
(a) Hepatitis A
(b) Hepatitis B
(c) Hepatitis C
(d) Hepatitis D
(e) Hepatitis E

QUESTION 144
A 36-year-old soldier serving in the Iraqi war has recently returned from service in Iraq for a brief visit to see his mother who was dying from cancer. He is fortunate to be alive as he was nearly killed by a roadside bomb 6 days ago which caused serious injuries to two other

servicemen. He was referred by his GP with suspected pneumonia which was preceded by flu-like symptoms 2 days ago.

On arrival he was confused, distressed and hypoxic with saturations of 79% on room air. He was cyanosed and had a respiratory rate of 36/min. Temperature was 37.4°C, heart rate 120/min and BP 135/88. He had normal heart sounds and crackles at the bases of both lungs. There was no rash or skin lesions.

He was commenced on high-flow oxygen via a rebreather mask, given 1.2 g of IV co-amoxiclav empirically and transferred to the intensive care unit.

Investigations
ABG on high-flow oxygen
pH 7.49
po_2 8.8 kPa
pco_2 5.9 kPa
FBC
Hb 14.6 g/dL
WCC 11.3×10^9/L (neutrophils 83%)
Plts 133×10^9/L
Clotting: normal
U + Es: normal
LFTs: normal
Portable CXR (AP view) widened mediastinum, mild streaking at the left base with a small left pleural effusion
ECG sinus tachycardia

36 hours later, the microbiology laboratory phones to inform you that they have identified Gram-positive rods from his blood cultures

Your next step should be:
(a) Inform public health
(b) Add in a macrolide antibiotic
(c) Add in ciprofloxacin
(d) Send repeat blood cultures
(e) Arrange transoesophageal echocardiogram

QUESTION 145
A 45-year-old man presents with a history of lethargy. His only past medical history is of irritable-bowel syndrome and an episode of pneumonia 6 months ago. As a businessman, he has spent much time abroad, including the Far East and Africa. The reason for attending his GP is that he now suffers from pleuritic chest pains, and has developed a cough.

On examination he has fever of 38.5°C, cervical and axillary lymphadenopathy and he has left-sided crackles in his chest. Pulse is 120/min, BP 80/40. Abdominal examination reveals a large liver and spleen. He is a heavy drinker, and smokes 20 cigarettes per day.

Initial blood tests show:

Hb 8.0 g/dL
WCC 35 × 10⁹/L (60% neutrophils, 10% metamyelocytes, 25% myelocytes, 1% promyelocytes, 2% nucleated red cells)
Platelets 30 × 10⁹/L
Na 132 mmol/L
K 3.6 mmol/L
Urea 19.6 mmol/L
Creatinine 251 μmol/L
CRP 350 mg/L
Bilirubin 86 μmol/L
ALT 251 U/L
ALP 499 U/L
INR 1.7
Albumin 23 g/L

What will you do next?
(a) Give broad-spectrum antibiotics
(b) Refer for allogeneic bone marrow transplant
(c) Arrange for bone marrow biopsy
(d) Refer for high-dose chemotherapy
(e) Arrange for a Mantoux test

QUESTION 146

A 71-year-old woman presented with headaches and blurred vision. She had a past medical history of ischaemic heart disease and hypertension, for which she took atenolol, aspirin and simvastatin. She had noticed that she had had less energy over the past 3 months, and the headaches started 3 weeks ago. She denied trauma to the head. She smoked 10 cigarettes per day. On direct questioning she admitted to very cold hands.

On examination, she appeared thin and pale. There was no jaundice or lymphadenopathy. Pulse 68/min, BP 155/95. Heart sounds were normal, JVP raised 3 cm. Chest was clear, abdominal examination revealed a palpable spleen, and her left leg was swollen. Tone, power, sensation and reflexes were normal, temporal arteries were pulsatile and non-tender,

and fundoscopy revealed bilateral retinal haemorrhages.

Results
Hb 9.2 g/dL
MCV 84 fl
WCC 3.2 × 10⁹/L
Platelets 104 × 10⁹/L
ESR 190 mm/h
Na 142 mmol/L
K 4.4 mmol/L
Urea 5.9 mmol/L
Creatinine 90 μmol/L
Protein 97 g/L
Albumin 34 g/L
Calcium 2.26 mmol/L
Urinalysis: protein +++, blood −
Protein electrophoresis: monoclonal band, 44 g/L IgM

How will you treat her?
(a) Plasmapheresis
(b) Melphalan
(c) Prednisolone
(d) Rituximab
(e) Prednisolone and cyclophosphamide

QUESTION 147

A 42-year-old woman presents with a tender swollen left leg. She is usually well, save for occasional abdominal pains and headaches. She has also had several episodes of painless haematuria, which her GP is investigating. Past medical history includes an episode of aplastic anaemia 2 years ago, for which she received blood product support but no bone marrow transplant.

On examination, she is apyrexial. No jaundice, anaemia, clubbing or lymphadenopathy. Pulse 75/min, BP 120/70. Cardiovascular and respiratory examination is normal. Abdominal examination reveals a 2-cm liver edge and a 3-cm spleen. Her left leg is swollen to the mid-calf with pitting oedema and venous congestion.

Investigations
Hb 9.6 g/dL
MCV 82 fL
WCC 2.4 × 10⁹/L
Platelets 71 × 10⁹/L
U + Es normal

INR 1.0
APTTR 1.1
Bilirubin 41 μmol/L
ALT 36 U/L
ALP 77 U/L

Which investigation is most likely to confirm the underlying diagnosis?
(a) Flow cytometry with CD59 labelling
(b) Antinuclear antibodies
(c) Bone marrow biopsy
(d) Parvovirus B19 titres
(e) Ultrasound of the abdomen

QUESTION 148

A 28-year-old man, known to inject heroin intravenously, presents with a rash over his lower legs. He had noted that his hands and feet had been tingling recently, which he put down to impurities in his heroin. He had also noted that his joints seemed stiff and sore recently. He had had several hospital admissions with skin abscesses and sepsis, as well as with heroin overdose. He denied cough or sputum production, but admitted to intermittent abdominal pains in between heroin doses.

On examination, he was unkempt and thin. There was no jaundice, clubbing or lymphadenopathy. Heart sounds were normal, chest was clear and peripheral pulses were palpable. Abdominal examination was normal, but a purpuric rash with small ulcers was noted over both lower limbs. Sensation was reduced in his hands and feet, and his knees, hips, ankles, wrists and finger joints were uncomfortable to move, though not swollen or tender. Tone, power and reflexes were normal, as was fundoscopy.

Investigations
Hb 10.3 g/dL
WCC 9.1 × 10⁹/L
Platelets 120 × 10⁹/L
ESR 120 mm/h
Na 133 mmol/L
K 4.7 mmol/L
Urea 14.1 mmol/L
Creatinine 180 μmol/L
Bilirubin 19 μmol/L

ALT 318 U/L
ALP 140 U/L
IgG 4.1 g/L
IgA 2.7 g/L
IgM 0.1 g/L
Rheumatoid factor: strongly positive
Urinalysis shows protein ++++, blood +. No Bence-Jones proteins

Which two investigations would be most likely to confirm his diagnosis?
(a) Echocardiography
(b) Hepatitis B titre
(c) HIV serology
(d) Hepatitis C titre
(e) ANCA
(f) ANA
(g) Cryoglobulins
(h) Abdominal ultrasound
(i) Mesenteric angiogram
(j) Urinary microscopy

QUESTION 149

A 58-year-old woman presented with tiredness, breathlessness and numbness in her feet. Her symptoms had come on gradually over the last year. She had been well for 7 years following a cholecystectomy, which was complicated by an episode of small-bowel obstruction 3 weeks postoperatively which required surgical intervention.

On examination, her temperature was 37.7°C. She looked pale. No icterus or lymphadenopathy was noted. Pulse 80 beats/min reg, BP 130/60 mmHg. Chest was clear, abdomen soft and non-tender. The spleen was just palpable. She had paraesthesia below the knees, absent ankle reflexes and extensor plantar response.

Investigations
Hb 7.4 g/dL
WCC 2.3 × 10⁹/L
Platelets 86 × 10⁹/L
MCV 112 fl
Reticulocytes 1%
Bilirubin 41 μmol/L
ALT 18 U/L
ALP 92 U/L
B₁₂ level 103 pg/L

Which investigation would be most likely to reveal the cause of her B_{12} deficiency?

(a) Upper GI endoscopy
(b) Hydrogen breath test
(c) Schilling test
(d) ^{75}SeCHAT test
(e) Gastric parietal cell antibodies

QUESTION 150

A 74-year-old man presents with symptoms of tiredness and bruising. He has not felt well for several months, but put this down to the fact that he was bereaved 8 months ago. He also suffers from prostatism, irritable-bowel syndrome and hypertension. He takes paroxetine, simvastatin, amlodipine and aspirin. He does not smoke or drink. On direct questioning, he admits to breathlessness on exertion and some indigestion. He denies change in bowel habit or blood in his stools.

On examination, he appears pale. There is no jaundice or lymphadenopathy. Pulse 80 reg, BP 165/80. He has several bruises over his forearms. Chest and heart examination are normal. Abdominal examination reveals no palpable liver, spleen or masses. Neurological examination is normal.

Bloods

Hb 8.0 g/dL
MCV 102 fl
WCC 2.0×10^9/L (neutrophils 50%, lymphocytes 40%, Pelger cells seen)
Platelets 50×10^9/L
Na 141 mmol/L
K 3.6 mmol/L
Urea 9.6 mmol/L
Creatinine 120 µmol/L
Bilirubin 9 µmol/L
ALT 23 U/L
ALP 151 U/L
ESR 21 mm/h
CRP 10 mg/L
Fe 24 µmol/L
Transferrin 2.17 g/L
Transferrin saturations 31%
Ferritin 67 µg/L
B_{12} 491 pg/L
Folate 6.8 µg/L
He declines a bone marrow biopsy

Question 1

What is the best way to treat him?

(a) Blood transfusion
(b) Iron and erythropoietin
(c) Hydroxycarbamide
(d) Upper GI endoscopy
(e) Melphalan

At his follow-up appointment a year later, he complains of sweats and easy bruising. He admits to having lost 13 kg (2 stone) in weight over the last 3 months. His repeat full blood count shows:

Hb 7.2 g/dL
MCV 99.6 fl
WCC 4.0×10^9/L (neutrophils 1.5×10^9/L, eosinophils 0.1×10^9/L, lymphocytes 0.5×10^9/L, monocytes 1.9×10^9/L)
Plts 16×10^9/L

Question 2

What has he developed?

(a) Idiopathic thrombocytopenic purpura
(b) Acute myeloid leukaemia
(c) Chronic myelomonocytic leukaemia
(d) Non-Hodgkin's lymphoma
(e) Folate deficiency

QUESTION 151

A 25-year-old Greek woman presents on routine antenatal screening with the following results:

Hb 11.5 g/dL
WCC 6.3×10^9/L
Platelets 250×10^9/L
MCV 65 fl
MCH 24 pg

She is usually fit and well, although she suffered from rheumatic fever as a child, and had an episode of brucellosis 3 years ago. She does not smoke or drink and takes no medications. She was brought up by her aunt as her parents were killed in a car crash.

On examination, she appears well. There is no jaundice or lymphadenopathy. Pulse 80 regular, BP 105/60. An ejection systolic murmur radiating to the neck is audible. Chest is clear, and abdominal examination reveals suprapubic distension.

Which test is most likely to reveal the cause for her abnormal blood results?
(a) Ferritin
(b) Iron and transferrin
(c) Bone marrow with iron staining
(d) Haemoglobin electrophoresis
(e) *Brucella* titres

QUESTION 152

A 23-year-old woman presents with a pulmonary embolism diagnosed on ventilation/perfusion scanning. She had a previous pulmonary embolism 3 years ago, and was found to have antiphospholipid syndrome. She is otherwise well, and denies rashes, joint pains or headaches. She smokes 20 cigarettes per day and drinks 10 units of alcohol per week. She takes 4 mg warfarin per day and occasional paracetamol.

On examination, she appears thin. She has no rashes, clubbing, cyanosis or lymph nodes. Pulse 95/min, BP 100/60. Oxygen sats 91% on air; respiratory rate 24/min. Chest, heart and abdominal examination are normal. Her admission blood results are as follows:

Hb 12.3 g/dL
WCC 5.1 × 10⁹/L
Platelets 82 × 10⁹/L
ESR 7 mm/h
INR 2.2
APTTR 1.6
ANA negative
VDRL positive
Na 140 mmol/L
K 4.1 mmol/L
Urea 2.3 mmol/L
Creatinine 47 μmol/L

What will you do?
(a) Change her warfarin to nicoumalone, aiming for an INR of 2.5
(b) Add in aspirin to her warfarin
(c) Start long-term low-molecular-weight heparin and discontinue warfarin
(d) Start heparin and raise her INR to > 3
(e) Insert an IVC filter

QUESTION 153

A 30-year-old Asian man returns from a 4-week trip abroad visiting family. Two weeks after arriving

home, he notices a lump on the side of his neck. He presents to his GP who notes that he has lymphadenopathy of the left neck and left axilla. The patient reports feeling somewhat feverish over the last few weeks. He smokes 20 cigarettes per day and has a chronic dry cough, but otherwise has no other medical problems.

On examination, his temperature is 37.8°C. Pulse is 90 regular, BP 115/60. Chest is clear, heart sounds are normal, and abdominal examination is unremarkable. Neurological examination is normal save for a right-sided ptosis.

Initial investigation shows:

Hb 12.0 g/dL
WCC 9.2 × 10⁹/L
Platelets 200 × 10⁹/L
ESR 35 mm/h
Na 135 mmol/L
K 4.0 mmol/L
Urea 8.0 mmol/L
Creatinine 100 μmol/L

The lump is biopsied under local anaesthetic, and histology confirms a high-grade non-Hodgkin's lymphoma, large B-cell type.

What investigation would help to define the prognosis better?
(a) Chest X-ray
(b) Chest CT
(c) Creatinine clearance
(d) Lactate dehydrogenase
(e) Beta-2 microglobulin

QUESTION 154

You are called to see a 47-year-old man on the oncology ward. He was diagnosed with high-grade non-Hodgkin's lymphoma a week ago, and underwent his first cycle of chemotherapy 2 days ago. He complains of feeling shivery, with aching joints and nausea. He denies a cough, sputum production or headache. He is usually fit and well, takes no medication, drinks 10 units of alcohol per week and has never smoked.

On examination, he looks unwell. Temperature 37.5°C, pulse 100 reg, BP 125/60. Rubbery lymph nodes are palpable in both supraclavicular fossae. Heart sounds are normal. Chest is clear, and abdominal examination reveals no organomegaly, masses or tenderness. His fluid chart reveals that he has had 1.2 litres of fluid over the last 12 hours, but has passed only 180 mL of urine.

Bloods
Hb 9.2 g/dL
WCC 4.1×10^9/L
Plts 188×10^9/L
Na 132 mmol/L
K 6.4 mmol/L
Urea 18.5 mmol/L
Creatinine 160 μmol/L
Calcium 1.88 mmol/L
Albumin 34 g/L
CXR: clear lung fields

What will you do next?
(a) Give fast IV fluids
(b) Start broad-spectrum antibiotics
(c) Start allopurinol
(d) Arrange for urgent ultrasound of the kidneys
(e) Give IV bicarbonate

QUESTION 155

A 63-year-old man presents with sudden-onset pain in his back which came on whilst he was opening a window. He complains of no weakness or numbness in his legs; bowel and bladder function are normal. He suffered a myocardial infarction 7 years ago, is known to be hypertensive and stopped smoking 7 years ago. He drinks 30 units of alcohol per week. He takes aspirin, a beta-blocker and a thiazide diuretic. He complains of no respiratory symptoms, but has been feeling tired for the last 3 months.

On examination, he is apyrexial but in some pain. Pulse 60 beats/min reg, BP 140/80 mmHg, JVP not raised, heart sounds are normal. Chest and abdominal examination are normal. There is no neurological deficit in the limbs. Spinal examination reveals marked tenderness at the T6 level.

Investigations
Hb 10.9 g/dL
MCV 86 fl
WCC 13.1×10^9/L
Platelets 423×10^9/L
Na 141 mmol/L
K 3.3 mmol/L
Urea 12.1 mmol/L
Creatinine 151 μmol/L
Calcium 2.81 mmol/L

Albumin 36 g/L
ESR 95 mm/h
CXR normal
Thoracic spine X-rays show a wedge fracture at T6

Which two investigations would best confirm the likely diagnosis?
(a) DEXA scanning
(b) 25-hydroxyvitamin D level
(c) Serum immunoglobulins
(d) Bone marrow biopsy
(e) Skeletal survey
(f) CT chest
(g) Serum ACE level
(h) Serum PTH
(i) Parathyroid MIBG scanning
(j) Bone scan

QUESTION 156

A 77-year-old woman presents with tiredness and breathlessness. She denies weight loss, change in bowel habit or indigestion. She complains of long-standing back and knee pain, for which she takes paracetamol and diclofenac. She does not drink or smoke, and lives alone with her cat. She walks with a stick and receives home help twice a week.

On examination, she appears thin. There are no palpable lymph nodes. She has crepitus and tenderness over both knees. Chest and cardiac examination are normal, and her abdomen is soft, non-tender, with no organomegaly. Her rectum is empty.

Bloods
Hb 9.2 g/dL
WCC 6.5×10^9/L
Plts 301×10^9/L
Na 134 mmol/L
K 4.1 mmol/L
Urea 8.7 mmol/L
Creatinine 147 μmol/L
Calcium 2.45 mmol/L
Albumin 35 g/L
ESR 56 mm/h
Protein electrophoresis: monoclonal IgA band, 2.7 g/L
Urine: negative for Bence–Jones proteins
Spine X-rays: sclerotic changes around L2/3

What will you do next?
(a) Stop diclofenac
(b) Organize a bone marrow biopsy
(c) Request iron studies
(d) Request upper GI endoscopy
(e) Give a trial of prednisolone

QUESTION 157

A 40-year-old man presented with recurrent diarrhoea of some years' duration which had always been treated effectively by the GP with metronidazole and loperamide. Past history revealed chest infections that required considerable absence from school. He had also been seen once by a local surgeon to treat a perianal abscess. He drinks 5 units of alcohol per week, does not smoke, and works as a plumber.

Examination revealed cervical lymphadenopathy, but no jaundice or clubbing. Pulse was 60 regular, BP 120/50. Heart sounds were normal and chest was clear. Abdominal examination revealed a palpable spleen.

Results

Hb 13.5 g/dL
WBC 5.5 × 10⁹/L
Platelets 340 × 10⁹/L
Na 140 mmol/L
K 4.0 mmol/L
Urea 6.5 mmol/L
Creatinine 100 μmol/L
Bilirubin 15 μmol/L
AST 30 U/L
ALP 150 U/L
Albumin 40 g/L
Total protein 61 g/L
Rheumatoid factor negative
HIV test negative
Stool culture negative

What investigation is most likely to clinch the diagnosis?
(a) Upper GI endoscopy and biopsy
(b) Sweat test
(c) Genotyping
(d) Immunoglobulin levels
(e) Lymph node biopsy

QUESTION 158

A 46-year-old woman presents with sudden onset of slurred speech and numbness in her face. She has never had any similar symptoms, and denies a headache prior to the slurring of her speech. She is able to move her arms and legs normally. She takes lisinopril for hypertension, smokes 10 cigarettes per day and drinks 20 units of alcohol per week. She admits to two abortions and two previous miscarriages.

On examination, there are no joint pains, jaundice, clubbing or lymphadenopathy. Pulse is 80 reg, BP 150/85. Heart sounds are normal with no murmurs; chest is clear. A faint purple net-like rash is evident over her arms. Abdominal examination is normal. She is dysarthric with a left-sided facial droop and tongue deviation to the left. Tone, power and sensation are normal in her arms and legs; plantars are downgoing.

Results

Hb 12.6 g/dL
WCC 7.7 × 10⁹/L
Plts 91 × 10⁹/L
Na 139 mmol/L
K 5.1 mmol/L
Urea 4.2 mmol/L
Creatinine 49 μmol/L
Calcium 2.19 mmol/L
Albumin 45 g/L
ESR 15 mm/h
INR 1.1
APTTR 1.6
Anticardiolipin antibody positive

ECG: sinus rhythm, 80/min
Echo: normal LV function; left atrium 3.5 cm, no thrombus seen. No mitral stenosis or regurgitation; no aortic stenosis or regurgitation

MRI of the brain confirms a lacunar infarct

What will you do next?
(a) Start warfarin
(b) Start aspirin and dipyridamole
(c) Request transoesophageal echocardiography
(d) Test for protein C and S
(e) Request Ham's test

QUESTION 159

A 72-year-old man is on treatment for polycythaemia rubra vera. He was diagnosed 6 months ago, at which time he had the following FBC:

Hb 19.5 g/dL
MCV 97 fl
WCC 5.5 × 10^9/L
Plts 590 × 10^9/L
B_{12} 682 pg/L
Folate 7.9 µg/L

He was commenced on hydroxycarbamide, which he takes along with paracetamol, ramipril, aspirin, sodium valproate and indapamide. He also has a history of hypertension and intracerebral haemorrhage, complicated by seizures.

On examination, he appears well, There is no jaundice or lymph nodes, chest and heart examination are normal, and there is no liver or spleen palpable in the abdomen

His repeat FBC shows:

Hb 15.2 g/dL
MCV 127 fl
WCC 4.1 × 10^9/L
Plts 330 × 10^9/L

What will you do?
(a) Check B_{12} levels
(b) Stop hydroxycarbamide
(c) Observe and see in 6 months
(d) Bone marrow biopsy
(e) Check phenytoin levels

QUESTION 160

A 27-year-old man known to have thalassaemia presents with dizziness and palpitations. He denies chest pain but admits to breathlessness on exertion. He receives regular blood transfusions, and takes desferrioxamine. He does not drink or smoke and is unemployed. He denies any cough, sputum production, bowel or urinary symptoms.

On examination, he is mildly jaundiced. Pulse 90 regular, BP 120/60 lying, 100/52 standing. JVP not raised, heart sounds are normal. Chest is clear, and abdominal examination reveals splenomegaly. Tone, power, reflexes, sensation and cranial nerve examination are normal.

Results

Hb 8.9 g/dL
MCV 61 fl
WCC 5.7 × 10^9/L
Plts 206 × 10^9/L
Na 136 mmol/L
K 4.6 mmol/L
Urea 5.0 mmol/L
Creatinine 101 µmol/L
Bilirubin 51 µmol/L
ALT 68 U/L
ALP 301 U/L
Albumin 31 g/L
ECG: left bundle branch block
CXR: clear lung field, normal heart size

What will you do?
(a) Request echocardiography
(b) Transfuse 2 units of blood
(c) Organize upper GI endoscopy
(d) Organize bone marrow biopsy
(e) Refer for splenectomy

QUESTION 161

A 64-year-old man presents to his GP complaining of itchiness. He first noted this 3 months ago; it tends to be worse on warm days. He has not noted a rash at any time. He takes metformin for type 2 diabetes, plus simvastatin, aspirin and ramipril. He also takes senna for long-standing constipation. He does not drink or smoke, and lives with his wife. He has no pets.

On examination, he appears well, with a ruddy complexion. There is no jaundice, cyanosis, clubbing or lymphadenopathy. Chest examination is normal, JVP not raised, heart sounds are normal and there is no ankle oedema. A spleen tip is palpable in the abdomen.

Results

Hb 19.6 g/dL
WCC 11.8 × 10^9/L
Plts 512 × 10^9/L
U + Es normal
LFTs normal
Calcium 2.47 mmol/L
Oxygen saturations 98% on air

341

What test would best confirm the diagnosis?
(a) Bone marrow biopsy
(b) Pulmonary function tests
(c) Red cell mass estimation
(d) Arterial blood gases
(e) Blood film

QUESTION 162

A 76-year-old woman presents with tiredness and breathlessness. She complains of feeling dizzy when she walks up stairs, and her symptoms have been getting slowly worse over the last 4 months. On direct questioning, she admits to some indigestion and has lost 2 kg in weight. She is usually fit and well, takes magnesium hydroxide and temazepam, does not smoke, and drinks 5 units per week of alcohol. She works part-time in the hospital volunteer café.

On examination, she is overweight. There is no jaundice, clubbing or lymphadenopathy. Pulse 80 reg, BP 135/70. Heart sounds are normal with no murmurs, chest is clear, and abdominal examination reveals no liver, spleen or masses. Rectal examination is normal.

Bloods

Hb 7.8 g/dL
MCV 72 fl
WCC 8.1 × 10^9/L
Plts 401 × 10^9/L
Na 143 mmol/L
K 3.9 mmol/L
Urea 5.1 mmol/L
Creatinine 89 µmol/L
LFTs normal
Ferritin 15 µg/L

What will you do next?
(a) Upper GI endoscopy
(b) Colonoscopy
(c) Upper GI endoscopy and colonoscopy
(d) Upper GI endoscopy and barium enema
(e) Trial of iron

QUESTION 163

An 81-year-old man is admitted with breathlessness, cough and sputum production. He gives a 6-month history of fatigue and reduced mobility, to the point where he is housebound

and has needed meals delivered. He has a past medical history of osteoarthritis, perforated duodenal ulcer requiring laparotomy, a myocardial infarction, chronic heart failure with systolic dysfunction, previous depression and a TIA. He takes aspirin, furosemide, ramipril, paroxetine, bisoprolol, co-codamol, senna and simvastatin. He does not drink or smoke, and uses a stick to help him around the house.

On examination, he appears pale. Pulse 90/min, BP 105/50. JVP elevated 3 cm. Heart sounds 1 + 2 with a pansystolic murmur at the apex. Left basal crackles are heard in the chest; his respiratory rate is 28 per minute and his oxygen saturations are 87% on air. Abdominal examination is unremarkable.

Results

Hb 8.2 g/dL
MCV 83 fl
WCC 16.5 × 10^9/L
Plts 491 × 10^9/L
Na 133 mmol/L
K 5.1 mmol/L
Urea 15.3 mmol/L
Creatinine 170 µmol/L
LFTs normal
Albumin 31 g/L
CRP 250 mg/L
CXR: left basal opacification

He receives IV antibiotics, oxygen and has his furosemide stopped. Over the next 5 days, he makes a good recovery. Further investigation of his anaemia reveals:

Iron 9
Transferrin 1.97 g/L
Transferrin saturations 17%
Ferritin 167 µg/L

How will you investigate his anaemia further?
(a) Upper GI endoscopy
(b) Trial of iron
(c) Bone marrow biopsy
(d) Erythropoietin level
(e) Blood film

QUESTION 164

A 23-year-old woman with sickle-cell anaemia presents having collapsed at home. She had had a cold for a couple of days, then developed increasing breathlessness and chest pain prior to admission. She takes no regular medications, does not drink, but smokes 10 cigarettes per day. She works in a supermarket.

On examination, she appears unwell with pale conjunctivae. She is distressed, sweaty and agitated. Pulse 120 reg, BP 90/50. Respiratory rate is 40/min, oxygen saturations 89% on 15 L oxygen. Heart sounds are normal; chest examination reveals bibasal crackles. Abdominal examination reveals a soft, non-tender abdomen.

Bloods

Hb 4.2 g/dL
MCV 82 fl
WCC 19.2 × 10^9/L
Plts 293 × 10^9/L
Na 147 mmol/L
K 4.8 mmol/L
Urea 3.4 mmol/L
Creatinine 53 μmol/L
Bilirubin 41 μmol/L
ALT 33 U/L
ALP 277 U/L
CRP 37 mg/L
CXR: patchy shadowing in the left lower and upper zones

ABGs

pH 7.32
$p\text{CO}_2$ 3.2 kPa
$p\text{O}_2$ 6.5 kPa
Bicarbonate 18 mmol/L
Base excess −6 mmol/L

She receives 100% oxygen, fluids and intravenous opiates. What will you do next?
(a) Arrange for blood transfusion
(b) Arrange for exchange transfusion
(c) Give low-molecular-weight heparin
(d) Start hydroxycarbamide
(e) Give broad-spectrum antibiotics

QUESTION 165

A 34-year-old woman with sickle-cell anaemia presents with a 6-hour history of abdominal pain. The pain came on after dinner and has worsened through the night. She takes the oral contraceptive pill; she does not drink or smoke. She has had no previous abdominal operations. She denies cough, sputum production or

haemoptysis, and has not been on any long journeys.

On examination, she appears unwell with pale conjunctivae. She is uncomfortable. Pulse 110 reg, BP 110/50. Respiratory rate is 28/min, oxygen saturations 96% on 35% oxygen. Heart sounds are normal; chest examination is clear. Abdominal examination reveals moderate right upper quadrant tenderness.

Bloods

Hb 8.2 g/dL
MCV 88 fl
WCC 13.1 × 10^9/L
Plts 293 × 10^9/L
Na 141 mmol/L
K 4.2 mmol/L
Urea 5.0 mmol/L
Creatinine 83 μmol/L
Bilirubin 25 μmol/L
ALT 78 U/L
ALP 257 U/L
CRP 185 mg/L
CXR: clear

What diagnostic test is most likely to confirm the diagnosis?
(a) Ventilation–perfusion lung scan
(b) Ultrasound of the abdomen
(c) Serum amylase
(d) Sickling test
(e) ^{99}Tc liver perfusion scan

QUESTION 166

A 71-year-old woman presents to her GP with low mood. She has been feeling tired and sleeping poorly for several months. She denies breathlessness, cough, sputum production or chest pain, and also denies change in bowel habit, indigestion or urinary symptoms. She admits to losing a couple of kilograms in weight. She has a past medical history of depression, hiatus hernia, hypertension and hypothyroidism. She takes ramipril, thyroxine and aspirin. She does not drink or smoke.

On examination, she is overweight. Pulse 70 regular, BP 165/95. Heart sounds are normal, chest is clear and no lymph nodes are palpable. Abdominal examination is normal with no organomegaly, and neurological examination reveals normal tone, power, reflexes and sensation.

Bloods

Hb 11.7 g/dL

WCC 17.4 × 10⁹/L (neutrophils 5.1 × 10⁹/L, lymphocytes 10.8 × 10⁹/L)

Plts 209 × 10⁹/L

Blood film: preponderance of small lymphocytes

ESR: 39 mm/h

Na 140 mmol/L

K 5.1 mmol/L

Urea 8.1 mmol/L

Creatinine 105 µmol/L

LFTs normal

Calcium 2.40 mmol/L

TSH 3.7 mU/L

Bone marrow confirms monoclonal lymphocytic infiltration with immature lymphocytes

How will you treat her?

(a) High-dose chemotherapy with CHOP

(b) Imantinib

(c) Chlorambucil

(d) Splenectomy

(e) Observe without treatment

ANSWERS TO SELF-ASSESSMENT QUESTIONS

13

QUESTION 1

(c) This is Eisenmenger's syndrome. Mortality rates in pregnancy are high, and thus pregnancy should be avoided.

QUESTION 2

(c) Eisenmenger's presenting in adulthood is usually due to an ASD, and here there is mixing at the atrial level. The high RV pressure points to Eisenmenger's; the low LV saturation suggests that shunting is occurring from right to left as well as left to right. The stroke was probably due either to hyperviscosity (polycythaemia caused by chronic cyanosis is common) or to a paradoxical embolus – there is more to this than a simple patent foramen however.

QUESTION 3

(d) This is infective endocarditis. The large vegetation and severe aortic regurgitation with signs of decompensated heart failure mean that urgent surgical referral is needed.

QUESTION 4

(b), (f) and (h). This is most likely to be infective endocarditis – he has signs of heart failure, a loud murmur and a fever. Vasculitis is another possibility, but blood cultures and echo need doing first given the clinical suspicion of endocarditis. Chest X-ray is needed given his respiratory symptoms regardless of whether you think this is endocarditis or vasculitis.

QUESTION 5

(e) He has severe AS, but is genuinely asymptomatic. A positive exercise test would be evidence in favour of selecting aortic valve replacement.

QUESTION 6

(c) He has mitral valve prolapse with mitral regurgitation, thus he is at high risk for endocarditis. Antibiotic prophylaxis differs between upper- and lower-body procedures. IV antibiotics are usually used for lower GI procedures – he is also penicillin-allergic.

QUESTION 7

(d) The catheter data show a step-up in oxygen saturation in the RA compared to the SVC. The timing of onset suggests that a secundum defect is more likely; atrial fibrillation could have precipitated his symptoms.

QUESTION 8

(d) The suspicion is that this lesion is an atrial myxoma. This requires urgent resection – referral for investigation at a cardiothoracic centre is probably the quickest way forward, although further imaging is probably needed.

QUESTION 9

(e) is probably the safest. He has features of HCM, but he also has Wolff–Parkinson–White syndrome. It is possible that his blackouts are due to AF conducted via an accessory pathway; verapamil may worsen this. Atenolol is contraindicated because of his asthma.

QUESTION 10

(a) The likely diagnosis is rheumatic fever – she has clinical evidence of carditis and arthritis (two major criteria) – all you lack is evidence of a streptococcal infection. Infective endocarditis is a possible alternative diagnosis, but considerably more evidence is required to confirm the diagnosis.

QUESTION 11

1 (c)

2 (a)

Isolated BHL in the absence of other nodal involvement, particularly the para-aortic nodes, makes sarcoidosis the most likely cause of this presentation. A sarcoid-like reaction can also occur in people who have been treated with chemotherapy in the past; it is however less common than sarcoid, particularly if extrapulmonary features are present. The patient is asymptomatic and therefore requires no immunosuppressive treatment at present but requires to be kept under surveillance with outpatient follow-up.

The following are the common indications for treatment in sarcoidosis:

Increasing symptoms, worsening CXR and PFTs
Cardiac and neurosarcoid
Sight-threatening ocular sarcoid
Hypercalcaemia
Lupus pernio
Splenic, hepatic and renal sarcoid

QUESTION 12

(d) There is evidence of neurosarcoidosis and therefore immunosuppressive treatment is indicated. This prednisolone regime is the commonest first-line option in clinical practice.

QUESTION 13

(c) This illustrates likely cystic fibrosis presenting in an adult with bronchiectasis.

QUESTION 14

(e) This illustrates a non-compliant CF patient who is probably not taking his pancreatin enzyme supplements to replace the exocrine function of the pancreas and subsequently suffers the complications of chronic pancreatitis.

QUESTION 15

1 (a)
2 (b)
Hypercalcaemia and hypophosphataemia in the setting of parathormone-related peptide secretion from squamous cell carcinoma. He needs urgent investigation for staging and tissue type and a staging CT chest is the most useful from the listed options.

QUESTION 16

1 (c)
2 (c)
This woman has bilateral community-acquired pneumonia, probably secondary to *Legionella pneumophila* in view of the severity, deranged liver enzymes, diarrhoea and return from holiday She requires a macrolide and co-amoxiclav or third-generation cephalosporin intravenously.

QUESTION 17

(b) This man has increasing breathlessness, a CXR that is non-diagnostic, fever and is on immunosuppression. PCP is high on the differential diagnosis list despite prophylactic Septrin and negative-induced sputum. Transbronchial biopsy might also clinch the diagnosis but pneumothorax risk is significant, particularly if there is underlying *Pneumocystis*.

QUESTION 18

(d) Basal emphysema in this young smoker probably indicates proteolytic imbalance secondary to alpha-1-antitrypsin deficiency.

QUESTION 19

1 (b)
2 (e)
Difficult question! In the absence of AFB from the sputum (only 30% diagnostic) and no associated B-symptoms, one would imagine the most likely scenario is *Aspergillus* filling an old TB cavity in the lung. The most useful steps in her management would be diagnostic bronchoscopy (fungal hyphae and AFB) and possibly therapeutic bronchoscopy or angiography and embolization if haemoptysis not settling.

QUESTION 20

1 (d)
2 (b)
This patient has many features suggestive of underlying obstructive sleep apnoea syndrome. There are lots of fancy tests available but in cases similar to this, one should always start with more basic investigations, namely overnight pulse oximetry, which is often diagnostic.

Heavy-goods vehicle licence-holders are one of the 'favoured' occupations as this job attracts many interesting issues and dilemmas. In this case the diagnosis has not been confirmed as yet and therefore general advice should suffice and an attempt at expediting further diagnostic tests should be attempted.

QUESTION 21

(c) This is a case of life-threatening hypersensitivity pneumonitis secondary to toluene diisocyanate paints. A facemask trial might be useful in normal circumstances but as this man's reaction was severe and life-threatening he should probably avoid painting as an occupation in view of the likelihood of recurrent exposure and relapse of the condition.

QUESTION 22

1 (d)

2 (b)

Clubbing in COPD patients is lung carcinoma until proven otherwise.

QUESTION 23

1 (d)

2 (b)

Clinical, CXR and HRCT features are very suggestive of a diagnosis of LCH in this smoker. Steroid therapy has not been shown to benefit this group of patients.

QUESTION 24

1 (c)

2 (e)

Lymphangioleiomyomatosis (LAM) is the most likely diagnosis in this middle-aged female with progressive breathlessness, no other features of asthma, hormonal disturbance and a retroperitoneal mass. High-resolution CT will show the typical features of the disease which is likely to involve all parts of the lung when compared to Langerhans-cell histiocytosis, which usually spares the bases.

QUESTION 25

(d), (f) and (g) He is dehydrated (large postural drop), and thus requires fluid. Given his low sodium and ascites, albumin would probably be the best fluid to give. The ascites suggests spontaneous bacterial peritonitis as a diagnosis; antibiotics are needed. He is encephalopathic;

bowel decontamination is indicated. Diazepam will worsen the encephalopathy. A central line and FFP may be required later; vitamin K should be tried first though. Increasing the spironolactone will worsen the dehydration and renal failure; giving IV potassium is a better solution to the low K.

QUESTION 26

(e) and (g) He has a high chance of having a variceal bleed, and thus needs early endoscopy. Terlipressin will reduce splanchnic blood flow and may thus reduce bleeding. FFP may not be necessary – you need to know his clotting first. Urinary catheter and central line will not help resuscitate him acutely, and an ascitic tap is also of lower priority. Vitamin K does need to be given as he is jaundiced, but this will take several hours to work. A Sengstaken tube will only be necessary if endoscopy cannot control the bleeding, or if he bleeds catastrophically before endoscopy can be arranged. Diazepam may be necessary to combat alcohol withdrawal, but may also further lower the blood pressure. Fluid resuscitation should be performed first. A nasogastric tube is not necessary and theoretically risks dislodging adherent clot on any varices.

QUESTION 27

(e) This is probably type 2 (proximal) renal tubular acidosis; although a raised urine bicarbonate and urine pH > 5.3 would be needed to confirm the diagnosis. The low potassium and glycosuria would fit with the diagnosis, and Wilson's disease is a known cause. Penicillamine usually causes proteinuria, which is absent in this case; it should not therefore be stopped. Although pregnancy can cause glycosuria, it does not usually cause low bicarbonate and low potassium.

QUESTION 28
Question 1

(b) and (d) Her albumin and clotting are normal; this is likely to be a variceal bleed, however, and thus terlipressin may be helpful in addition to rapid blood transfusion. A Sengstaken tube would only be needed if endoscopy was delayed and bleeding was so catastrophic that other measures had failed.

Question 2

(a) The high alkaline phosphatase, together with the female sex and low alcohol intake, suggest a diagnosis of PBC. Liver biopsy could also be used but is invasive and probably not necessary to make the diagnosis in this case.

QUESTION 29

(a) His history is suggestive of chronic pancreatitis, and his faecal fat collection confirms malabsorption. In this case, a pancreolauryl test is unlikely to add much; CT of the pancreas will show calcification and pseudocysts, and may show ductal dilatation.

QUESTION 30
Question 1

(b) This is acute Budd–Chiari syndrome (hepatic vein occlusion). This is often well shown on Doppler ultrasound, although venography may be required in some cases.

Question 2

(c) This would explain her prolonged APTTR and low platelets, as well as her Budd–Chiari and previous DVT. There is nothing else in favour of malignancy, and polycythaemia rubra vera is unlikely given the young age and only marginally elevated haemoglobin. Hepatic venous web is a possible cause, but is less likely given the other features.

QUESTION 31

(c) He may well have bacterial overgrowth – his anaemia is consistent with B_{12} deficiency, and his weight loss could be explained by malabsorption. The watery diarrhoea is often a feature. The diagnosis of Crohn's has already been made; thus a barium followthrough would only be useful to look for fistulae. Upper GI endoscopy is another possible investigation, but you are not given the option of jejunal aspiration in the question, which would be the most useful procedure to perform at endoscopy. It is unlikely

that massive bowel resection is to blame from the history, and the terminal ileum has been preserved. The low CRP militates against fulminant active Crohn's, as does the length of the history.

QUESTION 32

(a) The strongly positive ANA titre and high ESR points to autoimmune hepatitis, which can occasionally be fulminant in nature. There is no history to support mushroom poisoning or Weil's disease. Paracetamol poisoning is possible if the paracetamol was taken several days ago, but there is an alternative diagnosis here. Even fulminant hepatitis B infection is accompanied by positive serology in 95% of cases; a few patients clear the antigen very fast, but later develop antibodies against the virus.

QUESTION 33

(b) She has severe disease affecting extensive section of bowel as well as having a fistula. She has not responded to immunosuppression. She is therefore a candidate for infliximab. Surgery would be less appropriate – she is in poor health and has diffuse disease. She has already had extensive resection of small bowel – further extensive resection would run the risk of short-bowel syndrome.

QUESTION 34

(d) She almost certainly has primary biliary cirrhosis – although a biopsy would be needed to confirm the diagnosis fully. Her bilirubin, albumin and INR are normal, suggesting no liver failure and relatively early disease. As such, she does not require workup for transplantation yet. Ursodeoxycholic acid may slow down the disease process as well as improving symptoms and biochemistry.

QUESTION 35

(d) CT with contrast probably has the highest sensitivity and specificity for hepatocellular carcinoma, which is the likely diagnosis here. Ultrasound is less sensitive for small lesions, and FNA risks seeding along the needle track;

cytology alone without information about the architecture of the nodule may not be enough to make the diagnosis.

QUESTION 36

(b) He has pneumococcal septicaemia because of hyposplenism, as shown by the Howell–Jolly bodies. His coeliac disease is the aetiological agent for this. Lymphoma is possible, but there is no supporting evidence for this; similarly, there is no supporting evidence for HIV, and pneumococcal infection is not of itself an AIDS-defining illness. Long-term prophylactic penicillin, and vaccination against pneumococcus, *Haemophilus* and meningococcus are required.

QUESTION 37

(b) She has a recurrence of her autoimmune hepatitis, which is common on stopping steroids. Steroids should be first-line treatment, with a steroid-sparing agent (azathioprine or ciclosporin) added in once the disease is coming under control.

QUESTION 38

(b) Transferrin saturation would be the best first-line test, with genotyping being used as a confirmatory test. Genotyping alone for haemochromatosis would not confirm that iron overload was present and the cause of the symptoms.

QUESTION 39

(c) She has evidence of both iron and folate deficiency; duodenal biopsy is needed to exclude or diagnose coeliac disease, which would explain her symptoms and weight loss. Lower GI endoscopy may be needed if this investigation is negative.

QUESTION 40

(c) He has an exacerbation of his UC – he falls into the moderate category of severity and therefore does not require IV steroids. A course of oral steroids is required, probably with Predfoam enemas as well.

QUESTION 41

(b) This is likely to be primary sclerosing cholangitis. The intermittent pain and jaundice suggest the diagnosis; his UC is quiescent, making pericholangitis less likely. The lack of findings on ultrasound does not rule out the diagnosis.

QUESTION 42

(c) He has two factors precluding surgery – a hoarse voice, suggesting recurrent laryngeal nerve invasion, and distant lymph nodes. Biopsy of the lymph nodes is unlikely to alter the fact that surgery is precluded. Chemotherapy alone is of little use in oesophageal cancer, and a stent will at least relieve his dysphagia.

QUESTION 43

(b) You do not know the time between ingestion and presentation, but she has a significant level of paracetamol in her blood stream and would probably benefit from *N*-acetylcysteine – especially as the presence of enzyme-inducing antiepileptic medications will increase her risk. She may well have taken something else in addition to paracetamol to explain her drowsiness; supportive care will be needed, and further toxicology may occasionally be useful.

QUESTION 44

(b) It is unlikely that he has sustained severe liver damage – the INR can be raised by paracetamol without liver damage. Nevertheless, repeating the blood tests in 24 hours would ensure that the INR and ALT are returning to normal. He does not meet criteria for liver transplant, and it is too late for *N*-acetylcysteine to have any effect unless fulminant hepatic failure is in progress.

QUESTION 45

(c) She has a severe salicylate overdose – the levels are very high, she has a reduced conscious level, signs of pulmonary oedema and a severe metabolic acidosis. She requires dialysis.

QUESTION 46

(d) His normal pupils argue against a significant tricyclic overdose. Methanol and ethylene glycol would produce a much larger osmolar gap than seen here; he has no ketones or elevated blood glucose to substantiate the diagnosis of diabetic ketoacidosis.

QUESTION 47

(a) The tachycardia, hypotension and dilated pupils with a low GCS all fit with a tricylic overdose. Codeine would give small pupils; paroxetine is much less toxic than tricyclics, and benzodiazepines do not tend to dilate the pupils or produce an acidosis.

QUESTION 48

(c) He has severe tricyclic poisoning, as denoted by seizures, acidosis and ventricular arrhythmias. Sodium loading will help block the effect of tricyclics on sodium channels, and alkalinizing the blood will increase binding of tricyclics to proteins, thus reducing the amount of free tricyclic. Antiarrhythmics can be used (not class 1a or 1c agents) in refractory cases. Haemodialysis is ineffective.

QUESTION 49

Question 1

(e) Starting erythromycin has probably led to an increase in his digoxin level, which has produced nausea, bradycardia and a predisposition to ventricular arrthymias.

Question 2

(d) His potassium is within the normal range – further potassium may be dangerous. He has had a collapse, probably due to either VT or to heart block, plus documented VT on the monitor. This is probably enough to merit giving digoxin antibodies. DC cardioversion may lead to asystole, and although antiarrhythmics can be used, amiodarone is likely to delay metabolism of digoxin.

QUESTION 50

(d) The lack of focal signs and meningism are points against subarachnoid haemorrhage and encephalitis. They also do not explain the breathlessness and acidosis. Do not be fooled by the normal oxygen levels.

QUESTION 51

(e) Although she has a persistent headache, there are no neurological features to suggest an intracranial lesion. The symptoms coincide with a change of house – chronic carbon monoxide poisoning could explain all of her symptoms. If this is negative, brain scanning would be the next step.

QUESTION 52

(b) and (f). This is ethylene glycol poisoning. The severe acidosis, signs of pulmonary oedema, renal impairment and hypocalcaemia all fit with the diagnosis. Ethanol stops further metabolism of ethylene glycol to the toxic glycolic acid (which precipitates with calcium in the kidneys); haemodialysis can remove the ethylene glycol.

QUESTION 53

(a) The peripheral motor neuropathy, porphyrins and abdominal pain would fit with chronic lead poisoning – probably from stripping old paint. There is no rash or respiratory symptoms to go along with Churg–Strauss, which does not give rise to elevated porphyrin levels. Acute intermittent porphyria does not produce urinary coproporphyrins; although hereditary coproporphyria does, this is extremely rare and usually produces skin manifestations.

QUESTION 54

(c) His symptoms are typical of a nerve agent attack. Atropine and pralidoxime are the standard treatment for this – diazepam can also be added. Dicobalt edetate is a treatment for cyanide poisoning.

QUESTION 55

(b) He has several features of pesticide poisoning – bradycardia, hypoxia due to pulmonary oedema, loss of bowel control and excessive sweating. Plasma or erythrocyte cholinesterase can be measured and should be greatly reduced; treatment should not of course be delayed until this result is available!

QUESTION 56
Question 1
(e) His cerebellar signs are consistent with phenytoin toxicity – the duration of the symptoms is short and coincides with starting cimetidine, which may increase phenytoin levels. He does not have ophthalmoplegia, but Wernicke's is still worth considering here.

Question 2
(c) Toxicity is still possible with a normal-range phenytoin level – reduced protein binding can lead to elevated free phenytoin levels which are toxic. The best course of action is to stop the drug for a few days and see if clinical improvement occurs. If it does, the drug could be reintroduced at a lower dose. Halving the dose or changing to another medication is likely to muddy the waters and make the diagnosis less clear.

QUESTION 57
(d) She has a very high lithium level, with signs of severe toxicity. Haemodialysis is therefore the treatment of choice. Activated charcoal is not beneficial in lithium toxicity.

QUESTION 58
(a) He has hyperpyrexia, DIC, rhabdomyolysis and hyponatraemia, a constellation best explained by ecstasy overdose. Serotonin syndrome could also explain many of the features, but there is no history of depression or SSRI use to point in this direction.

QUESTION 59
(b) The picture is consistent with alcohol withdrawal, as is the timing. There are few clues to alcohol use here save for a low urea and low platelets, but the picture is not consistent with opiate overdose, and she does not meet the diagnostic criteria for thyroid storm. Haloperidol will lower the threshold for fits in alcohol withdrawal.

QUESTION 60
(d) Although his clinical state may be due to alcohol, the upgoing plantar is suspicious – CT scanning is therefore needed to look for intracranial bleeding. His GCS is very low and he has vomited; his airway needs to be secured as a first step before any further investigation.

QUESTION 61
1 (d)
2 (d)
The blood film picture coupled with the illustrated clinical features, which include neurological deficit, and the blood tests are suggestive of TTP. Platelet transfusion would be hazardous in this condition.

QUESTION 62
(e) This man has nephrotic syndrome from AA amyloid deposition. Trial of high-dose steroids can be useful in improving his proteinuria and reducing his symptoms. The suspicion has to be that his TB is the underlying driver for AA amyloid deposition, and thus antituberculous therapy is probably needed – especially if a trial of steroids is planned.

QUESTION 63
1 (c)
2 (b)
This woman has metastatic renal cell carcinoma. Resection is often advocated for palliative purposes in patients who can undergo surgery. Interferon-alpha can improve tumour regression. IL-2 can be used in those whose interferon-alpha therapy was unsuccessful.

QUESTION 64
1 (a)
2 (d)
She has a normal anion gap. Type 3 is exceedingly rare; hypokalaemia excludes type 4 and the raised urinary calcium supports type 1 and underlying osteomalacia.

QUESTION 65
1 (e)
2 (a)
White male, smoker with renal failure and pulmonary haemorrhage is likely to be suffering from one of the pulmonary renal syndromes. The likelihood of a positive ANCA or anti-GBM

antibody is high and would help support the diagnosis and initiate treatment. The CXR appearance is likely due to alveolar haemorrhage and a raised Kco would support this.

QUESTION 66

(b) This is likely to be SLE with antiphospholipid syndrome causing her DVT. Pointers to the diagnosis include arthralgia, renal impairment and pancytopenia – which would fit less well with endocarditis. PNH is a possibility but the renal impairment and proteinuria are less well explained by this.

QUESTION 67

(b) and (e). You have enough evidence to diagnose dermatomyositis – she has typical clinical features plus EMG evidence. Inflammation can be patchy and missed on biopsy. Prednisolone is the treatment of choice. Given her normal examination (including breast exam) and non-smoking status, further investigation for malignancy is probably not warranted unless new symptoms occur.

QUESTION 68

(d) She has an inflammatory process in her lungs – the severity and magnitude are suspicious for infection, rather than a rheumatoid-related process. She is immunosuppressed – *Pneumocystis* is therefore a possible diagnosis, and BAL is required to make the diagnosis.

QUESTION 69

(b) This is a scleroderma renal crisis. She requires dialysis as she is in established acute renal failure, but ACE inhibitors are needed to treat the underlying hypertensive process as it is driven by overactivity of the renin–angiotensin system in scleroderma.

QUESTION 70

(a) and (b) Lung biopsy is more likely to give a definitive histological diagnosis than renal biopsy in Wegener's granulomatosis. Having said this, it is more invasive and renal biopsy is more commonly performed in clinical practice.

QUESTION 71

(b) and (c) Oral ulcers, genital ulcers and uveitis suggest Behçet's disease given her ethnic background. Her TIA-like symptoms make this much more likely than Crohn's. The pathergy test would help to confirm the diagnosis. She probably requires steroids as she has neurological and eye involvement, but azathioprine can be used as a steroid-sparing agent. Thalidomide is effective against Behçet's ulcers, but given her sex and age, it would be contraindicated in case of pregnancy. Interferon-alpha, not beta, has been used to treat Behçet's.

QUESTION 72

(d) This is polyarteritis nodosa. High-dose steroids are needed, and he may need cyclophosphamide as well (not methotrexate). Hepatitis B (not C) is associated with the disease, and a positive hepatitis B test would be an indication to add in antivirals and consider plasmapheresis.

QUESTION 73

(b) and (g) He has a pulmonary-renal syndrome, and the rash is also suggestive of vasculitis. Wegener's, Churg–Strauss, microscopic polyarteritis and Goodpasture's are all likely possibilities here. Renal biopsy is likely to show glomerulonephritis, probably crescentic, but may not give the underlying cause.

QUESTION 74

(a) He has a number of features of Churg–Strauss disease, including an eosinophilia. Lung biopsy gives the most characteristic findings to confirm the diagnosis, but renal biopsy is an alternative. CT would add little – a tissue diagnosis is what is needed here.

QUESTION 75

(c) His pain may not be attributable to osteoarthritis, but it does not sound like PMR. Paget's is a distinct possibility given the raised ALP – a bone scan would help to confirm the diagnosis prior to starting bisphosphonates.

QUESTION 76

(b) and (d) Her clinical picture would certainly fit with giant cell arteritis (the headache makes this more likely than PMR). High-dose steroids are therefore required. Her lack of response to steroids is worrying – even though the dose is suboptimal – and a malignancy needs to be looked for. Myeloma is one possibility, and a liver ultrasound is also worthwhile in view of the raised ALP.

QUESTION 77

(c) He is having a relapse, as evidenced by his inflammatory markers, proteinase 3 titre and symptoms. Steroids and cyclophosphamide are needed to control this; co-trimoxazole can be used to reduce the frequency of relapses.

QUESTION 78

(a) You need to exclude septic arthritis in this woman. Patients with RA are at increased risk of septic arthritis, and her presentation requires that microscopy and culture take place before considering joint injection.

QUESTION 79

(c) Bosentan improves symptoms and exercise capacity in pulmonary hypertension, and may improve survival as well. There is no evidence of thromboembolic disease reported on her catheterization to suggest that warfarin is needed.

QUESTION 80

(b) She has had an ischaemic stroke, and although her inflammatory markers are raised, her CSF does not support a diagnosis of cerebral lupus. She does however have a murmur, and endocarditis (e.g. Libman–Sacks) is a possibility.

QUESTION 81

(b) Peripheral joint inflammation is the main problem here – sulfasalazine is effective for this in ankylosing spondylitis. Infliximab would be more appropriate if he had sacroiliitis not responding to other agents, including NSAIDs.

QUESTION 82

(e) He has a markedly obstructive set of PFTs. His lung volumes are not severely reduced, despite his kyphosis and fibrotic changes, suggesting that their effect is mild. He has only mild to moderate aortic regurgitation, without LV dilatation or loss of function.

QUESTION 83

(b) She has several features of Addison's – a postural drop, high potassium, low sodium and low glucose. The short Synacthen test is the best way to test for this.

QUESTION 84

(a) He has an adrenal crisis brought on by sudden steroid withdrawal – he may have a flare of Crohn's or obstruction that has precipitated the vomiting however. The priority is to resuscitate – IV steroid plus saline – then investigate with films. A random cortisol taken before giving steroid is often enough to confirm the diagnosis in acutely unwell individuals as it should show a high cortisol level; normal or low levels strongly suggest adrenocortical insufficiency. An alternative is to use dexamethasone, then perform a short Synacthen test.

QUESTION 85

(d) and (e) Her symptoms strongly suggest carcinoid syndrome. 5-HIAA levels will help confirm the diagnosis; CT will allow the presence of hepatic metastases and maybe the primary tumour to be localized. Echo will confirm right-sided valve involvement, but will not directly confirm the diagnosis of carcinoid.

QUESTION 86

(a) Octreotide relieves symptoms in up to 70% of patients with carcinoid syndrome. Chemotherapy is of little value; ^{131}I-MIBG therapy works in some tumours, but is not widely available. Given her relatively severe heart failure, her life expectancy is limited, and palliation is the focus. If octreotide fails to control the symptoms, other treatment modalities (interferon, embolization) could be considered.

QUESTION 87

(a) She has familial hypocalciuric hypercalcaemia – although her PTH is inappropriately high and her calcium is elevated, her urinary calcium level is much lower than would be expected in primary hyperparathyroidism. The disorder is asymptomatic and does not respond to parathyroidectomy.

QUESTION 88

(b) Although her PTH is slightly raised, this was taken at a time when her calcium level had fallen precipitously – thus triggering PTH release. She may not therefore have primary hyperparathyroidism, and the weight loss is worrying. Bone scanning is not affected by bisphosphonates, and is probably a useful first step in looking for malignancy. If her calcium level stabilizes but remains elevated, the PTH could be repeated to see if it is raised or suppressed.

QUESTION 89

(c) Her phenotype plus low calcium and elevated PTH strongly suggests pseudohypoparathyroidism, which can be confirmed by the Chase–Auerbach test. The Muller–Herzog test is fictional!

QUESTION 90
Question 1

(d) This man has acute intermittent porphyria. Morphine, pethidine and prochlorperazine are all safe to use; metoclopramide is not. Morphine is a better analgesic than pethidine; paracetamol is inadequate for this man's severe pain.

Question 2

(b) and (c) His acute intermittent porphyria requires treatment with haem arginate to shut off porphyrin synthesis – calories provided by intravenous dextrose will also help do this. He does not require surgery – this is likely to kill him.

QUESTION 91

(a) She has features of lung cancer and features that suggest Cushing's syndrome. A 24-hour urinary cortisol would be the first step in confirming the diagnosis of Cushing's – if there was doubt, a low-dose dexamethasone suppression test could be used. Although a bronchoscopy may well be needed, a chest X-ray might be a better first investigation for lung cancer!

QUESTION 92

(b) The high ACTH and suppressibility on high-dose dexamethasone testing suggest a pituitary origin for her Cushing's. MRI is needed to confirm the presence of a microadenoma; if surgery is planned, metyrapone can be given to block the effects of cortisol and improve blood pressure and wound healing prior to surgery.

QUESTION 93

(e) The likely diagnosis is diabetes insipidus – probably cranial due to head trauma 2 years ago. A water deprivation test will confirm the diagnosis; a response to DDAVP will confirm the cranial form of the condition.

QUESTION 94

(d) She starts the test with a low plasma osmolality, suggesting that she has drunk enough to dilute her plasma. As the test goes on, she is able to concentrate her urine, and does not lose very much weight (< 1 kg). Her results therefore suggest psychogenic polydipsia, not diabetes insipidus.

QUESTION 95
Question 1

(a) Her low calcium and raised alkaline phosphatase, along with the history, suggest osteomalacia – probably due to a combination of being house-bound, renal impairment and being on phenytoin.

Question 2

(c) Her calculated creatinine clearance is only 19 mL/min, which necessitates giving activated (1,25-hydroxy)vitamin D. Her PTH is elevated because of secondary hyperparathyroidism – she does not require parathyroidectomy.

QUESTION 96

(d) He has significant renal impairment and heart failure, thus metformin is relatively contraindicated. Similarly, the heart failure is a contraindication for glitazones. He therefore will require insulin. A dietetic review would be a useful adjunct, but is unlikely to be enough on its own.

QUESTION 97

(d) She is still producing a lot of ketones with consequent persisting acidosis. She therefore needs more insulin to switch off ketogenesis. In order to do this without becoming hypoglycaemic, she needs 10% dextrose. Lactate estimation is probably not necessary; she is improving slowly, there is little to suggest a serious underlying pathology, and the ketones in the urine explain the persisting acidosis.

QUESTION 98

(c) and (e) Her symptoms, plus the result of her fasting test, strongly suggest an insulinoma – CT of the pancreas is therefore required. The high calcium and highly active parathyroids suggest parathyroid hyperplasia. This combination suggests MEN type 1. Phaeochromocytoma and medullary thyroid carcinoma occur in type 2, not type 1 MEN. Prolactinoma is also common in MEN 1 and is screened for on a regular basis; prolactin levels would therefore be more useful than PTH, which would only serve to confirm the diagnosis of parathyroid overactivity. MRI pituitary is only needed if symptoms suggest an adenoma, or prolactin or growth hormone levels are elevated. There are no symptoms to suggest carcinoid.

QUESTION 99

(c) She has Addison's and diabetes mellitus; her macrocytic anaemia and slow pulse could well be due to hypothyroidism – making the diagnosis of APS type 2. It would be unusual to present with APS type 1 at such a late age; thus hypoparathyroidism is less likely.

QUESTION 100

(b) Addison's disease commonly presents by age 15 in patients with APS type 1 – this is the most dangerous condition to miss, and most guidelines recommend annual screening for this. Hyperthyroidism is not associated with APS type 1, thus thyroid peroxidase antibodies are not indicated. A full blood count is a better screen for pernicious anaemia, and glucose dipstick can be used to screen for diabetes.

QUESTION 101

(e) The administration of steroids has allowed him to excrete a water load – and unmasked his cranial diabetes insipidus. He has therefore passed a large amount of free water, producing dehydration and high sodium. Dextrose will replace the lost free water, and DDAVP will replace the missing vasopressin.

QUESTION 102

(d) He requires pituitary stress testing to see what other hormone deficiencies he has. His thyroid functions suggest pituitary disease; an inappropriately low TSH level for the thyroxine level, and his loss of hair suggests testosterone deficiency. He may have a lack of ACTH as well – this may be masked by low thyroxine levels, but starting thyroxine in this situation could lead to a pituitary crisis brought on by ACTH deficiency.

QUESTION 103

(d) He does not have acromegaly – his growth hormone level suppresses normally with a glucose load. He does have diabetes however; and his hypertension and diabetes would both be helped by losing some weight.

QUESTION 104

(d) Although she has significant comorbid disease, pituitary surgery offers her the best chance of cure – this will also help her diabetes and hypertension. If she declines surgery, radiotherapy or medical therapy could be used. Her organomegaly is almost certainly due to her acromegaly – especially given normal renal and liver function.

QUESTION 105

(d) She is suffering from thyroid storm – probably triggered by a chest infection on a background of not taking carbimazole. Fluids, beta-blockers and steroids are needed, plus propylthiouracil. This is then followed by Lugol's iodine. You should not wait for thyroid function tests before treating – delay may be fatal.

QUESTION 106

(b) Her symptoms are well controlled, and her T_4 is in the normal range. TSH often stays suppressed and is not a guide to the adequacy of treatment. There is no need for surgery or radioiodine at present; they may be needed if she relapses off therapy or does not wish to continue taking medication long-term.

QUESTION 107

(a) The clinical diagnosis is Klinefelter's syndrome; the small testes and tall stature are pointers. A pituitary tumour is less likely as the history is very long.

QUESTION 108

(a) She has a high creatinine, and may have a congenital renal malformation. Ultrasound, followed by further renal imaging, especially of the collecting system, is needed. There are no clinical signs of coarctation – investigation may be needed if her hypertension does not respond to weight reduction and antihypertensives. She does not need a glucose tolerance test, as her random glucose is normal.

QUESTION 109

(a) This is most likely to be a chronic subdural haematoma, which should show up on CT. Even if you wish to perform a lumbar puncture, CT is necessary first in this man as he has focal neurology and a reduced GCS.

QUESTION 110

(a) Her subdural haematomas are too small to evacuate; stopping aspirin may prevent them from getting bigger. MRI is unlikely to add to the diagnosis, and given her frailty, it is unlikely that neurosurgery would be an option even if the haematomas increased in size. Rescanning is therefore unlikely to change management.

QUESTION 111

(b) Large lungs with reduced Kco, together with a phaeochromocytoma, suggest neurofibromatosis – probably type 1. Although acoustic neuromas most often occur in type 2 NF, her sensorineural hearing loss suggests that an acoustic neuroma may be present; MRI would be the best way of diagnosing this.

QUESTION 112

(d) She has benign intracranial hypertension. Weight loss has proven effects in this condition; steroids can be used but may worsen weight gain. Loop diuretics, not thiazides, are usually used (acetazolamide is an alternative). Nalidixic acid is an antibiotic associated with the development of benign intracranial hypertension. Repeated LP is of little value, although shunting is of benefit.

QUESTION 113

(a) Although this may be benign intracranial hypertension, the history of previous DVT increases the chance that it is due to sagittal sinus thrombosis, which is more easily seen on MRI. This is probably the best initial investigation.

QUESTION 114

(b) He has myotonia, plus a number of other features (diabetes, cardiac conduction defects) that fit with myotonic dystrophy. An EMG will show repetitive firing on voluntary contraction; muscle biopsy is less specific; the gene defect can now be tested for.

QUESTION 115
Question 1

(a) He has features of normal-pressure hydrocephalus – a CT will show this. The CT will also show other differentials, such as a brain tumour, stroke or subdural haematoma.

Question 2

(e) Although he has hydrocephalus, and his CSF pressure is normal, there is no indication for shunting unless he improves functionally after removal of CSF at lumbar puncture.

357

QUESTION 116

(c) She has advanced disease and a pneumonia, but her MSQ suggests that her cognition is intact. In this circumstance, you must assume that she is competent to decide what treatment she accepts, and if she declines treatment you should not give it. If you believe that she lacks the capacity to make such a decision, legal advice and advice from a medical defence organization should be sought.

QUESTION 117

(c) There are symptoms and signs of bulbar palsy, but no limb features. Nevertheless, EMG may still be positive in clinically normal muscle in motor neurone disease. MRI spine is less helpful as the features are confined to cranial nerves.

QUESTION 118

(d) A COMT inhibitor would prolong the effect of each dose without increasing the overall dose of L-dopa. The chance of dyskinesia would therefore be minimized. Closer spacing of doses is another possible strategy; giving slow release at each dose would probably not work as the time to effect would be too long.

QUESTION 119

(a) Although she may have a mild degree of bradykinesia and a resting tremor, they are clearly not bothering her. As the aim of treatment in Parkinson's disease is to alleviate symptoms, there are no compelling reasons to start therapy straight away.

QUESTION 120

(c) She has a myasthenic crisis, triggered by the gentamicin. Plasmapheresis is an effective short-term treatment for this; steroids may worsen myasthenia gravis in the short term.

QUESTION 121

(b) Variable diplopia (especially when tired) suggests myasthenia – perhaps triggered by her penicillamine. AChR antibodies would help to confirm this diagnosis if positive, although sensitivity is low for ocular myasthenia. The other tests may be helpful to rule out less likely diagnoses, but would not confirm myasthenia.

QUESTION 122

(e) She has a rapidly progressive illness, with essentially normal investigations. The psychiatric symptoms near the time of onset are often seen in vCJD. Her LFTs are normal, which makes Wilson's disease less likely; no mention is made of basal ganglial symptoms. Spinocerebellar ataxias are usually less rapidly progressive, and the sensory and psychiatric symptoms are less well explained by this diagnosis.

QUESTION 123

(a) He has Friedreich's ataxia. Cardiomyopathy is common in this condition and is amenable to intervention to reduce outflow tract obstruction and treat arrhythmias. Diagnosis on echo could therefore improve his cardiac prognosis. MRI brain would confirm cerebellar atrophy – this alone would not change his outcome (unless a resectable lesion was found, which is unlikely given the history and other features).

QUESTION 124

(c) She has features of Guillain–Barré syndrome, supported by high protein levels in her CSF. Her FVC is very low, and she is at high risk of respiratory arrest. She should be transferred to ITU as a first step, then further treatment with IVIG can be instituted.

QUESTION 125

(e) and (j) She has ophthalmoplegia, ataxia and loss of reflexes after a respiratory tract infection – this is suggestive of the Miller–Fisher variant of Guillain–Barré syndrome. Lumbar puncture will show elevated protein levels, and anti-GQ1b antibodies are usually positive in this variant. Botulism is less likely; the time course is too long in this patient, and there is no history of ingesting a suspicious foodstuff.

QUESTION 126

(e) The snoring suggests that his airway is compromised; securing this should therefore be the first priority. Oxygen comes next, then when vital signs are stabilized, an urgent CT scan with a view to thrombolysis. He will probably need an insulin infusion as well; this is of lower priority.

QUESTION 127

(e) Her symptoms suggest a stroke. There is little in the history to suggest infection (e.g. encephalitis) as a cause for her symptoms. LP could be done to look for oligoclonal bands, but the history is rather rapid in onset for multiple sclerosis, there has been only one episode, and the MRI scan may help explore this differential as well.

QUESTION 128

(e) MRI is not an option due to her heart valve. Evoked potentials may give some evidence of demyelination to back up the clinical impression of optic neuritis; lumbar puncture could also be done (off warfarin) to look for oligoclonal bands. There are few features that suggest infective endocarditis here.

QUESTION 129

(b) Glatiramer or interferon may be indicated once she is over this acute episode, as she has frequent relapses. High-dose steroids may shorten this episode and allow her to regain mobility more quickly. MRI brain will add nothing, although MRI spine may be useful if there is any doubt as to whether MS or a mechanical cord compression is responsible for her symptoms.

QUESTION 130

(b) She has a progressive demyelinating polyneuropathy; the insidious course suggests chronic inflammatory demyelinating polyneuropathy, which is corroborated by the elevated CSF protein. Steroids or IV immunoglobulin are the usual first-line treatments; plasma exchange can also be used. Nerve biopsy is probably not necessary in this case given the other information available.

QUESTION 131

(d) She has a sensory axonal neuropathy, of which B_{12} deficiency is a cause. She also has a borderline elevated MCV, although MCV and haemoglobin can be normal in B_{12} neuropathy. Lumbar puncture would be more useful if a chronic demyelinating process was suspected; MRI spine would be useful if upper motor neurone signs were present.

QUESTION 132

1 (a)

2 (e)

A businessman and traveller to the Far East presenting with aseptic meningitis with extensor plantars and absent reflexes raises the suspicion of neurosyphilis. Fluorescence–*Treponema*–antibody–absorption test is more specific than VDRL. The clinical features complicating his progress the day after his admission are due to Jarisch–Herxheimer reaction.

QUESTION 133

1 (c)

Presentation of back pain over several months, with occupation exposure, mild neutropenia and deranged liver enzymes, suggests brucellosis.

QUESTION 134

1 (e)

2 (a)

Recent travel to a developing region, headache, high fever and relative bradycardia point towards *Salmonella typhi* enteric fever. After the first 10 days, bone marrow culture has the highest diagnostic yield.

QUESTION 135

1 (a)

2 (d)

She has evidence of TB exposure from her family history and chest X-ray appearance. The salt wastage from her biochemistry test is therefore likely due to chronic infection.

359

QUESTION 136

(a) This man has had three significant respiratory tract infections which are likely to be HIV-related and has a low CD4 count. He is stable at present and therefore better able to tolerate potential adverse effects from antiretroviral treatment. The golden rule in HIV therapy is to start early, ideally before the CD4 count falls below 200×10^6/L.

QUESTION 137

(d) This is a sexually active young woman who suffers from pelvic inflammatory disease, presumably complicated by sexually transmitted disease as she has attended the GU clinic. The acute presentation together with the deranged liver enzymes fits with perihepatitis secondary to gonococcal or, more commonly, chlamydial infection (Fitz-Hugh–Curtis syndrome).

QUESTION 138

1 (e)
2 (b)
Camping holiday, flu-like symptoms, rash and the lower motor neurone facial palsy are suggestive of Lyme disease.

QUESTION 139

(b) Mild anaemia, thrombocytopenia, jaundice, hepatosplenomegaly with a flu-like prodrome in the absence of rash and lymphadenopathy in a traveller should make you suspect malaria in spite of him completing his prophylactic antimalarial course. One set of blood films is not enough; serial films are needed. This is a common pitfall!

QUESTION 140

(a) This case is in keeping with toxic shock syndrome (fever, rash and hypotension) and the likely source of the toxin is the infected coil which needs to be removed as soon as possible by the gynaecologist.

QUESTION 141

1 (a)
2 (b)
Sepsis (note that he is on beta-blocker therapy and therefore the heart rate is probably underestimated) with hepatic and renal dysfunction in a vet should make you think of leptospirosis.

QUESTION 142

1 (e)
2 (e)
This is an acute descending paralysis and should therefore make you suspect a toxin to be the trigger. Tetanus usually manifests with tonic seizures and preserved consciousness. Normal blood parameters argue against intracranial abscess formation. Preserved sensation makes Guillain–Barré less likely. Botulism is therefore most likely and typical of this presentation and that is why this student who is struggling financially and likely to be resorting to canned food should receive antitoxin. Crucially, however, you need to get baseline ABGs and ask your intensive care colleagues to review him with a view to taking over his care.

QUESTION 143

1 (c)
2 (c)
There is evidence of liver damage. Factor VIII deficiency does not affect the extrinsic pathway; therefore the prolonged prothrombin time along with the low albumin reflects poor synthetic function of the liver. Hepatitis C is more likely as serological screening tests of blood products for hepatitis B came into clinical use much earlier.

QUESTION 144

(a) This is a case of suspected inhalational anthrax. The blood culture initial findings, CXR features and occupational history are supportive of this. One would assume that he should already be on IV penicillin and macrolide therapy in ITU and must immediately inform the relevant authorities of this notifiable disease.

QUESTION 145

(a) Although his blood film is consistent with leukaemia, it may also be due to overwhelming infection. Regardless of whether he has leukaemia, he has signs of a severe chest infection and requires antibiotics. He is not fit for chemotherapy – he has infection, renal failure and liver failure. TB is a cause of a leukaemoid reaction, but broad-spectrum antibiotics are the immediate priority here.

QUESTION 146

(a) She has Waldenström's macroglobulinaemia, with hyperviscosity syndrome, which requires plasmapheresis. Melphalan or other chemotherapy will then be needed to reduce the IgM level.

QUESTION 147

(a) This is paroxysmal nocturnal haemoglobinuria – the clues are the history of aplastic anaemia, the blood in urine and the presence of a probable DVT. Anti-CD59 and anti-CD55 flow cytometry shows the absence of these cell surface proteins and confirms the diagnosis. SLE (with antiphospholipid syndrome) is also possible but haematuria is unusual.

QUESTION 148

(d) and (g) The combination of rash, arthralgia, renal impairment and sensory symptoms would fit with cryoglobulinaemia – and his intravenous drug use is a strong risk factor for hepatitis C, the main cause. Hepatitis B is associated with PAN; this is also a possible diagnosis and shares many of the features. Rash and arthralgia are commoner in cryoglobulinaemia, however, as is a raised rheumatoid factor.

QUESTION 149

(c) The history of small-bowel resection suggests that she may have lost her terminal ileum; the Schilling test would detect this as even adding intrinsic factor would not lead to B_{12} absorption. There are no other malabsorptive symptoms to suggest bacterial overgrowth (hydrogen breath test); the SeHCAT test is for bile salt malabsorption.

QUESTION 150
Question 1

(a) His peripheral blood film is highly suggestive of myelodysplasia – although he has declined the bone marrow biopsy that would confirm the diagnosis. He has not got severe renal impairment and his iron stores are replete; iron is probably not therefore necessary (although EPO may sometimes be of benefit). The lack of iron deficiency argues against upper GI investigation. Transfusion will help his symptoms and is probably the best first-line therapy. Low-dose chemotherapy has little place except for palliation of CMML.

Question 2

(c) The rising monocyte count with worsening cytopenia suggests that he has developed CMML.

QUESTION 151

(d) She has a very low MCV for the level of haemoglobin; this and her Greek background suggest that beta-thalassaemia trait is more likely than iron deficiency. MCV often rises slightly in pregnancy.

QUESTION 152

(d) Recurrent thrombotic events on warfarin in antiphospholipid syndrome are best treated by increasing the INR to between 3 and 4. Although a filter would help protect against further PE, it would not prevent other potentially serious thrombotic events.

QUESTION 153

(d) The International Prognostic Index features for prognosis in NHL are: histology, stage (III/IV being adverse), LDH and performance status. Histology and performance status are known from the information that you are given; although a chest CT might be thought helpful, it would merely confirm disease on the same side of the diaphragm. Disease on both sides of the diaphragm is required for stage III to be diagnosed – an abdominal CT would be more helpful. LDH will however contribute new prognostic information.

QUESTION 154

(a) He has tumour lysis syndrome. Rapid IV fluids are probably most important – a good urine output

361

will help to reduce serum potassium and will prevent further deposition of urate in the renal tubules. Urinary alkalinization may also help prevent urate deposition, but may reduce serum ionized calcium still further. Allopurinol will be needed but will not be adequate therapy on its own.

QUESTION 155

(c) and (d) The combination of a wedge fracture in a youngish male, high ESR and high calcium make myeloma highly likely. Lung cancer is also a possibility, but the chest X-ray is clear, which diminishes the likelihood. Immunoglobulins and bone marrow biospy would give enough information to clinch the diagnosis; the bone scan is usually normal and although a skeletal survey might reveal further lytic lesions, this would not add diagnostically to the presence of a wedge fracture and hypercalcaemia.

QUESTION 156

(c) Her anaemia may be due to blood loss (NSAID, cancer) or to an inflammatory process. The small monoclonal band is not supported by other features of myeloma; it probably falls into the category of MGUS. Iron studies would allow a rational choice of further investigations – perhaps bone marrow if normal; stop diclofenac and pursue endoscopy if iron-deficient.

QUESTION 157

(d) The small gap between his total protein and albumin levels suggests low immunoglobulin levels. There is little going for coeliac disease or lymphoma on his blood tests – the disease is clearly long-standing since childhood.

QUESTION 158

(a) The anticardiolipin antibody, livedo rash, stroke and history of miscarriage all point to antiphospholipid syndrome. She therefore requires warfarin, despite being in sinus rhythm with no structural heart disease. Ham's test is no longer done to look for PNH, which is a much less likely diagnosis here.

QUESTION 159

(c) Hydroxycarbamide causes marked increases in MCV, and the reduced Hb and platelet counts suggest that it is working. His B_{12} level was fine 6 months ago and therefore does not need rechecking. Valproate can cause thrombocytopenia, but other cytopenias are rare.

QUESTION 160

(a) His symptoms, plus the presence of bundle branch block, suggest that he has a cardiac problem – probably due to iron overload. His LFTs suggest possible iron overload to the liver as well. Although he is anaemic, this is probably an appropriate level given the history of thalassaemia, and splenectomy probably won't improve his symptoms. Further transfusions should be minimized in view of his iron overload.

QUESTION 161

(c) He has polycythaemia, and the pruritis and splenomegaly are suggestive of polycythaemia rubra vera. A red cell mass estimation would confirm primary polycythaemia, and, if confirmed, the splenomegaly would reach diagnostic criteria for polycythaemia rubra vera.

QUESTION 162

(c) She has iron-deficiency anaemia, and in older people, it is common for upper and lower GI pathologies to coexist. She therefore needs investigation for both, and colonoscopy is the investigation of choice if she can tolerate it – she is usually fairly fit.

QUESTION 163

(e) His iron studies are difficult to interpret – his ferritin is high because of an acute-phase response, and his other iron studies do not fall neatly into either iron deficiency or anaemia of chronic disease. A blood film may show hypochromia or microcytic cells, or perhaps pencil cells. Failing this, a trial of iron may be necessary – at least until he is fit enough for further investigation.

QUESTION 164

(b) She has a severe chest crisis, and will probably require exchange transfusion to reduce the amount of sickled blood and boost her haemoglobin levels. Antibiotics may also be needed, but the low CRP suggests that she may not have pneumonia.

QUESTION 165

(b) She is most likely to have cholecystitis – gallstones are very common in patients with sickle-cell anaemia. This is more likely than lung infarction given her good oxygenation and normal chest X-ray.

QUESTION 166

(e) She has CLL, at a very early stage (no symptoms, no cytopenia, no lymph nodes). No treatment is therefore indicated at this stage.

NORMAL VALUES

BIOCHEMISTRY

Na 136–149 mmol/L
K 3.8–5.0 mmol/L
Urea 2.5–6.5 mmol/L
Creatinine 55–125 µmol/L
Total protein 65–80 g/L
Albumin 35–55 g/L
Bilirubin 2–13 µmol/L
ALT 5–27 U/L
ALP 30–130 U/L
GGT 0–30 U/L
Chloride 93–108 mmol/L
Bicarbonate 24–30 mmol/L
Calcium 2.15–2.65 mmol/L
Phosphate 0.8–1.4 mmol/L
Uric acid 0.1–0.4 mmol/L
CK 0–170 U/L
Plasma osmolality 285–295 mosmol/kg
Cholesterol 3.6–5.0 mmol/L
Triglyceride 0–2.0 mmol/L
Glucose 3.5–5.5 mmol/L
IgG 5–16 g/L
IgA 1.25–4.25 g/L
IgM 0.5–1.7 g/L
CRP 0–10 mg/L
Iron 16–30 µmol/L (males)
Iron 11–27 µmol/L (females)
TIBC 45–72 µmol/L
Vitamin B_{12} 200–900 pg/L
Mg 0.65–1 mmol/L
Faecal fat excretion < 6 g/24 hours
PSA 0–6 mg/L
Vitamin D 15–100 nmol/L

HORMONES

Cortisol 170–720 nmol/L (9 a.m.)
Cortisol 170–220 nmol/L (midnight)
Growth hormone < 10 ng/mL
Thyroxine 70–160 nmol/L
TSH 0.8–3.6 mU/L

HAEMATOLOGY

Hb 13.5–17.5 g/dL (males)
Hb 11.5–15.5 g/dL (females)
MCH 27–32 pg
MCHC 32–36 g/dL
MCV 76–98 fl
Reticulocyte count 0.2–2%
Platelet count 150–400 $\times$ 10^9/L
WCC 4–11 $\times$ 10^9/L
Neutrophils 2.5–7.5 $\times$ 10^9/L
Lymphocytes 1.5–3.5 $\times$ 10^9/L
Eosinophils 0.04–0.44 $\times$ 10^9/L
Basophils 0–0.1 $\times$ 10^9/L
Monocytes 0.2–0.8 $\times$ 10^9/L
ESR 0–10 mm/hour
Prothrombin time 12–15.5 seconds
Activated partial thromboplastin time 30–46
  seconds
Thrombin time 15–19 s
Bleeding time 2–8 minutes
Fibrinogen 2–4 g/L

CARDIOLOGY

RA 4 mmHg (3.2–4.8)
RV (end diastole) 4 (mean) mmHg
RV (systole) 25 (mean), (range 15–30) mmHg
PA (diastole) 10 (mean), (range 5–15) mmHg
PA (systole) 25 (mean), (range 5–30) mmHg
PAWP 10 (mean), (range 5–14) mmHg
LV (end diastole) 7 (mean), (range 4–12) mmHg
LV (systole) 120 (mean), (range 100–140)
  mmHg
Aorta (diastole) 70 (mean), (range 60–90) mmHg
Aorta (systole) 120 (mean), (range 90–140)
  mmHg

INDEX

Pagination in **bold** indicates a main diagnosis, in *italic* a differential diagnosis. Pagination for the question and answer section is prefixed by the Q or A number in brackets. Abbreviations are noted but not cross-referenced. For a list of abbreviations see pp. 272–6.